Cardiology: A Case Study Approach

Cardiology: A Case Study Approach

Editor: Remi Thompson

AMERICAN
MEDICAL PUBLISHERS
www.americanmedicalpublishers.com

AMERICAN
MEDICAL PUBLISHERS
www.americanmedicalpublishers.com

Cataloging-in-Publication Data

Cardiology : a case study approach / edited by Remi Thompson.
p. cm.
Includes bibliographical references and index.
ISBN 979-8-88740-591-9
1. Cardiology. 2. Cardiology--Case studies. 3. Heart--Diseases. I. Thompson, Remi.
RC667 .C37 2023
616.1--dc23

American Medical Publishers,
41 Flatbush Avenue,
1st Floor, New York,
NY 11217, USA

ISBN 979-8-88740-591-9 (Hardback)

Contents

Preface

Cardiology refers to the study of the diseases affecting heart and blood vessels. It is concerned with normal heart function and any deviations from a healthy heart. Many disorders affect the heart itself; whereas, some diseases occur outside of the heart and in the vascular system. These disorders include therosclerosis, aneurysm, stenosis, cardiomyopathy, high blood pressure, endocarditis, atrial fibrillation, and heart rhythm disorders. Cardiac MRI, stress tests, cardiac catheterization, coronary angiogram, electrocardiogram (EKG/ECG), and holter monitor test are some of the tests that are used to diagnose cardiovascular disorders and diseases. Cardiologists provide continual care to patients with cardiovascular diseases by performing certain diagnostic tests, and overseeing all the aspects of therapy including the administration of medications. This book aims to shed light on some of the unexplored aspects of cardiology. It presents case studies related to all contemporary topics of relevance to the field of cardiology. Those in search of information to further their knowledge will be greatly assisted by this book.

This book unites the global concepts and researches in an organized manner for a comprehensive understanding of the subject. It is a ripe text for all researchers, students, scientists or anyone else who is interested in acquiring a better knowledge of this dynamic field.

I extend my sincere thanks to the contributors for such eloquent research chapters. Finally, I thank my family for being a source of support and help.

Editor

1

Spontaneous Coronary Artery Dissection in a Patient with a Family History of Fatal Ascending Aortic Dissection: Case Report and Discussion of Diseases Causing Both Presentations

George Joy[1] **and Hany Eissa**[2]

[1]*Cardiology Department, St Bartholomew's Hospital, West Smithfield, London EC1A 7BE, UK*
[2]*Cardiology Department, Queen Elizabeth Queen Mother Hospital, St Peter's Rd, Margate CT9 4AN, UK*

Correspondence should be addressed to George Joy; georgejithinjoy@gmail.com

Academic Editor: Antonio de Padua Mansur

Background. Spontaneous coronary artery dissection (SCAD) is a rare cause of acute coronary syndrome (ACS). Aortic dissection and SCAD share common aetiologies such as a fibromuscular dysplasia (FMD), Marfan, Ehlers Danlos, and more rarely systemic lupus erythematosus and Loeys-Dietz; however, SCAD has never been known to have a familial association with aortic dissection. *Case Summary.* This case report describes a 48-year-old woman suffering from SCAD who had a mother who died from ascending aortic dissection in her 50s. *Discussion.* This is the first case report to our knowledge of a patient with SCAD with a first-degree relative with aortic dissection. Our case is interesting in that it shows that if predisposition to arterial dissection was inherited from mother to daughter, one of them suffered an extremely rare manifestation of their underlying disease. It also shows that a high index of suspicion is needed for SCAD in the presence of a patient with ACS and a family history of dissection elsewhere in the arterial tree.

1. Case Report

A 48-year-old woman was admitted to the emergency department with sudden onset severe chest tightness whilst doing yoga. This was associated with pins and needles in both arms, nausea, and abdominal discomfort. It lasted for 1 hour before it self-resolved and was not related to exertion. She reported being under increased emotional stress in the preceding month prior to presentation. She had no significant past medical history and was not on any regular medications.

She had a mother who died suddenly from an ascending aortic dissection in her 50s. Her mother was not hypertensive and suffered no symptoms or comorbidity suggestive of systemic illness.

The patient was hypotensive with a blood pressure of 90/60 mmHg and a heart rate of 80 bpm with no respiratory compromise or fever. Her troponin I (high-sensitivity assay) was 54 ng/dl, 79 ng/dl, and 27 ng/dl, respectively. Her electrocardiogram (ECG) showed sinus bradycardia with no ischaemic changes. A CT pulmonary angiogram was performed and excluded pulmonary embolus and showed no other cause for chest pain. An echocardiogram showed preserved biventricular function with no significant valvulopathy and normal ascending aorta dimensions. A coronary angiogram performed on day 2 of admission showed type 1 distal left anterior descending (LAD) coronary artery dissection with thrombolysis in antiplatelets and myocardial infarction (TIMI) 3 flow (Figure 1). She was initially managed with fondaparinux (factor Xa inhibitor) and dual antiplatelets with

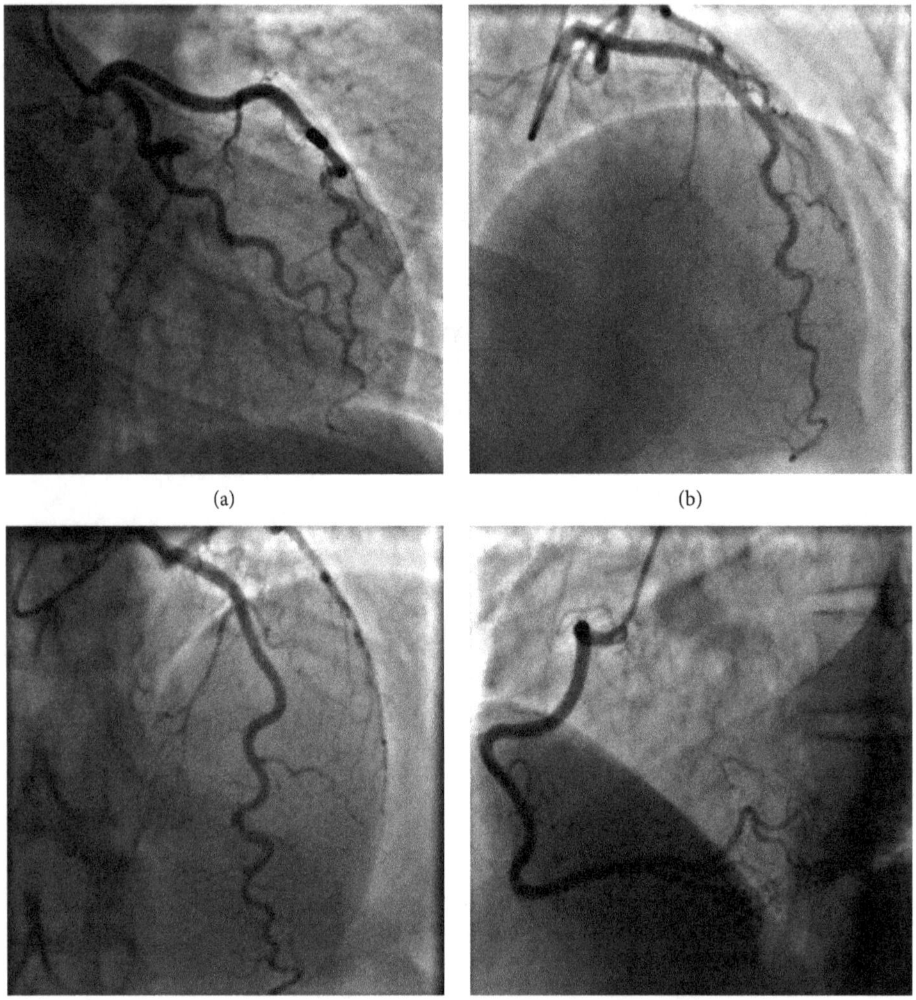

(a) (b) (c) (d)

Figure 1: (a–c) Type 1 spontaneous coronary artery dissection (SCAD) (contrast dye staining of the arterial wall with multiple arterial lumens) in the distal LAD. Increased arterial tortuosity* in all three epicardial vessels including RCA (d). *Coronary artery tortuosity is highly prevalent in patients with spontaneous coronary artery dissection and is associated with recurrence.

low-dose beta blocker long term once spontaneous coronary artery dissection (SCAD) was confirmed.

2. Discussion

Spontaneous coronary artery dissection (SCAD) is a cause of acute coronary syndrome (ACS) varying in severity from unstable angina to sudden cardiac death. This is the only case report to our knowledge of a patient with SCAD having a first-degree relative with aortic dissection. Twenty percent of patients with aortic dissection will have an underlying connective tissue disease [1]. We aim to discuss diseases that could link both presentations.

The incidence of patients with SCAD having fibromuscular dysplasia (FMD) has been reported as 74% [2]. Coronary FMD is rare and is characterised by dense intimal fibrous proliferation. Optical coherence tomography (OCT) may help establish the appearance of intima-media thickening; however, without this adjunctive imaging, FMD may only be diagnosed in extracoronary vessels in SCAD patients by CT or MRI [3]. A previous case report describing type B aortic dissection in a patient with FMD postulated this was more likely secondary to uncontrolled hypertension from renal FMD rather than primary arteriopathy in the aortic root [4]. Only three other case reports of aortic dissection from FMD have been described with one describing typical histopathologic features of FMD on the aortic root specimen postmortem [5]. Neither the patient nor her mother was hypertensive thereby making renal FMD less likely. Although overlaps with other connective tissue disease have been found, no definitive causative genes have been identified. The patient did not display any classical common clinical features of connective tissue disease, and she was unaware of the presence of these features in her mother [6]. Despite its rarity in aortic dissection, FMD appears to be the most likely culprit disease link between mother and daughter due to the lack of clinical features of other connective tissue disease outlined below.

Marfan syndrome (MFS) has an incidence of 1/10000 per year [7]. Isolated SCAD (i.e., not in association with aortic dissection) has been reported in Marfan syndrome and is extremely rare being described in five case reports to our knowledge occurring in young female patients with MFS. It is caused by cystic medial necrosis within the coronary artery leading to a predisposition to dissection [8]. Registry data has shown a prevalence of 4% of patients with ascending aortic dissection suffering from underlying Marfan disease [9]. Aortic dissection presents earlier in this group of patients within the 4th and 6th decade of life with a median age of 35. The aortic root is frequently more dilated prior to dissection (5.1 cm at the aortic root) causing an increased likelihood to suffer with aortic regurgitation prior to dissection [8]. Aortic dissection in MFS patients is more commonly not painful [1]. MFS is caused by autosomal dominant inheritance of FBN1 gene mutation encoding fibrillin 1 [7]. The patient did not meet diagnostic criteria for MFS including normal aortic dimensions, and therefore, MFS is unlikely to be the link between both patients.

Vascular Ehlers Danlos (vEDS) syndrome causing SCAD is extremely rare; we have identified seven case reports in the literature, including a patient in pregnancy with SCAD being the first presentation of vEDS [10–16]. Vascular EDS rarely affects the aorta, preferentially targeting first-order branch arteries. A review of 111 vEDS patients with vascular complications found only 10% suffering from aortic dissection [9]. vEDS is caused by autosomal dominant inheritance of COL3A1 mutation encoding for type 3 collagen and is commonly not diagnosed until vessel or hollow-organ rupture making it a suspect for the mother's presentation but would be an extremely rare manifestation in the daughter [17].

Some inflammatory conditions such as systemic lupus erythematosus (SLE) have been associated with SCAD in case reports, but this is highly uncommon; it is thought that 5% of SCAD have underlying inflammatory connective tissue disease [18]. Six case reports have described SCAD in association with SLE. A recent case report attributed SCAD as a first presentation of SLE, however without clinical criteria for SLE and positive ANA and anti-SMA [19]. Systematic review has identified 40 previous cases published of SLE with aortic aneurysm and or dissection [20]. Inflammatory causes are unlikely in our patient as blood tests a few months before her diagnosis were negative for ANA, rheumatoid factor, and ESR.

Loeys-Dietz syndrome is a rare connective tissue disorder that is caused by autosomal dominant inheritance of TGFBR-1 mutation that causes defects in elastogenesis leading to arterial tortuosity, aneurysm, and rupture. This affects any segment of the aorta, but has rarely been described in case reports to affect the coronary artery. Other associated features include cleft palate/uvula, hypertelorism, craniosynostosis, and other congenital heart defects such as ASD or bicuspid aortic valve [21]. The absence of these features makes Loeys-Dietz unlikely in our patient or her mother.

3. Conclusion

Our case shows a presentation of SCAD with an unusual family history. The main learning points from this case are that a high index of suspicion of SCAD is needed in a young patient presenting with ACS and that connective tissue disease and extracoronary arterial screening needs to be considered in these situations. There is no obvious disease that links both presentations although we propose FMD as the most likely culprit. It is clear from literature review that if the predisposition to dissection was inherited from mother to daughter, one of them suffered a rare manifestation of their underlying disease. SCAD is a life-changing event for the patient due to the complications of myocardial infarction and the threat of lifelong recurrence.

Consent

Consent has been obtained from the patient prior to submission for publication.

References

[1] C. M. Pearman, "Ehlers-Danlos with disease of the aorta and mitral valve," *Journal of Acute Medicine*, vol. 2, no. 4, pp. 128–130, 2012.

[2] D. Adlam, A. Wood, and A. al-Hussaini, "Editorial on "Characteristics of extension and de novo recurrent spontaneous coronary artery dissection"," *Eurointervention*, vol. 13, no. 12, pp. e1381–e1383, 2017.

[3] N. Moulson, J. Kelly, M. B. Iqbal, and J. Saw, "Histopathology of Coronary Fibromuscular Dysplasia Causing Spontaneous Coronary Artery Dissection," *JACC Cardiovascular Interventions*, vol. 11, no. 9, pp. 909-910, 2018.

[4] J. H. Man, A. Rothstein, P. J. Patel, and C. J. Lee, "Endovascular management of an acute type B aortic dissection in a patient with fibromuscular dysplasia," *Journal of Vascular Surgery Cases and Innovative Techniques*, vol. 4, no. 2, pp. 76–79, 2018.

[5] T. Tasaki, K. Hatanaka, M. Kirishima et al., "Aortic fibromuscular dysplasia complicated by dissection: a case report and review of literature," *Cardiovascular Pathology*, vol. 31, pp. 41–46, 2017.

[6] E. K. Brinza and H. L. Gornik, "Fibromuscular dysplasia: advances in understanding and management," *Cleveland Clinic Journal of Medicine*, vol. 83, suppl 2, pp. S45–S51, 2016.

[7] A. O. Caglayan and M. Dundar, "Inherited diseases and syndromes leading to aortic aneurysms and dissections," *European Journal of Cardio-Thoracic Surgery*, vol. 35, no. 6, pp. 931–940, 2009.

[8] C. Sato, K. Wakabayashi, and H. Suzuki, "Natural course of isolated spontaneous coronary artery dissection in Marfan syndrome," *International Journal of Cardiology*, vol. 177, no. 1, pp. 20–22, 2014.

[9] H. W. L. de Beaufort, S. Trimarchi, A. Korach et al., "Aortic dissection in patients with Marfan syndrome based on the IRAD data," *Annals of Cardiothoracic Surgery*, vol. 6, no. 6, pp. 633–641, 2017.

[10] H. Eltchaninoff, A. Cribier, and B. Letac, "Peripheral and coronary artery dissections in a young woman. A rare case of type IV Ehlers-Danlos syndrome," *Archives des maladies du coeur et des vaisseaux*, vol. 90, no. 6, pp. 841–844, 1997.

[11] A. F. Cereda, P. A. Canova, and F. S. Soriano, "Spontaneous coronary artery dissection after pregnancy as first

manifestation of a vascular Ehlers-Danlos syndrome," *The Journal of Invasive Cardiology*, vol. 29, no. 6, pp. e67–e68, 2017.

[12] C. V. Hampole, F. Philip, A. Shafii et al., "Spontaneous coronary artery dissection in Ehlers-Danlos syndrome," *The Annals of Thoracic Surgery*, vol. 92, no. 5, pp. 1883-1884, 2011.

[13] L. C. Ades, R. D. Waltham, A. A. Chiodo, and J. F. Bateman, "Myocardial infarction resulting from coronary artery dissection in an adolescent with Ehlers-Danlos syndrome type IV due to a type III collagen mutation," *Heart*, vol. 74, no. 2, pp. 112–116, 1995.

[14] M. Nakamura, J. Yajima, Y. Oikawa et al., "Vascular Ehlers-Danlos syndrome: –all three coronary artery spontaneous dissections," *Journal of Cardiology*, vol. 53, no. 3, pp. 458–462, 2009.

[15] A. M. Athanassiou and M. A. Turrentine, "Myocardial infarction and coronary artery dissection during pregnancy associated with type IV Ehlers-Danlos syndrome," *American Journal of Perinatology*, vol. 13, no. 3, pp. 181–183, 1996.

[16] V. Catanese, P. Venot, F. Lemesle, F. Delille, I. Runge, and B. Kuchly, "Myocardial infarction by spontaneous dissection of coronary arteries in a subject with type IV Ehlers-Danlos syndrome," *Presse medicale*, vol. 24, no. 29, pp. 1345–1347, 1995.

[17] P. H. Byers, J. Belmont, J. Black et al., "Diagnosis, natural history, and management in vascular Ehlers–Danlos syndrome," *American Journal of Medical Genetics Part C: Seminars in Medical Genetics*, vol. 175, no. 1, pp. 40–47, 2017.

[18] S. N. Hayes, E. S. H. Kim, J. Saw et al., "Spontaneous coronary artery dissection: current state of the Science: A Scientific Statement From the American Heart Association," *Circulation*, vol. 137, no. 19, 2018.

[19] S. Reddy, T. Vaid, N. C. Ganiga Sanjeeva, and R. K. Shetty, "Spontaneous coronary artery dissection as the first presentation of systemic lupus erythematosus," *BMJ Case Reports*, 2016.

[20] S. M. Yuan, "Aortic aneurysm and dissection in systemic lupus erythematosus," *Zeitschrift für Rheumatologie*, vol. 78, no. 3, pp. 287–294, 2019.

[21] A. Agrawal, S. Baaj, J. Schwartz, and J. J. Lopez, "Spontaneous coronary artery dissection in Loeys-Dietz syndrome: role of optical coherence tomography in diagnosis and management," *The Journal of Invasive Cardiology*, vol. 27, no. 9, pp. e196–e198, 2015.

2

Quadricuspid Aortic Valve: Report of Two Cases and Brief Review

Oreoluwa Oladiran,[1] **Ifeanyi Nwosu**,[2] **Rashmi Dhital**,[1] **and Gbujie Ezioma**[3]

[1]*Reading Hospital, Tower Health System, West Reading, Pennsylvania, USA*
[2]*Leighton Hospital NHS Trust, Crewe, Cheshire, UK*
[3]*Saint Peter's University, New Brunswick, New Jersey, USA*

Correspondence should be addressed to Oreoluwa Oladiran; oreoluwa.oladiran@towerhealth.org

Academic Editor: Assad Movahed

Quadricuspid aortic valve (QAV) is a rare congenital cardiac defect characterized by the presence of four aortic valve leaflets of equal or varying sizes. Even rarer is its clinical presentation with aortic stenosis. Diagnosis of QAV could be challenging but is of great importance as patients often present with progressive aortic regurgitation. We present 2 cases of QAV presenting differently: one with aortic stenosis requiring valve replacement and the other with aortic regurgitation requiring close monitoring.

1. Case 1

62-year-old woman with medical history significant for aortic stenosis and chronic atrial fibrillation presented to the emergency department with fatigue and progressively worsening shortness of breath with minimal exertion. She was asymptomatic at rest and denied chest pain, orthopnea, paroxysmal nocturnal dyspnea, leg swelling, presyncope, or syncope. She was incidentally found to have a systolic murmur during her pregnancy 20 years prior to this presentation. Notably, she had been offered aortic valve replacement in the past but declined.

Vital signs were normal with blood pressure of 110/60 mmHg, pulse rate of 79/min, temperature of 97.2°F, and respiratory rate of 16 breaths/min with normal oxygen saturation of 100% on ambient air. Physical examination was significant for irregularly irregular heart rhythm, and ejection systolic murmur was loudest in the aortic area with radiation to the carotids. Her lungs were clear to auscultation, and no pedal edema was noted. Electrocardiogram revealed atrial fibrillation with voltage criteria for left ventricular hypertrophy. Her most recent transthoracic echocardiogram revealed a thickened calcified aortic valve with decreased excursion with 4.6 m/s velocity suggesting a peak of 86 mmHg and mean of 36 mmHg suggestive of severe aortic stenosis. No other significant valvular abnormalities noted. Cardiac catheterization revealed widely patent coronary arteries.

Based on the presence of worsening symptoms and the risk of sudden cardiac death, the decision was made to proceed with surgical aortic valve replacement. Given her history of chronic atrial fibrillation, she was also planned for left atrial appendage exclusion and Cox Maze IV procedure simultaneously with the aortic valve replacement. Intraoperative transesophageal echocardiogram revealed quadricuspid aortic valves confirmed during surgical exploration (Figure 1). The native stenotic quadricuspid aortic valve leaflets were excised, and a 21 mm Saint Jude Medical Trifecta valve was implanted. The left atrial appendage was excised, and Cox Maze IV procedure was performed. Postoperatively, she remained in junctional rhythm and underwent uneventful placement of the dual chamber pacemaker on postoperative day 3. She recovered without further complications and was discharged on the eight postoperative day.

2. Case 2

53-year-old female with past medical history of aortic regurgitation and hypertension presented to the cardiology office for routine follow-up. She denied chest pain, shortness of breath, orthopnea, dyspnea, or leg swelling. Physical examination revealed normal vital signs. Cardiac auscultation

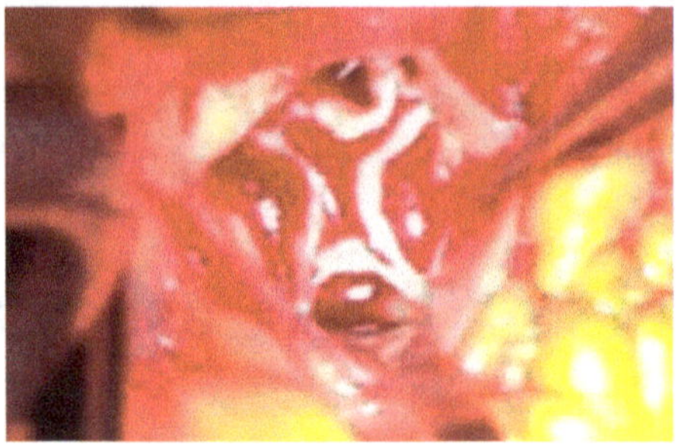

Figure 1: Intraoperative image showing quadricuspid aortic valve: Hurwitz type C/Nakamura type IV.

revealed diastolic murmur loudest at the 3rd left intercostal space. The remainder of physical examination was unremarkable. Transthoracic echocardiogram (TTE) 3 months earlier revealed a trileaflet aortic valve with moderate aortic insufficiency. TTE also noted a poorly defined subaortic membrane which prompted further assessment of valve anatomy by transesophageal echocardiogram (TEE) which confirmed the presence of quadricuspid aortic valve with severe aortic regurgitation from incomplete coaptation of the valve leaflets. Given that she was asymptomatic, we planned to continue surveillance by clinical and echocardiographic monitoring.

3. Discussion

The normal aortic valve is trileaflet and with the pulmonary valve represents the two semilunar heart valves. The leaflets, namely, right coronary, left coronary, and noncoronary cusps, are named based on their relationship to the coronary arteries [1]. Anatomical variations of the aortic valve have been documented notably, the unicuspid, bicuspid, and quadricuspid valves. Of these variants, the bicuspid valve is the commonest followed by unicuspid valve [2]. Quadricuspid aortic valve (QAV) is a rare congenital anomaly with documented incidence of 0.008% by autopsy, 0.043% by transthoracic echocardiogram, and 1% intraoperatively during aortic valve surgery [3, 4]. While both of our patients were female, it has been shown to have a slightly higher male preponderance [5] with mean age of presentation between 46 and 50 years. The embryology of QAV remains poorly understood, but it is believed to result from aberrant division of one of the three mesenchymal ridges that normally gives rise to three aortic valve cushions [6, 7]. Acquired heart diseases such as infective endocarditis and rheumatic fever may contribute to the development of a false QAV, but the absence of corpus arantii (nodules of semilunar cusps) helps to distinguish true congenital from an acquired QAV [8].

Hurwitz and Roberts described the seven (A–G; Figure 2) most common anatomic variants of QAV based on the size of the valve leaflets [9]. Type A has 4 equal cusps, type B has 3 normal cusp and a small accessory cusp, and type C has 2 large cusps and 2 small cusps. Types A and B represent about 73% of all the cases of QAV [10]. Other classification systems exist based on the position of the accessory cusps as described by Nakamura et al. [11] (Figure 3). In type I, the supernumerary cusp lies between the left and right coronary cusps. In type II, it lies between the right and noncoronary cusps. In type III, it lies between the left and noncoronary cusps, and in type IV, the supernumerary cusp cannot be identified as there are 2 equal sized smaller cusps. It is important to note that the position of the accessory cusp has no effect on the severity of the valvular insufficiency [4, 12]. Based on these classifications, our first patient had Hurwitz type C and Nakamura type IV while the second patient likely has Hurwitz type A and Nakamura type I quadricuspid aortic valve.

Quadricuspid aortic valve (QAV) usually presents as an isolated congenital anomaly, but other associated cardiac anomalies have been reported in about 18-32% of cases including aortic root dilatation [13], tetralogy of Fallot [14], patent ductus arteriosus [15], atrial and ventricular septal defects [16, 17], and anomalous origin of the coronary arteries [12].

Clinical presentation varies being mostly asymptomatic in the young, recall that both patients were asymptomatic until adulthood. The symptomatic patients will present with palpitations, dyspnea, fatigue, chest pain, and feature of congestive heart failure. Cases of ischemic stroke as an initial presentation has been reported [18]. Patients with QAV mostly present with aortic insufficiency and less commonly aortic stenosis [5]. More than half will present in adulthood with features of aortic insufficiency and more than 50% will require aortic valvular replacement in the sixth and seventh decade of life due to worsening aortic regurgitation [2, 19]. Infective endocarditis occurs in 1.4% of these patients [8] depending on the Hurwitz classification and its effect on dynamics of blood flow across the valve as mechanical stress on the abnormal valves [20] is thought to play a key role.

The routine use of echocardiography in suspected cases of valvular heart disease has allowed for early and accurate diagnosis of QAV. Although transthoracic echocardiography is often used in clinical settings, transesophageal echocardiography provides a more accurate assessment of valvular anatomy [8]. Magnetic resonance imaging and computerized tomography can also aid diagnosis, although not generally used solely for this purpose [18, 21]. In the absence of symptoms as described above, patients with QAV should be followed up closely. For symptomatic patients, treatment options range from valve repair to valve replacement. Repair may be feasible in some patients, but most will require valve replacement. Valve replacement, which could be surgical as in the first case described or transcatheter, is preferred in patients with severe aortic valvular dysfunction. Tricuspidalization is a preferred repair option in patients with Hurwitz types A, B, and C QAV [4].

4. Conclusion

Quadricuspid aortic valve is a rare congenital cardiac defect usually diagnosed incidentally. While most patients develop aortic regurgitation later in life, some as reported in the first case develop aortic stenosis while others remain asymptomatic. Although there are no guideline-based approach to management, it is prudent to regularly follow up these patients for early signs of aortic valve dysfunction.

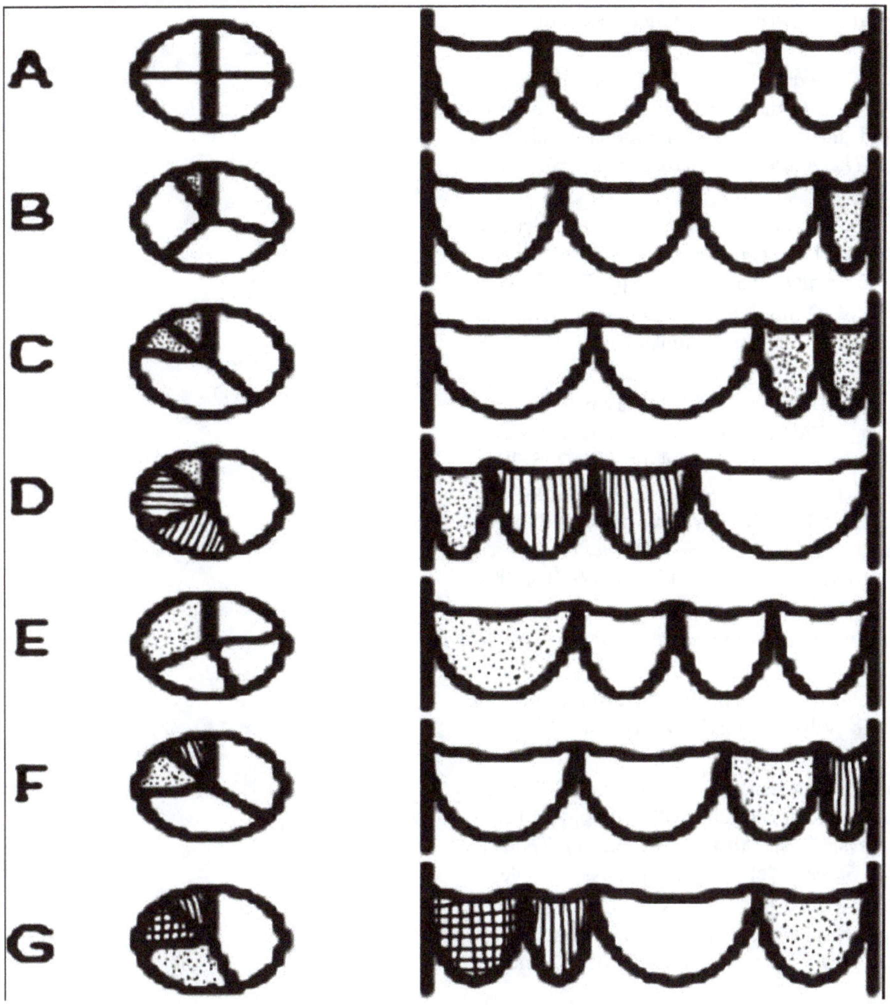

FIGURE 2: Hurwitz and Roberts classification of quadricuspid aortic valve.

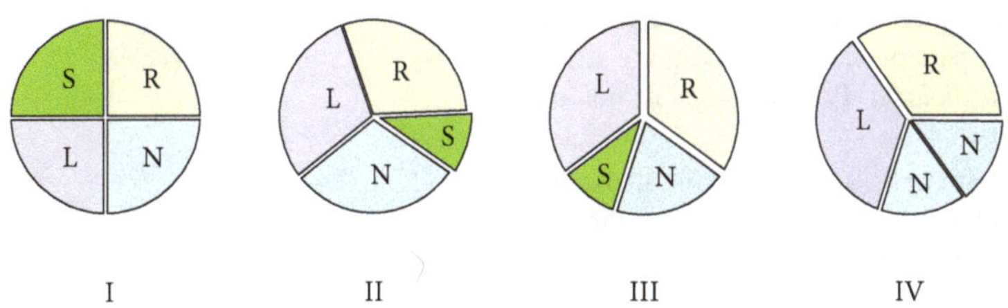

FIGURE 3: Nakamura et al. classification of quadricuspid aortic valve. L = left coronary cusp; N = noncoronary cusp; R = right coronary cusp; S = supernumerary cusp.

References

[1] N. Monigari, R. R. Poondru, H. Kareem, and T. Devasia, "Quadricuspid aortic valve: a rare congenital cardiac anomaly," *Case Reports*, vol. 2014, no. 1, 2014.

[2] O. Tutarel, "The quadricuspid aortic valve: a comprehensive review," *The Journal Heart Valve Disease*, vol. 13, no. 4, pp. 534–537, 2004.

[3] B. J. Feldman, B. K. Khandheria, C. A. Warnes, J. B. Seward, C. L. Taylor, and A. J. Tajik, "Incidence, description and functional assessment of isolated quadricuspid aortic valves," *The American Journal of Cardiology*, vol. 65, no. 13, pp. 937-938, 1990.

[4] M. Y. C. Tsang, M. M. Abudiab, N. M. Ammash et al., "Quadricuspid aortic valve: characteristics, associated structural cardiovascular abnormalities, and clinical outcomes," *Circulation*, vol. 133, no. 3, pp. 312–319, 2016.

[5] B. Fernández, A. C. Durán, A. Martire, D. López, and V. Sans-Coma, "New embryological evidence for the formation of quadricuspid aortic valves in the Syrian hamster

(*Mesocricetus auratus*)," *Journal of Comparative Pathology*, vol. 121, no. 1, pp. 89–94, 1999.

[6] B. Fernández, M. C. Fernández, A. C. Durán, D. López, A. Martire, and V. Sans-Coma, "Anatomy and formation of congenital bicuspid and quadricuspid pulmonary valves in Syrian hamsters," *The Anatomical Record*, vol. 250, no. 1, pp. 70–79, 1998.

[7] K. Savino, E. Quintavalle, and G. Ambrosio, "Quadricuspid aortic valve: a case report and review of the literature," *Journal of Cardiovascular Echography*, vol. 25, no. 3, pp. 72–76, 2015.

[8] L. E. Hurwitz and W. C. Roberts, "Quadricuspid semilunar valve," *The American Journal of Cardiology*, vol. 31, no. 5, pp. 623–626, 1973.

[9] A. Malviya, P. Kumar, J. Mishra, and P. Srivastava, "Quadricuspid aortic valve – A case report and literature review," *The Egyptian Heart Journal*, vol. 68, no. 4, pp. 271–275, 2016.

[10] Y. Nakamura, I. Taniguchi, M. Saiki, K. Morimoto, and T. Yamaga, "Quadricuspid aortic valve associated with aortic stenosis and regurgitation," *The Japanese Journal of Thoracic and Cardiovascular Surgery*, vol. 49, no. 12, pp. 714–716, 2001.

[11] S.-M. Yuan, "Quadricuspid aortic valve: a comprehensive review," *Brazilian Journal of Cardiovascular Surgery*, vol. 31, no. 6, 2016.

[12] L. Williams, P. Peters, and P. Shah, "Tricuspidization of quadricuspid aortic valve," *Annals of Thoracic Surgery*, vol. 95, no. 4, pp. 1453–1455, 2013.

[13] Y. Suzuki, K. Daitoku, M. Minakawa, K. Fukui, and I. Fukuda, "Congenital quadricuspid aortic valve with tetralogy of Fallot and pulmonary atresia," *The Japanese Journal of Thoracic and Cardiovascular Surgery*, vol. 54, no. 1, pp. 44–46, 2006.

[14] S.-H. Seol, U. Kim, H.-J. Cho, D.-K. Kim, D.-I. Kim, and D.-S. Kim, "Quadricuspid aortic valve with patent ductus arteriosus," *Texas Heart Institute Journal*, vol. 37, no. 6, pp. 726-727, 2010.

[15] L. Sousa, F. Pinto, G. Nogueira, S. Kaku, and A. M. Antunes, "Quadricuspid aortic valve and atrial septal defect," *Revista portuguesa de cardiologia*, vol. 20, no. 3, pp. 329-330, 2001.

[16] S. Demirkol, S. Balta, Z. Arslan, M. Unlu, U. Kucuk, and A. Iyisoy, "Association of quadricuspid aortic valve and ventricular septal defect in a patient who had undergone atrial septal defect surgery," *Kardiologia Polska*, vol. 71, no. 5, p. 546, 2013.

[17] M. Spartalis, E. Tzatzaki, E. Spartalis et al., "Ischemic stroke in a patient with quadricuspid aortic valve and patent foramen ovale," *Cardiology research*, vol. 8, no. 4, pp. 169–171, 2017.

[18] J. Zhu, J. Zhang, S. Wu, Y. Zhang, F. Ding, and J. Mei, "Congenital quadricuspid aortic valve associated with aortic insufficiency and mitral regurgitation," *Journal of Cardiothoracic Surgery*, vol. 8, no. 1, 2013.

[19] P. P. Bassareo, T. Hasan, M. Bonvicini, and G. Mercuro, "Quadricuspid aortic valve and anomalous origin of the left circumflex coronary artery in a young man with Down syndrome," *Clinical Case Reports*, vol. 3, no. 4, pp. 271–273, 2015.

[20] K. Kajinami, N. Takekoshi, and H. Mabuchi, "Images in cardiology. Non-invasive detection of quadricuspid aortic valve," *Heart*, vol. 78, no. 1, p. 87, 1997.

[21] J. J. Idrees, E. E. Roselli, A. Arafat et al., "Outcomes after repair or replacement of dysfunctional quadricuspid aortic valve," *The Journal of Thoracic and Cardiovascular Surgery*, vol. 150, no. 1, pp. 79–82, 2015.

3

Right Coronary Artery to Coronary Sinus Fistula Post Endomyocardial Biopsy

Aniket S. Rali,[1] Farhad Sami,[2] Andrew Sauer,[1] and Zubair Shah[1]

[1]*Department of Cardiovascular Medicine, The University of Kansas Health System, USA*
[2]*Department of Internal Medicine, The University of Kansas Health System, USA*

Correspondence should be addressed to Zubair Shah; zshah2@kumc.edu

Academic Editor: Kuan-Rau Chiou

Endomyocardial biopsy (EMB) continues to remain the gold standard for surveillance of rejection post orthotropic heart transplantation (OHT). It can be performed under fluoroscopic or echocardiographic guidance. In the hands of an experienced operator, the complications of EMB are uncommon with <1% chance of any serious acute complications. Most common complications of EMB include access site-related complications, namely, venous thrombosis, carotid cannulation, hematoma, air embolism, and pneumothorax. We present a case of a rare complication of EMB in a patient with OHT causing a coronary sinus to right coronary artery (RCA) fistula.

1. Introduction

Endomyocardial biopsy (EMB) continues to remain the gold standard for surveillance of rejection post orthotropic heart transplantation (OHT). ACC/AHA and ESC recommend EMB as a diagnostic tool in the evaluation and treatment of unexplained cardiomyopathy encompassing 14 different clinical scenarios [1, 2]. Since the first intravascular approach of EMB described in 1962 by Sakakibara and Konno [3], significant evolution in techniques and approaches has taken place [4]. Currently, EMB is done via an internal jugular or femoral vein (or the femoral artery if getting left heart biopsy) utilizing transcatheter insertion of a bioptome to biopsy the endocardium of the interventricular septum. It can be performed under fluoroscopic or echocardiographic guidance. In the hands of an experienced operator, the complications of EMB are uncommon with <1% chance of any serious acute complications [5, 6]. Most common complications of EMB include access site-related complications, namely, venous thrombosis, carotid cannulation, hematoma, air embolism, and pneumothorax [7, 8]. Cardiac specific complications have also been described and include self-limited arrhythmias, myocardial perforation, pericardial tamponade, pulmonary embolization, and tricuspid valve damage [5]. We present a case of a rare complication of EMB in a patient with OHT causing a coronary sinus to the right coronary artery (RCA) fistula.

2. Timeline

A 63-year-old male patient underwent heart transplantation on for Stage D heart failure due to ischemic cardiomyopathy. The patient continued to have unremarkable hospital course posttransplant and was discharged to home. Over the next 12 months, the patient continued to have an uncomplicated course with normal EMBs free of rejection. At our institute, we perform weekly biopsies for the first month posttransplant and then start spacing them out monthly for the first year. Per our institutional protocol, the patient presented for a coronary angiography, right heart catheterization, and EMB one year after transplant. We perform all our EMBs for transplanted hearts under fluoroscopy guidance. During this visit, he was noted to have a large RCA with the arteriovenous fistula to coronary sinus on coronary angiography. Follow-up coronary CTA confirmed a RCA to coronary sinus fistula. A retrospective review of all the EMB specimens obtained till date was performed and showed one of the biopsy samples containing blood vessel tissue.

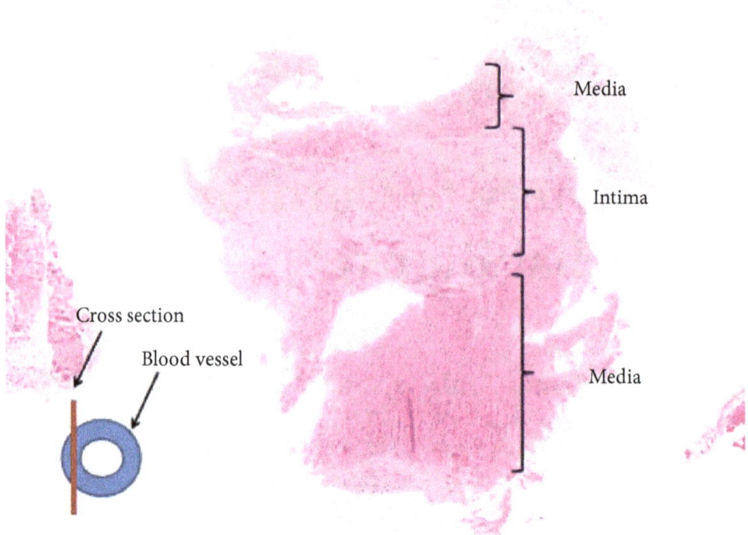

FIGURE 1: EMB pathology specimen confirming a blood vessel.

3. Case Presentation

Our patient is a 63-year-old male who underwent heart transplantation for stage D heart failure with reduced ejection fraction (HFrEF) due to ischemic cardiomyopathy. The patient's postoperative course was unremarkable, and there was no evidence of allograft rejection on the 12 biopsies obtained within first six months posttransplantation. He presented for an outpatient right heart catheterization (RHC), coronary angiography, and EMB for his routine one year posttransplantation evaluation. Coronary angiography revealed a very large RCA measuring 5 mm with a fistulous connection from posterolateral branch to possibly the right atrium (Supplemental Video 1-2). There was no "step-up" in venous saturations suggestive of an intracardiac shunt. Hemodynamics were unremarkable with a pulmonary artery pressure of 29/18, a pulmonary capillary wedge pressure of 12 mmHg, and a cardiac output of 5.6 L/min. The patient's transthoracic echocardiogram (TTE), two months posttransplant, was suggestive of a very subtle right coronary artery to right atrial shunt which was not noted on the initial read (Supplemental Video 3). This anomaly was not present on the donor heart TTE immediately pretransplant. A retrospective systematic review of all EMB slides revealed a blood vessel sample present on one of the prior biopsies (Figure 1). This particular biopsy was obtained via a transjugular venous access and under fluoroscopy guidance. We also pursued a coronary CTA that revealed an ectatic RCA measuring approximately 6 mm in diameter and an ectatic posterolateral branch measuring 4.5×5.5 mm with a fistulous communication to a dilated coronary sinus (Supplemental Videos 4-5). The fistula was not hemodynamically significant as the patient had continued to remain asymptomatic, with normal right atrial and right ventricular dimensions and normal filling pressures on RHC. Hence, the patient did not undergo any interventions for this fistula. Despite this anomaly, the patient remained asymptomatic with improving exercise capacity on a 6-month follow-up from his heart angiogram. He was managed conservatively with good follow-up.

4. Discussion

The right ventricle to coronary artery fistulas are previously reported complications of EMB [9–12]. The solitary case of fistula between the coronary artery and coronary sinus has also been described [13], but in general, fistulas to cardiac veins as complication of EMB are very rare. We report a unique case of fistulous connection between the RCA and the RA via a coronary sinus. We hypothesize that in our patient, the bioptome was advanced deep into the coronary sinus and this was confused to be the right ventricular outflow tract (RVOT) on 2D fluoroscopy images. This begets a discussion about the current techniques used for EMBs, especially in light of an increased number of EMBs performed annually in the United States in recent years [6].

EMB is usually performed under fluoroscopic or 2D echocardiographic guidance with each having its advantages and pit falls [14, 15]. Owing to single plane imaging systems, most fluoroscopy techniques provide limited information about the anteroposterior movement of the bioptome tip. Furthermore, soft tissue structures are not visualized on fluoroscopy. While 2D echocardiography provides better visualization of soft tissue, it is most likely to be affected by artifacts when trying to visualize the bioptome tip. Technical advances, including 3-dimensional imaging, may allow better visualization of cardiac structures and biopsy instrumentation [16, 17]. However, the currently available data is limited and unable to definitely demonstrate superiority of one technique over the other. Imamura et al. have recommended the use of guide wire and right ventriculogram to deliver the bioptome more precisely at the site of biopsy; however, theirs is a single-center retrospective analysis with small sample size [18].

Our patient experienced a rare complication of EMB while undergoing a routine surveillance biopsy using a standard of care techniques. He was managed conservatively without any interventions for the fistula as he was asymptomatic without any evidence of right sided volume or pressure overload. However, if the fistula proved to be hemodynamically significant, we were planning on treating it with a covered stent in the coronary sinus. Although it did not prove to be clinically significant in our patient, such a fistula could ultimately lead to right sided volume overload and adverse remodeling.

Our report presents a rare and potentially hemodynamically significant complication of a routine surveillance endomyocardial biopsy. This further demonstrates the importance of careful evaluation of the biopsy site each time and using all available imaging modalities to avoid such complications.

Authors' Contributions

Aniket S. Rali and Farhad Sami contributed equally to this work.

References

[1] M. K. Bennett, N. A. Gilotra, C. Harrington et al., "Evaluation of the role of endomyocardial biopsy in 851 patients with unexplained heart failure from 2000-2009," *Circulation Heart Failure*, vol. 6, no. 4, pp. 676–684, 2013.

[2] L. T. Cooper, K. L. Baughman, A. M. Feldman et al., "The role of endomyocardial biopsy in the management of cardiovascular disease: a scientific statement from the american heart association, the American College of Cardiology, and the European Society of Cardiology," *Journal of the American College of Cardiology*, vol. 50, no. 19, pp. 1914–1931, 2007.

[3] S. Sakakibara and S. Konno, "Endomyocardial biopsy," *Japanese Heart Journal*, vol. 3, pp. 537–543, 1962.

[4] K. R. Melvin and J. W. Mason, "Endomyocardial biopsy: its history, techniques and current indications," *Canadian Medical Association Journal*, vol. 126, no. 12, pp. 1381-1386, 1982.

[5] A. M. From, J. J. Maleszewski, and C. S. Rihal, "Current status of endomyocardial biopsy," *Mayo Clinic Proceedings*, vol. 86, no. 11, pp. 1095–1102, 2011.

[6] Z. Shah, A. Rali, and K. Gupta, "National trends and procedural complications from endomyocardial biopsy: results from the National Inpatient Sample, 2007-2014," *Cardiology*, vol. 142, no. 4, p. 223, 2019.

[7] C. Baraldi-Junkins, H. R. Levin, E. K. Kasper, B. K. Rayburn, A. Herskowitz, and K. L. Baughman, "Complications of endomyocardial biopsy in heart transplant patients," *The Journal of Heart and Lung Transplantation*, vol. 12, 1, Part 1, pp. 63–67, 1993.

[8] F. Saraiva, V. Matos, L. Gonçalves, M. Antunes, and L. A. Providência, "Complications of endomyocardial biopsy in heart transplant patients: a retrospective study of 2117 consecutive procedures," *Transplantation Proceedings*, vol. 43, no. 5, pp. 1908–1912, 2011.

[9] M. J. Henzlova, H. Nath, R. P. Bucy, R. C. Bourge, J. K. Kirklin, and W. J. Rogers, "Coronary artery to right ventricle fistula in heart transplant recipients: a complication of endomyocardial biopsy," *Journal of the American College of Cardiology*, vol. 14, no. 1, pp. 258–261, 1989.

[10] D. H. Fitchett, C. Forbes, and A. J. Guerraty, "Repeated endomyocardial biopsy causing coronary arterial-right ventricular fistula after cardiac transplantation," *The American Journal of Cardiology*, vol. 62, no. 10, pp. 829–831, 1988.

[11] T. Lefevre, G. Gosselin, M. Carrier, T. K. Leung, I. Dyrda, and R. Bonan, "Coronary artery-right ventricular fistula in a patient with heart transplantation. A complication of endomyocardial biopsy," *Archives des Maladies du Coeur et des Vaisseaux*, vol. 83, no. 11, pp. 1713–1718, 1990.

[12] T. J. Locke, S. S. Furniss, and C. G. McGregor, "Coronary artery-right ventricular fistula after endomyocardial biopsy," *British Heart Journal*, vol. 60, no. 1, pp. 81-82, 1988.

[13] R. W. Lowry, J. B. Young, H. S. Kleiman, and W. A. Zoghbi, "Transesophageal echocardiographic demonstration of right coronary artery—to—coronary sinus fistula in a heart transplant recipient," *Journal of the American Society of Echocardiography*, vol. 6, no. 4, pp. 449–452, 1993.

[14] C. Blomström-Lundqvist, A.-M. Noor, J. Eskilsson, and S. Persson, "Safety of transvenous right ventricular endomyocardial biopsy guided by two-dimensional echocardiography," *Clinical Cardiology*, vol. 16, no. 6, pp. 487–492, 1993.

[15] L. W. Miller, A. J. Labovitz, L. A. McBride, D. G. Pennington, and K. Kanter, "Echocardiography-guided endomyocardial biopsy. A 5-year experience," *Circulation*, vol. 78, 5, Part 2, pp. Iii99–Ii102, 1988.

[16] M. E. Amitai, I. Schnittger, R. L. Popp, J. Chow, P. Brown, and D. H. Liang, "Comparison of three-dimensional echocardiography to two-dimensional echocardiography and fluoroscopy for monitoring of endomyocardial biopsy," *The American Journal of Cardiology*, vol. 99, no. 6, pp. 864–866, 2007.

[17] D. Platts, M. Brown, G. Javorsky, C. West, N. Kelly, and D. Burstow, "Comparison of fluoroscopic versus real-time three-dimensional transthoracic echocardiographic guidance of endomyocardial biopsies," *European Journal of Echocardiography*, vol. 11, no. 7, pp. 637–643, 2010.

[18] T. Imamura, K. Kinugawa, D. Nitta et al., "Is the internal jugular vein or femoral vein a better approach site for endomyocardial biopsy in heart transplant recipients?," *International Heart Journal*, vol. 56, no. 1, pp. 67–72, 2015.

4

Pyoderma Gangrenosum following Pacemaker Implantation

Noura Ayoubi,[1] Zaydi Javeed,[1] Raymond Cutro,[2] and Brooke T. Baldwin[3]

[1]*Morsani College of Medicine, University of South Florida, Tampa, Florida, USA*
[2]*Department of Cardiology, James A. Haley Veterans' Hospital, Tampa, Florida, USA*
[3]*Department of Dermatology, James A. Haley Veterans' Hospital, Tampa, Florida, USA*

Correspondence should be addressed to Noura Ayoubi; nayoubi@health.usf.edu

Academic Editor: Aiden Abidov

Pyoderma gangrenosum (PG) is a rare neutrophilic dermatosis characterized by noninfectious, inflammatory, ulcerating lesions. Pathergy can be seen in these patients, whereby minor trauma or surgery can result in the development of PG ulcerations. Here, we present a case of PG following pacemaker implantation. A 76-year-old male with a history of rheumatoid arthritis presented to the cardiology team with symptomatic bradycardia. Indications for implantation were met, and the procedure was performed in a routine fashion. The patient returned to clinic for follow-up four days later, complaining of pain at the incision site, coupled with erythema and purulent drainage. Consultations with an infectious disease specialist and a dermatologist were requested, and the diagnosis of pyoderma gangrenosum was considered. The patient underwent device removal and received systemic corticosteroids at a dose of 1 mg/kg prednisone with complete lesion healing in 3 weeks. While being maintained on steroids, the patient underwent reimplantation of a new pacemaker on the contralateral side without complication and had a normal postoperative course. We present this case report, along with the review of literature, in order to highlight the multidisciplinary approach to management, which requires dermatologic treatment in order to achieve pacemaker success.

1. Introduction

Pyoderma gangrenosum (PG) is a rare neutrophilic dermatosis characterized by noninfectious, inflammatory, ulcerating lesions [1]. Lesions occur most commonly on the lower legs, but any part of the skin can be involved. The most common age of presentation is between 40 and 60 years, with less common cases occurring in children or older adults [1, 2]. While the exact etiology is unknown, the neutrophilic reaction is hypothesized to occur due to the interplay between neutrophilic dysfunction, genetic risk factors, and systemic inflammation. Ulcerative colitis, Crohn's disease, rheumatoid arthritis, and chronic active hepatitis are commonly involved inflammatory disorders [1]. Pathergy can be seen in these patients, whereby minor trauma or surgery can result in the development of PG ulcerations [1].

Here, we present a case of PG following pacemaker implantation in a patient with rheumatoid arthritis. This rare complication has only been reported in the literature in 6 cases [3–8]. We will be presenting our case as well as reviewing the literature in order to characterize cases of PG complicating pacemaker implantation and how dermatologic and cardiac conditions were concomitantly managed.

2. Case Report

A 76-year-old male with a history of rheumatoid arthritis presented to the cardiology team with symptomatic bradycardia. Indications for implantation of a dual-chamber pacing system were met, and the procedure was performed in a routine fashion in the left prepectoral area by the cardiac electrophysiologist. Standard postoperative precautions were

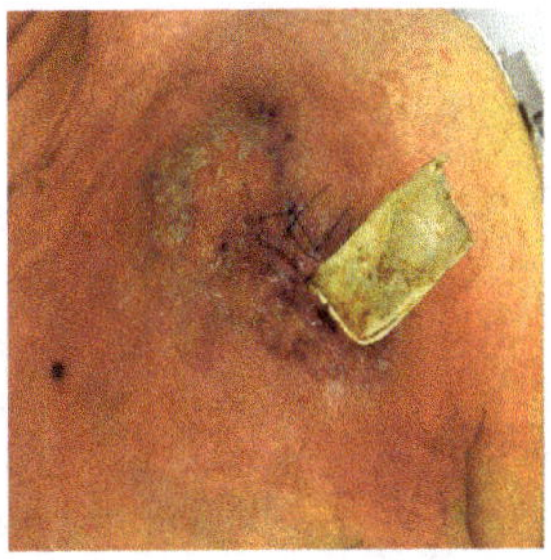

Figure 1: Purulent ulcer with dusky, violaceous borders on a background of erythema.

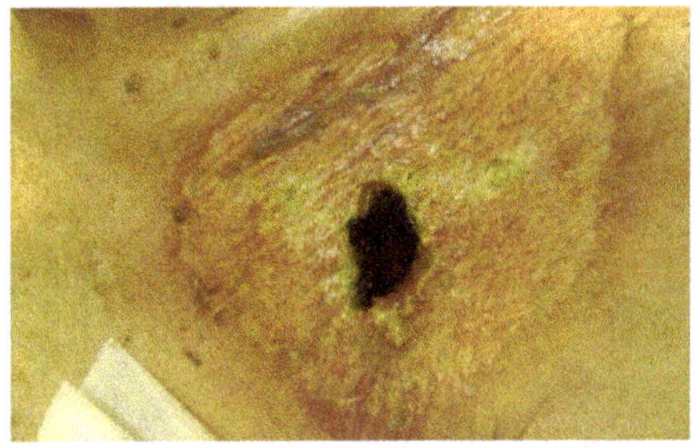

Figure 2: Healing ulcer with black central crusting and a rim of erythema.

taken, and the patient was discharged uneventfully the following day. A course of prophylactic antibiotics was prescribed, consisting of doxycycline 100 mg PO twice daily.

The patient returned to the pacemaker clinic for follow-up four days later, complaining of pain at the incision site, coupled with erythema and purulent drainage (Figure 1). Signs and symptoms were suspicious for a pocket infection, and the patient was admitted for parenteral antibiotics (vancomycin and piperacillin/tazobactam) and scheduled for device removal. A complete blood count (CBC) revealed a mildly elevated white blood cell count (10.9×10^3/microliter) and a neutrophil count within normal limits. Swabs of the purulent material in the pacemaker pocket at the time of device explantation were sent for aerobic and anaerobic cultures and were negative for bacterial growth. Three sets of blood cultures were also negative.

Consultations with an infectious disease specialist and a dermatologist were requested, and the diagnosis of pyoderma gangrenosum was strongly considered. Skin biopsy was performed, revealing massive neutrophilic infiltration and necrosis consistent with pyoderma gangrenosum. The patient underwent device removal and received systemic corticosteroids at a dose of 1 mg/kg prednisone with complete lesion healing in 3 weeks (Figure 2). While being maintained on steroids, the patient underwent reimplantation of a new pacemaker on the contralateral side without complication and had a normal postoperative course. Steroids were then tapered gradually over 3 months with no recurrence of disease 1 year later.

3. Discussion

PG has been associated with systemic inflammation, surgery, or minor trauma. However, most cases are of unknown etiology. PG lesions often begin as tender, inflammatory papules or pustules with an indurated, dusky red peripheral rim [1]. As necrosis ensues, an ulcer forms a pustular base with a violaceous border. Less commonly, PG can present with bullous, vegetative, or pustular predominance [9]. Postoperative PG can be seen following surgery, whereby ulcers present at the surgical site within 2 weeks following the operation [10]. This presents as severe pain out of proportion to physical exam along with erythema and wound dehiscence [10].

Diagnosis of PG is often difficult to make, given the nonspecific clinical and histopathological manifestations. Clinical findings may mimic primary cutaneous infection, vasculitis, drug-induced tissue injury, or other inflammatory disorders [1]. Biopsy often reveals nonspecific findings that can include granulomatous dermatitis, folliculitis, and leukocytoclastic vasculitis [1]. Workup for underlying etiologies of PG should be considered. This includes CBC, erythrocyte sedimentation rate (ESR), liver function tests (LFTs), protein electrophoresis, antineutrophil cytoplasmic antibodies (ANCA), and cryoglobulins [1]. In many cases, an underlying etiology is not found.

The first-line treatment of PG is systemic corticosteroids (0.5-2.0 mg/kg/day), along with local wound management [1, 8]. Addition of oral cyclosporine to systemic steroids may be required when initial disease is severe [1]. Mycophenolate mofetil, cyclophosphamide, chlorambucil, and azathioprine have also been effective in corticosteroid-resistant cases [1, 11]. Once systemic corticosteroid is tapered, maintenance with immunosuppressant agents can be considered. Commonly used immunosuppressants are cyclosporine and antitumor necrosis factor (TNF) agents, which include infliximab and etanercept [8].

Presentation of PG following pacemaker implantation has been reported in 6 cases, 4 of which were initially managed as infectious complications and treated with antibiotics (Table 1). Following continued necrosis and ulceration, further workup revealed a diagnosis of pyoderma gangrenosum. In all cases, systemic corticosteroids resulted in local improvement of PG ulcers. In some of the cases, reimplantation of the pacemaker with the use of cyclosporine allowed cardiologists to manage the cardiac condition while preventing recurrence of PG.

We present this case report, along with the review of literature, in order to highlight the multidisciplinary approach to management, which requires dermatologic treatment in order to achieve pacemaker success. Given the rare nature of the complication, cardiologists are unlikely to encounter it in practice. However, when it does occur, it is likely that an infectious nature be the highest on the list of differential diagnoses simply due to the clinical presentation. Nevertheless, it is important for cardiologists to consider PG and have a lower threshold for a dermatologic consult or biopsy in cases where antibiotics have been ineffective. This can prevent delayed diagnosis, reducing the risk of more severe

Table 1: Pyoderma gangrenosum following pacemaker implantation.

Author, year	Patient characteristics	Onset	Presentation	Outcome
Lo et al. [3], 2002	85 F with monoclonal gammopathy and polymyalgia rheumatica	Not discussed	Ulcer with erythematous border on the left anterior chest	Initial treatment as infection led to pacemaker extraction; healing occurred with systemic corticosteroids.
Gebska et al. [4], 2005	71 M	Recurrent skin lesions at the site of pacemaker implantation in the upper thorax	Not discussed	Steroid therapy resulted in improvement and abdominal implant was considered instead.
Kaur et al. [5], 2006	71 F with syncope	3 weeks following pacemaker implantation	Red, indurated, and partially open ulcer at the site of implant	Patient was started on antibiotics and pacemaker was removed. Two more trials of pacemaker insertion were done with continued ulceration in both cases. Topical steroids were ineffective. Prednisolone (20 mg/day) for 10 days resulted in improvement. Remained well-controlled on cyclosporine for two months without recurrence.
Cosio et al. [6], 2006	70 F with monoclonal gammopathy, diabetes, and 2 : 1 atrioventricular block	Postoperative day 7	Painful, necrotic lesion at the implant site	Prednisone (60 mg daily) led to healing within 3 weeks. Patient developed concomitant heart failure and nephrotic syndrome, which led to death 1 month following admission.
Duncan et al. [7], 2009	64 M with second-degree heart block	15 months following pacemaker implantation	Unrelated trauma to the implant site led to cystic swelling and subsequent ulceration	Pacemaker broke down following ulceration. Antibiotics failed to benefit. Prednisolone (60 mg/day) led to improvement. This was followed by recurrence after steroids taper. Restarting prednisolone with cyclosporine (3 mg/kg) led to complete healing. Patient remained controlled on cyclosporine.
Marzak et al. [8], 2019	72 M with 2 : 1 atrioventricular block	Postoperative day 4	Inflammatory, infiltrative, necrotic ulcer at the implant site	Initial treatment with antibiotics led to continued necrosis; local healing occurred with systemic corticosteroids. On postoperative day 45, patient developed septic shock secondary to infection of prior PG lesion. Removal and reimplantation of new pacemaker were done. IV infliximab (5 mg/kg), colchicine (1 mg/day), corticosteroids (1 mg/kg), and antibiotics were prophylactically given. One-year follow-up was uneventful.
Ayoubi et al., 2019	76 M with rheumatoid arthritis	Postoperative day 4	Pain at the incision site, coupled with erythema and purulent drainage	Initial treatment with antibiotics was ineffective. Swabs of purulent material revealed negative cultures for bacterial growth. Systemic prednisone (1 mg/kg) resulted in complete healing in 3 weeks. Steroid maintenance allowed for reimplantation of new pacemaker without complications.

complications such as actual infection. Furthermore, prophylaxis against PG can allow for reimplantation of the pacemaker by cardiologists, allowing patients to receive the requirement operation that prompted this condition in the first place.

Abbreviations

PG: Pyoderma gangrenosum
CBC: Complete blood count
ESR: Erythrocyte sedimentation rate
LFT: Liver function tests
ANCA: Antineutrophil cytoplasmic antibodies
TNF: Tumor necrosis factor.

References

[1] T. P. Habif, *Clinical Dermatology: A Color Guide to Diagnosis and Therapy*, Elsevier Inc, 2016.

[2] E. Ruocco, S. Sangiuliano, A. G. Gravina, A. Miranda, and G. Nicoletti, "Pyoderma gangrenosum: an updated review," *Journal of the European Academy of Dermatology and Venereology*, vol. 23, no. 9, pp. 1008–1017, 2009.

[3] T. S. N. Lo, M. Griffith, and M. E. Heber, "Pyoderma gangrenosum presented as a refractory wound infection following permanent pacemaker implantation," *Heart*, vol. 87, no. 5, p. 414, 2002.

[4] E. Gebska, M. Pindycka-Piaszczyńska, W. Zajecki, B. Filipowska, D. Sabat, and J. Jarzab, "Pyoderma gangrenosum after a pacemaker implantation–case report," *Polski Merkuriusz Lekarski*, vol. 18, no. 103, pp. 92–95, 2005.

[5] M. R. Kaur, J. E. Gach, H. Marshall, and H. M. Lewis, "Recurrent postoperative pyoderma gangrenosum complicating pacemaker insertion," *Journal of the European Academy of Dermatology and Venereology*, vol. 20, no. 4, pp. 466-467, 2006.

[6] F. G. Cosío, C. G. Herrada, A. Monereo, A. Pastor, and A. Núñez, "Pyoderma gangrenosum complicating pacemaker implant," *Europace*, vol. 8, no. 12, pp. 1068-1069, 2006.

[7] A. Duncan, A. Bharati, J. Wu, P. Currie, and S. I. White, "Pyoderma gangrenosum following pacemaker insertion," *Clinical and Experimental Dermatology*, vol. 34, no. 3, pp. 444-445, 2009.

[8] H. Marzak, J. J. von Hunolstein, D. Lipsker, M. Chauvin, O. Morel, and L. Jesel, "Management of a superinfected pyoderma gangrenosum after pacemaker implant," *HeartRhythm Case Reports*, vol. 5, no. 2, pp. 63–65, 2019.

[9] C. Schadt, "Pyoderma gangrenosum: Pathogenesis, clinical features, and diagnosis," 2019, https://www.uptodate.com/contents/pyoderma-gangrenosum-pathogenesis-clinical-features-and-diagnosis?search=pyoderma%20gangrenosum&source=search_result&selectedTitle=1~92&usage_type=default&display_rank=1.

[10] S. N. Tolkachjov, A. S. Fahy, D. A. Wetter et al., "Postoperative pyoderma gangrenosum (PG): the Mayo Clinic experience of 20 years from 1994 through 2014," *Journal of the American Academy of Dermatology*, vol. 73, no. 4, pp. 615–622, 2015.

[11] U. Wollina and G. Haroske, "Pyoderma gangraenosum," *Current Opinion in Rheumatology*, vol. 23, no. 1, pp. 50–56, 2011.

5

A Case Report of Accidental Intoxication following Ingestion of Foxglove Confused with Borage: High Digoxinemia without Major Complications

Maria Silvia Negroni,[1] Arianna Marengo,[2] Donatella Caruso,[3] Alessandro Tayar,[1] Patrizia Rubiolo,[2] Flavio Giavarini,[3] Simone Persampieri,[1] Enrico Sangiovanni,[3] Franca Davanzo,[4] Stefano Carugo,[1] Maria Laura Colombo,[2] and Mario Dell'Agli[3]

[1]*Division of Cardiology, San Paolo Hospital, Department of Health Sciences, University of Milan, Via A. Di Rudini 8, Milan, Italy*
[2]*Department of Drug Science and Technology, Università degli Studi di Torino, Via Pietro Giuria 9, Turin, Italy*
[3]*Department of Pharmacological and Biomolecular Sciences, Università degli Studi di Milano, Via Balzaretti 9, Milan, Italy*
[4]*Poison Control Centre of Milan, Niguarda Ca' Granda Hospital, Milan, Italy*

Correspondence should be addressed to Mario Dell'Agli; mario.dellagli@unimi.it

Academic Editor: Kuan-Rau Chiou

Foxglove (*Digitalis purpurea* L.) leaves are frequently confused with borage (*Borago officinalis* L.), which is traditionally used as a food ingredient. Due to the presence of the cardiac glycosides, mostly digitoxin, foxglove leaves are poisonous to human and may be fatal if ingested. A 55-year-old Caucasian woman complaining weakness, fatigue, nausea, and vomiting was admitted to the Emergency Department. Her symptoms started following consumption of a home-made savory pie with 5 leaves from a plant bought in a garden nursery as borage. Digoxinemia was high (10.4 μg/L). The patient was admitted to the cardiac intensive care unit for electrocardiographic monitoring. Two days after admission, a single episode of advanced atrioventricular (AV) block was recorded by telemetry, followed by a second-degree AV block episode. Plasma samples at day 11 were analysed by LC-MS spectrometry, and gitoxin was identified suggesting that this compound may be responsible for the clinical toxicity rather than digoxin. In the case of *Digitalis* spp. poisoning, laboratory data should be interpreted according to the clinical picture and method of analysis used since a variety of glycosides, which are chemically similar to the cardioactive glycosides but without or with fewer cardiac effects, may be incorrectly recognized as digoxin by the test, giving misleading results.

1. Introduction

Intoxication due to misleading identification of plants is increasing especially among consumers of natural products. Among frequent cases already described in the literature are those in which foxglove (*Digitalis purpurea* L.) is picked up and consumed as wild borage (*Borago officinalis* L.).

Borage is an annual herbaceous plant whose young leaves are widely consumed in several countries as a traditional food ingredient; young leaves are widely used in traditional Italian cuisine.

Foxglove is an herbaceous biennial or short-lived plant with flowers arranged in a terminal elongated cluster; flowers are typically purple, but some species may have pink, yellow, or white flowers. Due to the presence of the cardiac glycosides, mostly digitoxin, foxglove leaves are poisonous to human and may be fatal if ingested. However, pure compounds, digitoxin and digoxin, are currently used as drug in patients with congestive heart failure.

Borage leaves resemble those of foxglove, and cases of confusion between the two plants have already been reported in literature [1, 2]. The wrong identification may occur especially before flowering since the flowers of the two plants, often blue, but sometimes pink for borage and the rose tubular flowers of foxglove make them clearly distinguishable [3]. The mistake is also due to the hairiness of the leaves which

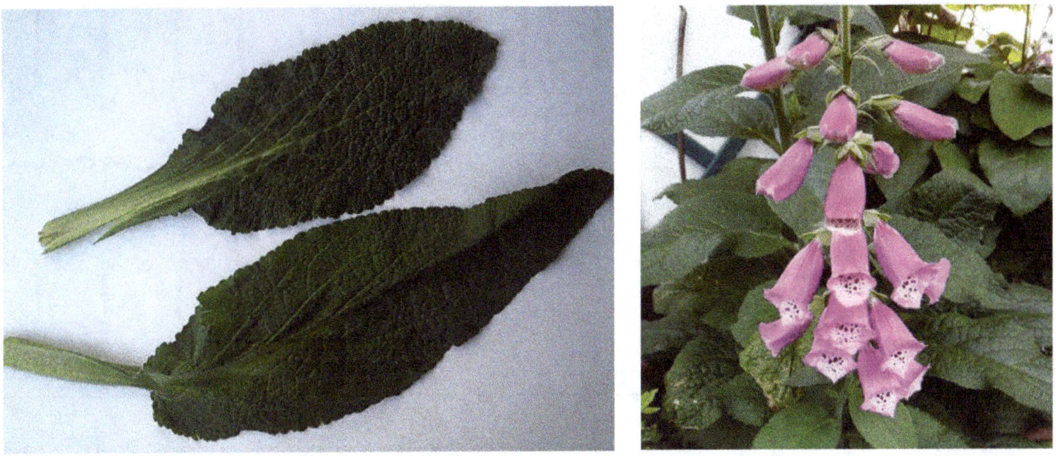

(a) (b)

FIGURE 1: (a) Two fresh leaves belonging to a plant responsible for the intoxication. Samples were deposited at the Poison Centre of Niguarda Hospital, Milan, Italy. The leaves were subjected to macro and microscopic analyses suitable for the identification by a botanist. Then, the leaves were dried and used for phytochemical analyses. (b) Plant during flowering.

present similar characteristics, although borage leaves are covered with rough and bristly hairs whereas foxgloves leaves are provided with soft hairs similar to velvet.

2. Case Report

A 55-year-old Caucasian woman was admitted to the Emergency Department (ED) with generalized discomfort including weakness and fatigue, nausea, and vomiting. Her symptoms had started 4 hours after lunch following consumption of a home-made savory pie with a potato, an egg, and 5 leaves from a plant bought 1 year before in a garden nursery, labelled and sold as "Borage," a well-known edible plant in Italy.

The Poison Control Centre of Niguarda Hospital (Milan, Italy) was consulted, and a sample consisting of two fresh leaves was sent to the aforementioned centre for the botanical identification (Figure 1(a)). The leaves were subsequently identified as a plant belonging to the *Digitalis* genus. At admission to emergency department (ED), vital signs, initial laboratory tests, and physical examination were normal. She only complained moderate epigastric pain. An electrocardiogram (ECG) showed sinus arrhythmia with nonspecific abnormalities of ventricular repolarization (VR). She was treated with intravenous (IV) metoclopramide and was maintained under observation in ED. Due to persisting symptoms, an abdominal ultrasound scan was performed, with no detection of liver or pancreas morphofunctional abnormalities.

A second ECG was performed, showing sinus rhythm (SR) at 70 bpm with normal AV conduction and worsening of VR, characterized by diffuse ST segment depression with down-up sloping, i.e., a "scooping" pattern. Transthoracic echocardiography revealed normal morphology and functional left ventricle.

The patient denied drug ingestion except for low dose methimazole, prescribed for a history of inveterate hyperthyroidism. Due to the symptoms and the electrocardiographic anomalies compatible with cardiac glycosides intoxication and bearing in mind the recent ingestion of plant leaves, blood samples were collected to dose serum digoxin levels using the multiple-point immune-rate test (VITROS DGXN) as standard procedure of the hospital laboratory. Digoxinemia was high (10.4 μg/L, with the therapeutic range from 0.8 to 2.0 μg/L). The patient was admitted to the cardiac intensive care unit for monitoring. Hydration treatment with electrolytic solution and potassium supplements was carried on. Diuresis was forced with IV furosemide.

The Poison Control Centre was contacted, and appropriate procedures were suggested for the case and support of the patient.

Two days after admission, a single episode of advanced AV block (two consecutive P waves not followed by a QRS complex) was recorded by telemetry, followed by a second-degree AV block episode (Figure 2(a)). Three days after admission, a transient appearance of late bigeminal ventricular ectopic beats was observed. On the fourth day, a single run of accelerated idioventricular rhythm (8 beats at 72 bpm) was detected (Figure 2(b)). Serum potassium levels were constantly normal. Gastric symptoms resolved after 2 days with IV antiemetic and oral proton pump inhibitor. Telemetry showed a persistent SR with occasional episodes of sinoatrial block and a slow regression of the VR intoxication signs. Serum digoxinemia were still considered toxic (2.4 μg/L) on day 12 (Figure 3).

After discharge at day 12, the patient returned to her home and sent us a picture of the plant on his balcony, which in the meantime bloomed. The typical purple tubular flowers confirmed that it was a plant belonging to the *Digitalis* genus (Figure 1(b)).

Samples obtained at day 11 were subjected to extraction and injected in liquid chromatography-mass spectrometry (LC-MS) system to identify individual metabolites. Mass spectrometry is considered the best methodology to detect toxic components from poisonous plants giving unequivocal identification. In brief, molecules are subjected to ionization

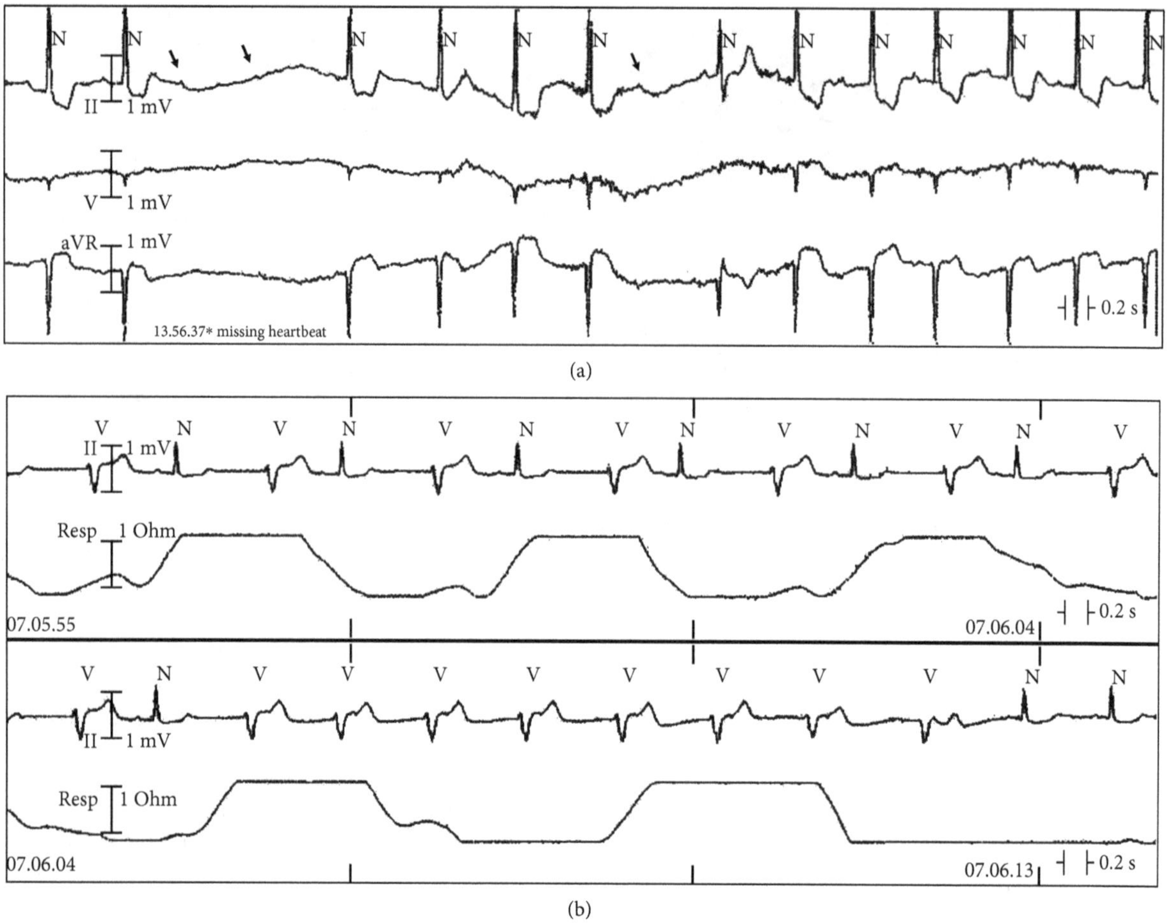

Figure 2: (a) Telemetry recordings showing sinus rhythm with a single episode of advanced AV block (two consecutive P waves not followed by a QRS complex—arrows) followed by second-degree AV block episode. Note diffuse ST segment depression with down-up sloping typical of digitalis intoxication. (b) Telemetry recordings showing bigeminal ventricular ectopic beats and a run of accelerated idioventricular rhythm (8 beats at 72 bpm). Reduction of the intoxication signs.

and separated according to their mass-to-charge (*m*/*z*) ratio. Retention time (RT) represents the measurement of the time taken by a molecule from injection to detection; a variety of factors may influence this parameter including the mobile and stationary phases.

As shown in Figure 4, plasma contained traces of gitoxin identified in comparison to the authentic peak (b) whereas digitoxin and digoxin were not detectable. Peak at retention time (RT) 3.87, with 825 *m*/*z* and fragmentation at 779 *m*/*z* was also present in the plasma; although fragmentation was similar to other cardioactive glycosides, unequivocal identification was not possible.

3. Discussion

Botanical identification is a prerequisite essential to confirm cardiac glycoside intoxication. According to the typical morphology, leaves were identified as inserted on the stem; these leaves are without petiole, ever smaller and long lanceolate, with the rounded base, margin crenate, and subacute apex; they are rather coarsely reticulated-veined, covered (both sides) with soft white glandular trichomes, short, unicellular stalk, and bicellular head. There are also covering trichomes, uniseriate, and multicellular (3–5 cells) with collapsed cells. From the set of observations made at the time of admission to the hospital, it was reasonably agreed that the patient had ingested *Digitalis* instead of borage leaves.

To confirm botanical identification and provide key information on the presence of specific cardiac glycosides in the plant, leaf extract was analysed by HPLC-PDA-ESI-MS/MS system. A comparison between the leaf extract profile with those of the different commercially available standard compounds was performed. The overlap of the retention times and spectral information (UV and MS fragmentation pattern) confirmed the presence of digitoxin and gitoxin in the leaf extract while digitonin, digoxin, and lanatoside C were not detected.

The amounts of digitoxin and gitoxin were 0.41 μg/mg (RSD% = 0.6) and 0.197 μg/mg (RSD% = 8.2) (dried plant material), respectively, according to the data reported in the literature [4].

Phytochemical analysis unequivocally identified a plant of genus *Digitalis* as responsible for the intoxication; however, it was important to identify the cardiac glycosides present in the plasma of the woman.

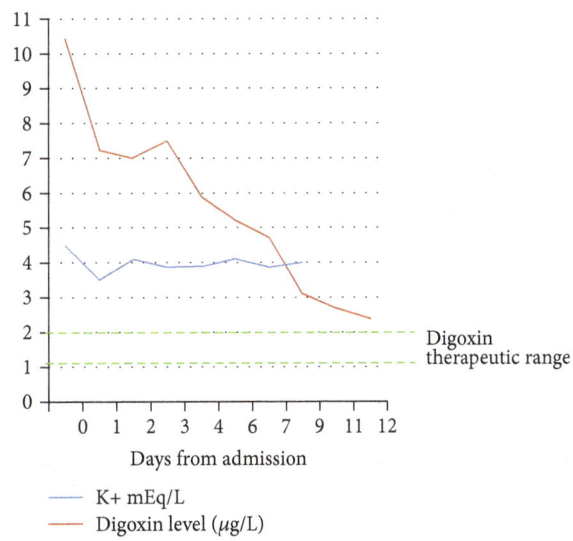

FIGURE 3: Graphical representation of potassium and digoxin serum levels measured in the study patient from day 0 up to day 12.

The leaves from the plant sold to the patient as borage resulted as belonging to the genus *Digitalis* after morpho-botanical and phytochemical analysis. Accidental or suicidal ingestion of plants containing cardiac glycosides may cause several clinical manifestations with a possible fatal outcome [5].

The severity of the poisoning may depend on the amount of plant ingested and on the clinical condition of the subject. Episodes of *Digitalis* toxicity due to overdose or accumulation of the drug in chronically treated patients are also well described in literature. However, there is no linear correlation between arrhythmias from *Digitalis* intoxication and serum digoxin levels [6]. Episodes of clinical intoxication associated with plasma concentrations in the therapeutic range may be explained by the narrow therapeutic window of the drug. In addition, natural sources of cardiac glycosides contain a multitude of metabolites in varying proportions and with different chemical, biological, and pharmacokinetic properties.

In general, a suspected diagnosis of *Digitalis* intoxication is based on anamnestic data, typical clinical manifestations (gastrointestinal, cardiac, neurological, ocular), and electrocardiographic patterns and is confirmed by laboratory tests. However, digoxin dosage in case of plant poisoning may vary according to the method of analysis used [7].

The multiple-point immune-rate test (VITROS DGXN) is based on an antigen-antibody reaction coupled with an enzymatic reaction. The antigen competes with the enzyme for binding to the antibody. The enzyme mediates the oxidation of colorless leuco dye thus forming a dye. The rate of dye formation is inversely proportional to the digoxin concentration in the sample.

In the clinical case described, the digoxinemia determined with this method was particularly high (10.4 μg/L, while plasma levels of digoxin greater than 10 μg/L are considered potentially lethal) despite modest early gastrointestinal symptoms and mild cardiac manifestations (short-term arrhythmias with spontaneous resolution). Once clinically stable and with no specific antidote administration, a slow and gradual reduction in serum digoxin levels was also observed in the patient.

Taking into account digoxin-like glycoside cross-reactivity (as declared by the immuno-enzymatic test manufacturer), and the fact that *Digitalis purpurea* L. generally does not contain digoxin but digitoxin and gitoxin in the leaves and gitalin in the seeds (while digoxin is contained in the leaves of *Digitalis lanata* L., the source of the human drug), we carried out a more specific qualitative analysis of both the different components of the plant and patient plasma. Thus, liquid chromatography coupled with mass spectrometry (LC-MS) was used to analyse a sample of the leaves ingested by the patient, and the plasma collected at day 11. In the leaves, the presence of digitoxin and gitoxin was confirmed, while digitonin, digoxin, and lanatoside C were not detected. Plasma sample was extracted, and peaks compared with commercially available standards; chromatographic profile by LC-MS (SCIEX Triple Quad™ 3500, AB Sciexsrl, Italy) revealed traces of gitoxin whereas digitoxin was undetectable. A peak at R.T. 3.87 with fragmentation typical of cardiac glycosides but still unknown was also detected (Figure 4).

Digitoxin has a longer half-life (5-7 days) than digoxin (36-48 hours) and gitoxin; toxic effects, which are similar to those of digoxin, may last longer. However, just low amount of gitoxin were detected in the plasma 11 days after intoxication. As reported in Figure 4, the patient at day 11 showed digoxinemia at levels considered toxic (2.4 μg/L); the high value without serious symptoms could be due to the method, which measures all glycosides occurring in the plant also those without potential toxicity. However, toxic effects due to the presence of digitoxin in the first days following intoxication cannot be excluded.

Literature describes episodes of intoxication with homemade digitalis extracts with a favourable evolution without administration of digoxin antibody fragments (Fab) [8] or characterized by an intoxication duration period not

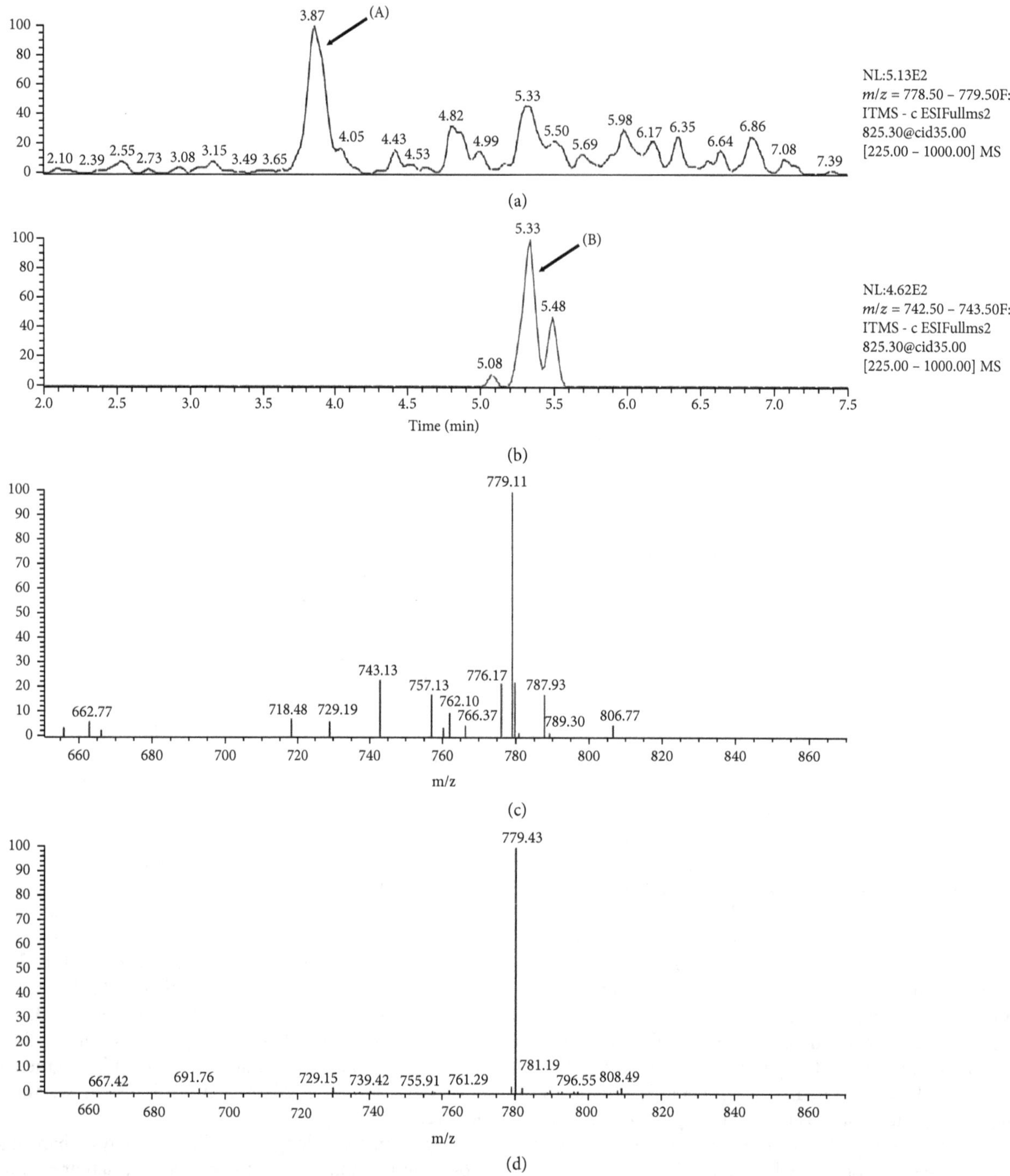

Figure 4: Plasma analysis by LC-MS. (a) Plasma profile with peak (A) corresponding to a glycoside unidentified; (b) authentic standard of gitoxin, which allowed to identify the compound in plasma sample; (c) fragmentation of gitoxin with typical fragment at 743 m/z; and (d) fragmentation of unknown compound with a fragment at 779 m/z.

significantly reduced by antidote therapy (as would be expected in cases of drug intoxication instead) [9]. Foxglove acute intoxication is the result of the additive effects of the various cardiac glycosides contained in the plant.

The indication of a specific treatment remains within the discretion of the emergency physician at present and is based mainly on the manifestations and severity of the clinical picture.

In the case of *Digitalis* spp. poisoning, whose active principles are used as drugs (i.e., digitoxin or digoxin), laboratory data should be interpreted according to the method of analysis used taking into consideration that a variety of glycosides chemically similar to cardioactive glycosides but without or with fewer cardiac effects may be recognized as digoxin by the test, giving misleading results.

Acknowledgments

This research was partially supported by grants from MIUR "Progetto Eccellenza."

References

[1] L. Bonfanti, G. Lippi, I. Ciullo et al., "In the kingdom of "tortelli" (ravioli-like pasta) plant poisoning is still a threat. A case report of near-fatal poisoning from Digitalis purpurea accidentally confused with Borago officinalis," *Acta Biomed*, vol. 87, no. 3, pp. 353–357, 2017.

[2] S. Maffè, L. Cucchi, F. Zenone et al., "Digitalis must be banished from the table: a rare case of acute accidental Digitalis intoxication of a whole family," *Journal of Cardiovascular Medicine*, vol. 10, no. 9, pp. 727–732, 2009.

[3] T. Brigham, M. Schroder, and W. Cocksedge, *Good Practices for Plant Identification*, Agriculture and Agri-Food, Canada, 2004.

[4] H. J. Kwon, H. J. Sim, S. I. Lee, Y. M. Lee, Y. D. Park, and S. P. Hong, "HPLC method validation for *Digitalis* and its analogue by pulsed amperometric detection," *Journal of Pharmaceutical and Biomedical Analysis*, vol. 54, no. 1, pp. 217–221, 2011.

[5] S. L. Ramlakhan and A. K. Fletcher, "It could have happened to van Gogh: a case of fatal purple foxglove poisoning and review of the literature," *European Journal of Emergency Medicine*, vol. 14, no. 6, pp. 356–359, 2007.

[6] W. Shapiro, "Correlative studies of serum digitalis levels and the arrhythmias of digitalis intoxication," *The American Journal of Cardiology*, vol. 41, no. 5, pp. 852–859, 1978.

[7] L. M. Castello, S. Negro, F. Santi et al., "Accidental digitoxin intoxication: an interplay between laboratory and clinical medicine," *Biochemia Medica*, vol. 22, no. 3, pp. 380–384, 2012.

[8] S. Thierry, F. Blot, J. C. Lacherade, Y. Lefort, P. Franzon, and C. Brun-Buisson, "Poisoning with foxglove extract: favorable evolution without fab fragments," *Intensive Care Medicine*, vol. 26, no. 10, p. 1586, 2000.

[9] S. A. Rich, J. M. Libera, and R. J. Locke, "Treatment of foxglove extract poisoning with digoxin-specific Fab fragments," *Annals of Emergency Medicine*, vol. 22, no. 12, pp. 1904–1907, 1993.

6

Percutaneous Balloon Pericardiotomy (PBP) Revisited

Raed Aqel[1] **Muawiyah Elqadi,**[2] **Ahmad Hammouri,**[2] **and Mohammad S. Alqadi**[3]

[1]*National Center for Diabetes, Endocrinology and Genetics Center, Amman, Jordan*
[2]*Al-Quds University, Faculty of Medicine, Jerusalem, State of Palestine*
[3]*Al-Ahli Hospital, Hebron, State of Palestine*

Correspondence should be addressed to Raed Aqel; raed.aqel@yahoo.com

Academic Editor: Assad Movahed

Background. A Percutaneous Balloon Pericardiotomy (PBP) procedure is a reemerging nonsurgical technique that helps in preventing the reaccumulation of pericardial effusion. It is done percutaneously without general anaesthesia. It has been proved to be effective in alleviating and preventing recurrent pericardial effusion. *Case Presentation.* We reported a 52-year-old male with stage IV adenocarcinoma causing recurrent pericardial effusion. The patient experienced a worsening shortness of breath. A surgical pericardial window was denied by the surgery team secondary to severe respiratory distress; subsequently, the patient underwent Percutaneous Balloon Pericardiotomy. *Conclusion.* Percutaneous Balloon Pericardiotomy is efficacious and safe when done by well-trained physicians. We think it should be considered as a preferred treatment modality in most sicker patients with recurrent pericardial effusion.

1. Background

Recurrent large hemodynamically significant pericardial effusions, whether inflammatory or noninflammatory, remain a major health risk that can be life-threatening. Almost exclusively, these patients end in critical care units (CCU or ICU) undergoing emergency pericardial fluid aspiration mostly through catheter-based pericardiocentesis and sometimes through surgical aspiration and pericardial window creation [1].

Percutaneous Balloon Pericardiotomy (PBP) procedure is a reemerging older procedure; it is a nonsurgical technique that helps in preventing reaccumulation of pericardial effusion [1]. It is done percutaneously in the Cath suite avoiding heavy sedation and anaesthesia required for surgical window creation [2]. Initially, it was proposed by Palacios et al. in 1991 [3], after which being adopted and improved by many others [4]. Herein, we revisit this topic through a case report of PBP and review of literature.

2. Case Presentation

A 52-year-old male with stage IV adenocarcinoma of unknown primary, with lung and liver metastasis, presented with a worsening shortness of breath. TTE showed a large pericardial effusion pending tamponade for which he underwent emergency pericardiocentesis where 1 L of haemorrhagic fluid was drained, the drain was left in place for 48 hours then stopped, and the patient was discharged home after 48 hours. Fluid analysis showed exudative nature but no malignant cells.

Three months later, the patient presented again with a worsening shortness of breath and respiratory distress. Transthoracic echocardiogram (TTE) showed a reaccumulation of large 2.6 cm concentric pericardial effusion, with no evidence of tamponade.

A surgical pericardial window was denied by the surgery team secondary to severe respiratory distress. The patient underwent PBP. A drain was left for 24 hours after which

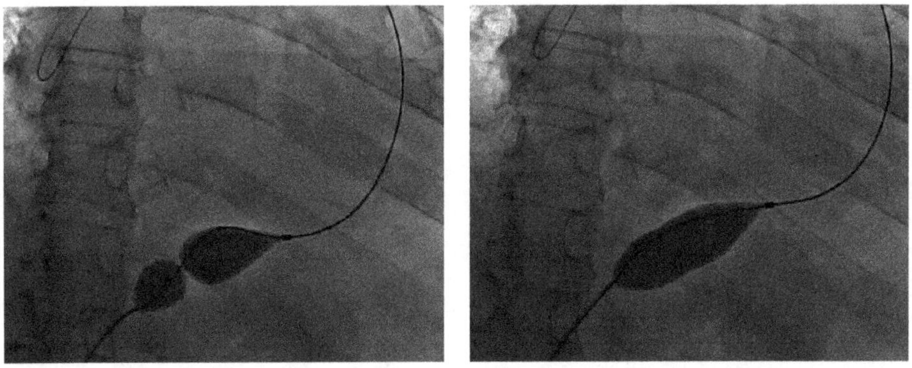

(a) (b)

FIGURE 1: (a) Fluoroscopically showing the pericardiotomy balloon by the pericardium. (b) After balloon inflation, the balloon waist disappeared.

the patient was discharged home. His subsequent clinic and TTE evaluation at 3 and 6 months revealed no more pericardial effusion accumulation.

3. Procedure

After administration of local anaesthesia, pericardiocentesis was performed using the classic subxiphoid approach; after aspiration of 700 cc of haemorrhagic fluid utilizing a pigtail, a stiff wire exchange was performed. Under fluoroguidance, a $2.0 * 20\,\text{mm}$ Z MED balloon, Medtronic manufacture, was placed at the pericardial edge; the balloon was inflated twice until the balloon waist disappeared (Figure 1), and a drain was left in place for 24 hours after the procedure.

Intraprocedure echocardiography showed intact cardiac champers. Follow-up CXR and TTE after 24 hours showed a mild increase in the left pleural effusion with no pericardial effusion.

4. Discussion

Recurrent pericardial effusion can complicate many inflammatory and noninflammatory disorders, including infectious diseases, systemic inflammatory disorders, endocrine system diseases, and chronic renal failure [5]. Moreover, disseminated malignancy can cause large pericardial effusions and can lead to cardiac tamponade [6]. Large pericardial effusions with and without tamponade is considered a clinical emergency as they might lead to progressive development of hemodynamic instability, rendering prompt diagnosis and initiation of treatment extremely essential [2].

The optimal management of pericardial effusion with tamponade remains controversial and is highly dependent on its etiology [1]. Pericardiocentesis with drainage is considered to be one of the mostly used nonsurgical treatment modalities, which can be accompanied by the installation of chemotherapeutic or sclerosing agents within the pericardial cavity [7]. Surgical approach can be used for resistant cases by the creation of a pericardial window to prevent reaccumulation [6]. The recurrence rate after pericardiocentesis is 13% to 50%, whereas it is just 4.9% after subxiphoid surgical windowing of the pericardium [7].

PBP (Percutaneous Balloon Pericardiotomy) was introduced in 1991 by Palacios et al. [3]. It provided a less invasive method than the surgical windowing with lower recurrence rates of effusion when compared with pericardiocentesis and sclerosing agents' instillation [7]. As it does not require general anaesthesia, it can be a preferred treatment modality in malignant pericardial effusions where the patients are extremely sick to undergo surgical pericardial window [8].

Despite its high success rate, which was reported to be 93% in a multicentre study of 50 patients by Ziskind et al. [7], balloon pericardiotomy has never gained a wide-spectrum acceptance because of its technical difficulty and the lack of training. Literature review revealed many case reports describing many different-etiologies large pericardial effusions treated successfully with this modality.

PBP involves the creation of a localized window or stoma between the small pericardial cavity and the spacier left pleural cavity using a percutaneous balloon-dilating catheter. The aim is to create a channel between the two cavities in an attempt to prevent the reaccumulation of fluid within the constraint pericardium [6]. This modality of treatment has proved its effectiveness in patients who present with recurrent moderate to large pericardial effusions secondary to a variety of inflammatory or noninflammatory disorders; in fact, it was even described in large recurrent pericardial effusion secondary to severe pulmonary hypertension [9]. It is generally contraindicated in infected pericardial effusions and seldomly used in this scenario [10]. This modality of treatment provides a long-term relief of pericardial effusion by shunting the fluids from the smaller pericardial space, to the bigger more forgiving pleural cavity [5].

PBP procedure is as safe as pericardiocentesis if it is done by a well-trained personnel. However, an extra caution is to be considered upon placing and inflating the pericardioplasty balloon to avoid cardiac chamber injury.

5. Conclusion

PBP is a safe and very effective procedure in treating and preventing the recurrence of pericardial effusion in certain groups of patients. Extra hands-on training is very essential.

Consent

The patient's consent was obtained from the patient himself.

Authors' Contributions

Study concept or design was done by Raed Aqel. Data collection was done by Muawiyah Elqadi, Ahmad Hammouri, and Mohammad S. Alqadi. Writing the paper was done by Raed Aqel, Ahmad Hammouri and Muawiyah Elqadi.

References

[1] M. Imazio and Y. Adler, "Management of pericardial effusion," *European Heart Journal*, vol. 34, no. 16, pp. 1186–1197, 2013.

[2] M. Galli, A. Politi, F. Pedretti, S. Zerboni, and B. Castiglioni, "Percutaneous balloon pericardiotomy for malignant pericardial tamponade," *Chest*, vol. 108, no. 6, pp. 1499–1501, 1995.

[3] I. F. Palacios, E. Murat Tuzcu, A. A. Ziskind, J. Younger, and P. C. Block, "Percutaneous balloon pericardial window for patients with malignant pericardial effusion and tamponade," *Catheterization and Cardiovascular Diagnosis*, vol. 22, no. 4, pp. 244–249, 1991.

[4] R. Aqel, N. J. Al-Khatib, G. H. Ra'ed et al., "Case report first percutaneous balloon pericardiotomy (PBP) or pericardioplasty in Jordan: a case report and review of literature," *Jordan Medical Journal*, vol. 44, no. 4, 2010.

[5] O. Bertrand, V. Legrand, and H. Kulbertus, "Percutaneous balloon pericardiotomy: a case report and analysis of mechanism of action," *Catheterization and Cardiovascular Diagnosis*, vol. 38, no. 2, pp. 180–182, 1996.

[6] N. Swanson, I. Mirza, N. Wijesinghe, and G. Devlin, "Primary percutaneous balloon pericardiotomy for malignant pericardial effusion," *Catheterization and Cardiovascular Interventions*, vol. 71, no. 4, pp. 504–507, 2008.

[7] A. A. Ziskind, A. C. Pearce, C. C. Lemmon et al., "Percutaneous balloon pericardiotomy for the treatment of cardiac tamponade and large pericardial effusions: description of technique and report of the first 50 cases," *Journal of the American College of Cardiology*, vol. 21, no. 1, pp. 1–5, 1993.

[8] R. Bhardwaj, W. Gharib, W. Gharib, B. Warden, and A. Jain, "Evaluation of safety and feasibility of percutaneous balloon pericardiotomy in hemodynamically significant pericardial effusion (review of 10-years experience in single center)," *Journal of Interventional Cardiology*, vol. 28, no. 5, pp. 409–414, 2015.

[9] R. A. Aqel, W. Aljaroudi, F. G. Hage, J. Tallaj, B. Rayburn, and N. C. Nanda, "Left ventricular collapse secondary to pericardial effusion treated with pericardiocentesis and percutaneous pericardiotomy in severe pulmonary hypertension," *Echocardiography*, vol. 25, no. 6, pp. 658–661, 2008.

[10] R. Aqel, D. Mehta, and G. J. Zoghbi, "Percutaneous balloon pericardiotomy for the treatment of infected pericardial effusion with tamponade," *The Journal of Invasive Cardiology*, vol. 18, no. 7, pp. E194–E197, 2006.

7

Catheter-Directed Thrombectomy: An Alternative in Massive Pulmonary Embolism

Andres Cordova Sanchez[1], **Mostafa Vasigh**,[2] **Oluwateniola Olatunde**,[2] **and Debanik Chaudhuri**[2]

[1]*Department of Medicine, SUNY Upstate Medical University, Syracuse, NY 13210, USA*
[2]*Division of Cardiology, SUNY Upstate Medical University, Syracuse, NY 13210, USA*

Correspondence should be addressed to Andres Cordova Sanchez; cordovaa@upstate.edu

Academic Editor: Yigit Canga

Massive pulmonary embolism (PE) is a life-threatening condition. The mainstay treatment is thrombolysis. Catheter-directed thrombectomy involves a group of new techniques that appear to have relatively low complications and mortality. These techniques have so far been studied mostly in submassive PE. We present a patient with massive PE that was successfully treated with catheter-directed thrombectomy.

1. Introduction

Massive PE is defined as acute PE with systolic blood pressure<90 mmHg for >15 minutes, ≥40 mmHg drop from baseline, or requiring hemodynamic support [1]. It has a mortality risk of 43% to 62% compared to around 15% for nonmassive PE [2].

Its management consists of early anticoagulation plus thrombolysis or thrombectomy. The mainstay treatment is thrombolysis, although it has several contraindications.

Catheter-directed therapies can be divided into directed thrombolysis and embolectomy. Catheter-directed thrombectomy is a reasonable option when there are contraindications for thrombolysis. The available systems are Flowtriever, Penumbra Indigo, and AngioVac. These thrombectomy systems are still being studied. Most studies so far have focused on submassive PE. To our knowledge, there are no studies focusing on massive PE.

We present a patient with massive PE and cardiac arrest that underwent a successful percutaneous embolectomy with a Penumbra Indigo Cat 12 device.

2. Case

A 73-year-old man with past medical history significant for upper gastrointestinal bleed 1 month ago and ischemic stroke with residual aphasia and right-sided hemiplegia 3 months before admission, respectively. He was transferred from an outside hospital for sudden acute hypoxic respiratory failure requiring 5 liters of oxygen via nasal cannula and cardiogenic shock on epinephrine and norepinephrine support. A computed tomography angiography of the chest showed a saddle PE with large thrombus burden in both right and left pulmonary arteries, leftward septal deviation, right ventricle (RV) 52.56 mm, left ventricle (LV) 27.55 mm, and RV/LV ratio of 1.9 (Figure 1). He was started on a heparin drip. En route to our hospital, he became pulseless and unresponsive. Cardiopulmonary resuscitation was started; return of spontaneous circulation was obtained after 2 rounds of epinephrine. Postarrest, he regained baseline mental status.

He was not a candidate for TPA given recent cerebral infarct and gastrointestinal bleeding; thus, he was planned for thrombectomy.

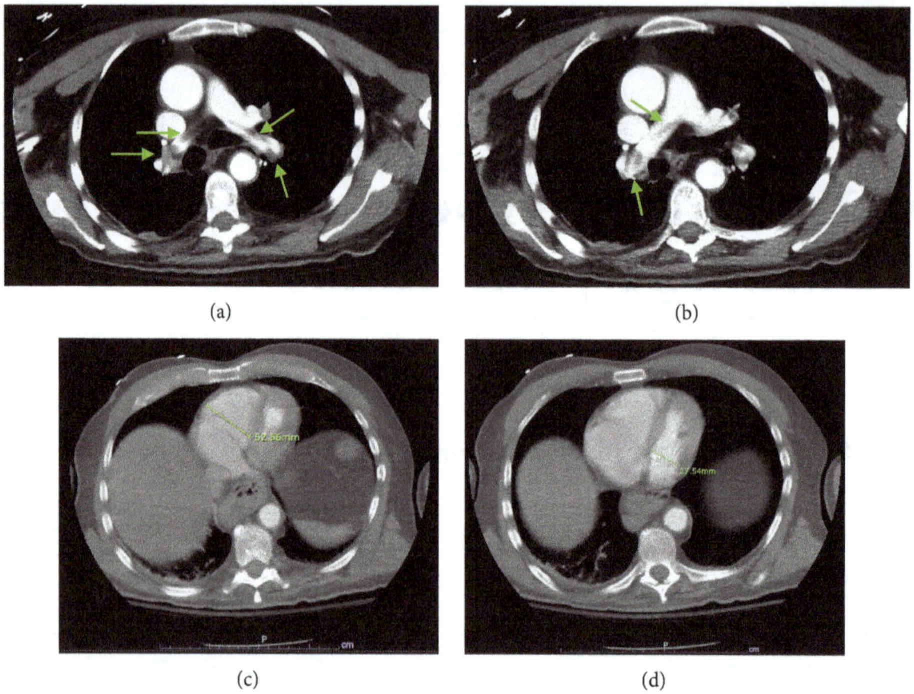

(a) (b) (c) (d)

FIGURE 1: (a, b) Pulmonary embolism on the left and right pulmonary arteries. (c, d) RV and LV measurement demonstrating an RV/LV diameter of 1.9, septal bowing to the left further supports right ventricular strain.

On arrival, he was still on obstructive shock, requiring two pressor support. He was requiring 4 liters of oxygen via nasal cannula to saturate above 90%. Soon after arrival, percutaneous thrombus aspiration with a Penumbra Indigo embolectomy CAT 12 device was done. Pulmonary angiogram after the procedure showed near-complete resolution of thrombus burden. A small residual thrombus remained despite multiple passes with the device. No complications occurred during the procedure. Postthrombectomy systolic pulmonary artery pressure dropped to 43 mmHg from 47 mmHg prethrombectomy. The patient was successfully weaned off pressors and oxygen shortly after. Doppler ultrasound of the lower extremities showed a right lower extremity deep vein thrombosis. An echocardiogram done approximately 10 hours after thrombectomy was a normal study with an ejection fraction of 70%, normal left and right ventricular function, and estimated pulmonary arterial pressure of 23 mmHg.

He remained hemodynamically stable during the rest of his hospitalization, was eventually transitioned to apixaban, and discharged on the 5th day of hospitalization.

3. Discussion

Massive PE is a life-threatening condition that requires time-sensitive management and carries high mortality risk. When thrombolysis has failed or in cases with absolute contraindications, catheter or surgical embolectomy is to be considered [1].

The Penumbra Indigo system uses a catheter connected to a suction device. To date, there is only one prospective study investigating this device, the EXTRACT-PE trial. However, it was done almost exclusively in submassive PE and had only one patient enrolled with massive PE. They found a mean reduction of RV/LV ratio of 0.43, all-cause mortality at 30 days of 2.5%, and a median introduction to removal time of 37 minutes, and major bleeding was seen in approximately 1.7% [3] compared to 10% to 11.5% with thrombolysis [4, 5]. Of the 119 patients included in the study, there was one patient death and one device-related distal artery perforation [3]. The FLARE trial looked at the use of the Flowtriever system in patients with submassive PE; it demonstrated a reduction of the RV/LV ratio of 0.38, 3.8% of major complications, and an average procedural time of 94 minutes [6].

Surgical embolectomy is an invasive procedure that classically requires median sternotomy, cardiopulmonary bypass, and pulmonary trunk excision. A minimally invasive procedure also exists [7]. Operative time appears to be similar in both classical and minimally invasive approaches at 160 minutes to 251 minutes [8]. Mortality has been reported at 6% to 23.7% for massive and 3.6% to 9.1%for submassive [9–11].

Given these results, it appears that catheter embolectomy is a safe and fast approach in patients with submassive PE. However, to our knowledge, no studies have focused on massive PE.

Catheter-directed thrombolysis uses low dose thrombolytic infusion directly into the PE and is an option for patients with pulmonary embolism that have relative contraindication to systemic thrombolysis [1]. Preliminary results from the PERFECT registry showed the use of catheter-directed thrombolysis in eight patients with absolute contraindications for systemic thrombolytics without any major bleeding events [12]. We considered that, in our case, the risk of a major bleeding event was too high on the account

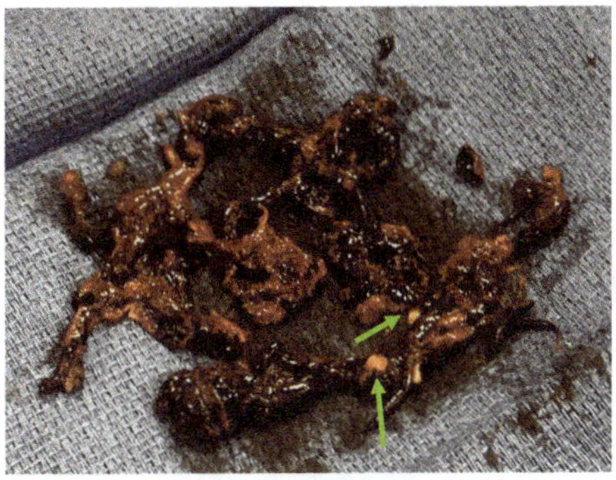

FIGURE 2: Thrombus removed during thrombectomy. White appearing thrombus (arrows) suggesting chronically organized thrombus.

of recent gastrointestinal bleeding and cerebrovascular event. Thus, only catheter embolectomy without the use of any thrombolytics was done.

Our patient presented with massive PE and high risk of bleeding. He was treated with catheter embolectomy using a Penumbra Cat 12 device with excellent results. A small residual thrombus remained despite several passes with the device; this could have been a chronically organized thrombus attached to the vessel wall, which was supported by the presence of white, chronically appearing aspirate (Figure 2).

4. Conclusions

Catheter-directed embolectomy could be considered a safe and fast alternative for the management of massive PE in patients that have failed or are not candidates for thrombolysis. These findings will need to be confirmed in randomized controlled trials.

The presence of chronically organized thrombus in patients with acute massive PE could complicate the use of catheter-directed thrombectomy.

References

[1] B. Rivera-Lebron, M. McDaniel, K. Ahrar et al., "Diagnosis, treatment and follow up of acute pulmonary embolism: consensus practice from the PERT consortium," *Clinical and Applied Thrombosis/Hemostasis*, vol. 25, 2019.

[2] N. Kucher, E. Rossi, M. de Rosa, and S. Z. Goldhaber, "Massive pulmonary embolism," *Circulation*, vol. 113, no. 4, pp. 577–582, 2006.

[3] A. K. Sista, J. M. Horowitz, V. F. Tapson et al., "Indigo aspiration system for treatment of pulmonary embolism: results of the EXTRACT-PE trial," *JACC: Cardiovascular Interventions*, vol. 14, no. 3, pp. 319–329, 2021.

[4] G. Piazza, B. Hohlfelder, M. R. Jaff et al., "A prospective, single-arm, multicenter trial of ultrasound-facilitated, catheter-directed, low-dose fibrinolysis for acute massive and submassive pulmonary embolism: the SEATTLE II study," *JACC: Cardiovascular Interventions*, vol. 8, no. 10, pp. 1382–1392, 2015.

[5] G. Meyer, E. Vicaut, T. Danays et al., "Fibrinolysis for patients with intermediate-risk pulmonary embolism," *New England Journal of Medicine*, vol. 370, no. 15, pp. 1402–1411, 2014.

[6] T. Tu, C. Toma, V. F. Tapson et al., "A prospective, single-arm, multicenter trial of catheter-directed mechanical thrombectomy for intermediate-risk acute pulmonary embolism: the FLARE study," *JACC: Cardiovascular Interventions*, vol. 12, no. 9, pp. 859–869, 2019.

[7] A. Iaccarino, G. Frati, L. Schirone et al., "Surgical embolectomy for acute massive pulmonary embolism: state of the art," *Journal of Thoracic Disease*, vol. 10, no. 8, pp. 5154–5161, 2018.

[8] C. Pasrija, A. Shah, E. Sultanik et al., "Minimally invasive surgical pulmonary Embolectomy," *Innovations: Technology and Techniques in Cardiothoracic and Vascular Surgery*, vol. 12, no. 6, pp. 406–410, 2017.

[9] R. C. Neely, J. G. Byrne, I. Gosev et al., "Surgical embolectomy for acute massive and submassive pulmonary embolism in a series of 115 patients," *The Annals of Thoracic Surgery*, vol. 100, no. 4, pp. 1245–1252, 2015.

[10] W. B. Keeling, T. Sundt, M. Leacche et al., "Outcomes after surgical pulmonary embolectomy for acute pulmonary embolus: a multi-institutional study," *The Annals of Thoracic Surgery*, vol. 102, no. 5, pp. 1498–1502, 2016.

[11] M. Leacche, D. Unic, S. Z. Goldhaber et al., "Modern surgical treatment of massive pulmonary embolism: results in 47 consecutive patients after rapid diagnosis and aggressive surgical approach," *Journal of Thoracic and Cardiovascular Surgery*, vol. 129, no. 5, pp. 1018–1023, 2005.

[12] W. T. Kuo, A. Banerjee, P. S. Kim et al., "Pulmonary embolism response to fragmentation, embolectomy, and catheter thrombolysis (PERFECT): initial results from a prospective multicenter registry," *Chest*, vol. 148, no. 3, pp. 667–673, 2015, PMID: 25856269.

8

Seizure: An Adverse Effect of Regadenoson in Myocardial Perfusion Imaging

Sohab S. Radwan and Owen G. Schwartz

Department of Internal Medicine, MedStar Washington Hospital Center, USA

Correspondence should be addressed to Sohab S. Radwan; sohab_radwan@hotmail.com

Academic Editor: Assad Movahed

Regadenoson is a selective adenosine 2a (A2a) receptor agonist that is used in cardiac stress testing to evaluate for ischemic heart disease and has largely replaced adenosine in the modern era. Since adenosine receptors are involved in synaptic transmission between neurons throughout the central nervous system (CNS) including the cerebral cortex, hippocampus, and other structures as well, regadenoson can lower the seizure threshold in susceptible individuals. Epileptogenic activity is an uncommon yet potentially severe adverse effect of regadenoson use, and therefore, more awareness is required in screening patients at risk and evaluating alternate ways to investigate coronary artery disease (CAD) in susceptible individuals.

1. Introduction

Regadenoson is a selective A2a receptor agonist that acts on coronary artery smooth muscle to promote vasodilatation, increasing myocardial blood flow. It is widely used in rest-pharmacological stress myocardial perfusion imaging (MPI) as part of cardiac testing to evaluate for CAD, especially in patients with limited exercise capacity. It has largely replaced adenosine in MPI due to a better safety profile. However, adenosine receptors and their subtypes are present in several extracardiac tissues resulting in cross reactivity and potential toxicity. One example is that adenosine receptors play a role in neuroregulation and excitatory glutamatergic transmission; thus, regadenoson can lower seizure threshold through A2a receptor stimulation. We hereby present a case of seizure provoked by regadenoson administration and subsequently discuss the underlying mechanism.

2. Case Presentation

A 74-year-old female with a past medical history of hypertension, diabetes mellitus type 2, CAD status post coronary artery bypass grafting, and ischemic stroke with residual left-sided weakness presented to the emergency department with a one-day history of retrosternal chest pain radiating to her left shoulder. On presentation she was normotensive, and electrocardiogram (EKG) revealed sinus rhythm with a heart rate of 72 beats per minute, left axis deviation, and T wave inversion in leads I and aVL which were unchanged from a prior EKG several months ago. Initial troponin I was negative. Based on her risk factor profile and pretest probability for CAD, she was scheduled for a rest-pharmacological stress MPI test. While at rest, the patient was injected intravenously with 99mTc-tetrofosmin and images were acquired approximately 45-60 minutes later with 180-degree single-photon emission computerized tomography (SPECT). Subsequently, the patient was injected with 0.4 mg of regadenoson over 15-20 seconds while being monitored by12-lead EKG. Approximately 30 seconds after regadenoson injection, the patient was injected with 99mTc-tetrofosmin and 180-degree SPECT images were taken approximately 45 minutes later. The gated SPECT images revealed normal rest and stress tetrofosmin perfusion, as well as a normal left ventricular function. Approximately 120 minutes after regadenoson administration, the patient developed a generalized tonic-clonic seizure that lasted for 3 minutes. On initial assessment, she was hemodynamically stable and not hypoxic. She received 2 mg of lorazepam and 1 g of levetiracetam intravenously, which aborted the seizure. She did not receive aminophylline. On physical examination after she regained consciousness, she was confused and not oriented. Cranial nerves were intact, and motor strength was unchanged from baseline (5/5 at the right upper and lower extremities and 4/5 at the left upper and lower extremities). Initial blood work revealed sodium of 142 mmol/L, potassium 3.8 mmol/L, glucose 5.82 mmol/L, calcium 2.17 mmol/L, and magnesium 0.78 mmol/L. Due to concern for a new cerebrovascular accident in setting of prior history and this acute event, she underwent an emergent brain magnetic resonance imaging (MRI) study which did not reveal any acute changes. She was started on levetiracetam 500 mg orally twice daily. An electroencephalogram (EEG) was performed and revealed no epileptiform abnormalities or epileptogenic foci. Of note, she was not taking any antidepressants such as bupropion or other medications that may lower seizure threshold. She was discharged home 4 days later, with a diagnosis of regadenoson-induced seizure.

3. Discussion

Regadenoson is a selective A2a receptor agonist, which is predominant in coronary artery smooth muscle. However, it is also a weak agonist at A1a receptors with negligible affinity to A2b and A3a receptors as well [1]. It is commonly used as a pharmacological stress test agent to assess coronary blood flow in patients with limited functional capacity who cannot undergo exercise stress testing. When compared to adenosine, regadenoson was associated with a greater and more rapid peak in heart rate and demonstrated noninferiority in detecting perfusion defects with a better safety profile [2, 3]. However, given the wide range of adenosine receptors and their subtypes, a diverse adverse effect profile of regadenoson has been reported including nausea, vomiting, dyspnea, and headache [4]. Other side effects such as atrioventricular block, bronchoconstriction, and flushing have been attributed to its agonistic effects on A1a, A2b, and A3a receptors, respectively, despite low affinity [1, 5].

Seizure is one of the recently recognized adverse effects of regadenoson with increasing incidence. As of June 2018, a total of 148 cases of seizures and 10 cases of seizure-like phenomena were reported to the US Food and Drug Administration as adverse effects of regadenoson. Of note, the population size exposed to regadenoson, as well as the average time from injection to seizure onset, and past history of seizures or strokes in those patients have not been reported to the FDA [4]. A2a receptors are widely distributed in the CNS including the cerebral cortex, striatum, nucleus accumbens, and hippocampus [6]. Adenosine, specifically, through A2a receptors plays a role in glutamate outflow tracts and thus is involved in excitatory neurotransmission between neurons [7]. Several animal models, specifically rodents, have been studied regarding the role of A2a receptors in neuronal interaction, as well as the clinical application of adenosine receptor antagonists in treatment of seizures. One study investigated the consequences of deleting the A2a receptor in mice by comparing the incidence of electroshock-induced seizures in A2a-knockout mice versus controls [8]. Results showed that A2a-knockout mice demonstrated lower percentage as well as intensity of seizures than controls [8]. In another study, bilateral striata of rats were lesioned using the excitotoxin quinolinic acid, and this was followed by the administration of SCH 58261 (potent A2a receptor antagonist) [7]. Those who received SCH 58261 showed significantly lower motor, electroencephalographic, and neuropathologic changes secondary to excitotoxin [7]. Despite such findings, the clinical application of adenosine receptor antagonists in the treatment of epilepsy is still under investigation.

Regarding the pharmacokinetics of regadenoson, the elimination half-life follows a 3-compartment model [9]. The half-life of the initial phase is approximately 1-4 minutes, followed by an intermediate phase which has a half-life up to 30 minutes [9]. The final and terminal phase has a half-life lasting up to 2 hours [9, 10]. Most adverse effects begin soon after regadenoson administration and resolve usually within 15 minutes; though of those reported, the majority involves bronchospasm and cardiac conduction blocks [11]. Moreover, a case series by Page et al. demonstrated 3 cases of regadenoson-induced seizures that developed within 2-5 minutes of administration [12]. Two cases had a prior medical history of seizures and were receiving antiepileptic drugs, while one had no prior seizure history which however displayed hemodynamic instability prior to seizure onset [12]. On the other hand, it has been reported that seizure onset following regadenoson administration may be delayed as well, but no specific time onset was defined [13, 14]. For such reasons, aminophylline, a nonselective adenosine receptor antagonist, has been used to prevent delayed adverse effects, especially in patients at higher risk, such as a prior history of seizures [14]. Although it potentially antagonizes adenosine receptors, aminophylline is not a good option for reversal of regadenoson-induced seizures, as it may be sometimes ineffective in such setting and may even lower seizure threshold further and thus provoke seizures [12].

While the exact incidence of regadenoson-induced seizures is unknown, more cases are being reported as discussed above. We believe that the seizure in our patient may have been provoked by regadenoson, since other organic and structural causes were ruled out. The American Society of Nuclear Cardiology (ASNC) recommends avoiding regadenoson in patients with a medical history of seizures and structural brain disease and lists it as a relative contraindication to this medication [15]. We believe that our case adds to the available literature describing this uncommon but potentially severe adverse effect of regadenoson. It also advocates for increased physician awareness in screening patients at risk and providing prompt detection and appropriate management. It is also imperative to remember that aminophylline should be used with caution in reversal of regadenoson-induced seizure as indicated above. Additionally, nuclear medicine physicians and technicians need to be aware of such adverse events, and appropriate acute seizure termination measures should be always easily accessible.

Authors' Contributions

This case report was written by SSR and OGS. Both doctors were involved in the diagnosis and treatment of the said patient.

References

[1] National Center for Biotechnology Information, "PubChem compound database; CID=219024," https://pubchem.ncbi.nlm.nih.gov/compound/219024.

[2] A. E. Iskandrian, T. M. Bateman, L. Belardinelli et al., "Adenosine versus regadenoson comparative evaluation in myocardial perfusion imaging: results of the ADVANCE phase 3 multicenter international trial," *Journal of Nuclear Cardiology*, vol. 14, no. 5, pp. 645–658, 2007.

[3] K. P. Garnock-Jones and M. P. Curran, "Regadenoson," *American Journal Cardiovascular Drugs*, vol. 10, no. 1, pp. 65–71, 2010.

[4] "openFDA Dashboard, U.S. Food & Drug Administration," https://openfda.shinyapps.io/dash/.

[5] S. G. Johnson and S. Peters, "Advances in pharmacologic stress agents: focus on regadenoson," *Journal of Nuclear Medicine Technology*, vol. 38, no. 3, pp. 163–171, 2010.

[6] S. Sheth, R. Brito, D. Mukherjea, L. P. Rybak, and V. Ramkumar, "Adenosine receptors: expression, function and regulation," *International Journal of Molecular Sciences*, vol. 15, no. 2, pp. 2024–2052, 2014.

[7] P. Popoli, C. Frank, M. T. Tebano et al., "Modulation of glutamate release and excitotoxicity by adenosine A_{2A} receptors," *Neurology*, vol. 61, no. 11, Supplement 6, pp. S69–S71, 2003.

[8] M. El Yacoubi, C. Ledent, M. Parmentier, J. Costentin, and J.-M. Vaugeois, "Adenosine A_{2A} receptor deficient mice are partially resistant to limbic seizures," *Naunyn-Schmiedeberg's Archives of Pharmacology*, vol. 380, no. 3, pp. 223–232, 2009.

[9] G. M. Bengalorkar, K. Bhuvana, N. Sarala, and T. N. Kumar, "Regadenoson," *Journal of Postgraduate Medicine*, vol. 58, no. 2, pp. 140–146, 2012.

[10] W. Al Jaroudi and A. E. Iskandrian, "Regadenoson: a new myocardial stress agent," *Journal of the American College of Cardiology*, vol. 54, no. 13, pp. 1123–1130, 2009.

[11] *Product Information: LEXISCAN(TM) IV injection, regadenoson IV injection*, Astellas Pharm US Inc, Deerfield, IL, USA, 2008.

[12] R. L. Page, P. Spurck, J. L. Bainbridge, J. Michalek, and R. A. Quaife, "Seizures associated with regadenoson: a case series," *Journal of Nuclear Cardiology*, vol. 19, no. 2, pp. 389–391, 2012.

[13] Rapiscan, "INN-regadenoson - European Medicines Agency - Europa EU. Summary of product characteristics," https://www.ema.europa.eu/en/documents/product-information/rapiscan-epar-product-information_en.pdf.

[14] F. Mettler and M. Guiberteau, *Essentials of Nuclear Medicine and Molecular Imaging*, Elsevier, 7th edition, 2019.

[15] M. J. Henzlova, W. L. Duvall, A. J. Einstein, M. I. Travin, and H. J. Verberne, "ASNC imaging guidelines for SPECT nuclear cardiology procedures: stress, protocols, and tracers," *Journal of Nuclear Cardiology*, vol. 23, no. 3, pp. 606–639, 2016.

9

Gag Reflex-Mediated Restoration of Sinus Rhythm during TEE Probe Insertion for Atrial Fibrillation: A Word of Caution

Zeid Nesheiwat,[1] Marcel Ghanim,[1] Joseph Eid,[1] Neha Patel,[1] Cameron Burmeister,[1] and Ehab Eltahawy[2]

[1]*Department of Internal Medicine, The University of Toledo Medical Center, Toledo, Ohio, USA*
[2]*Department of Cardiology, The University of Toledo Medical Center, Toledo, Ohio, USA*

Correspondence should be addressed to Zeid Nesheiwat; nesheiwatzeid@gmail.com

Academic Editor: Assad Movahed

It is recommended to attempt vagal maneuvers as initial therapy in various types of supraventricular tachycardia. While various forms of vagal techniques have been described, a gag reflex-mediated vagal technique, to the best of our knowledge, has not been. We present a case of gag reflex-mediated restoration of sinus rhythm in a patient with atrial fibrillation and rapid ventricular response upon transesophageal probe insertion. This case is unique due to the mechanism of vagally mediated cardioversion. It emphasizes that operators must be cautious regarding the risk of embolization of a potential thrombus from vagal-mediated cardioversion with unknown thrombus burden.

1. Introduction

Supraventricular tachycardias (SVTs) are narrow complex tachyarrhythmias with QRS complex of less than 100 milliseconds [1]. It has been shown that parasympathetic input to the heart results in slowing of the heart rate through various pathways. Parasympathetic stimulation causes the release of acetylcholine, which then slows the atrioventricular node conduction velocity while increasing the refractory period and decreasing the rate of impulse through the sinus node [2]. Vagal maneuvers are used as an initial attempt to decrease heart rate in SVTs.

Atrial fibrillation is an SVT associated with increased risk for atrial thrombus formation and embolization. Transesophageal echocardiogram (TEE) is frequently performed to rule out the presence of atrial thrombi before elective cardioversion of atrial fibrillation to reduce the risk of stroke upon restoration of normal sinus rhythm. The success and risk of less invasive maneuvers, such as vagal stimulation, has not been thoroughly explored.

2. Case Presentation

We present a 44-year-old male with no significant past medical history who arrived at the emergency department with sudden onset retrosternal chest pain of a 4-hour duration. The chest pain was described as heavy in nature and nonradiating, with associated dyspnea, diaphoresis, and dizziness. At initial evaluation, the patient was hemodynamically stable. Initial electrocardiogram revealed sinus tachycardia with no ischemic changes. Troponins were negative. However, during his stay, the patient suddenly developed palpitations and was found to be in atrial fibrillation with rapid ventricular response with a heart rate ranging from 130 to 150 (Figure 1).

The patient was initially placed on a diltiazem infusion to control the heart rate. The patient then underwent an echocardiogram which was unremarkable. A subsequent cardiac catheterization revealed severe, thrombotic stenosis of the mid left anterior descending coronary artery, which was successfully treated by balloon angioplasty and SYNERGY drug-eluting stent placement.

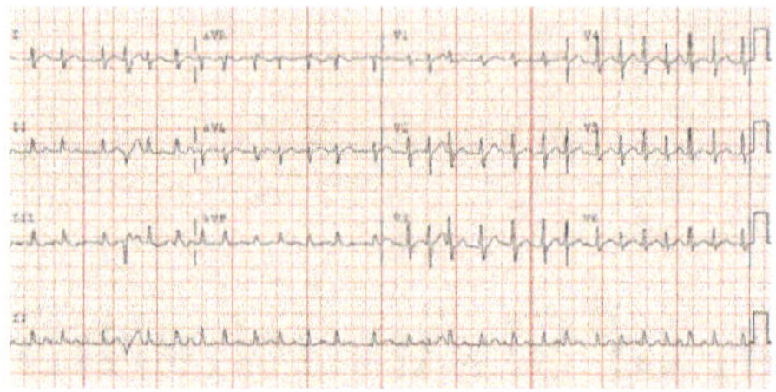

FIGURE 1: Precardioversion electrocardiogram showing atrial fibrillation with rapid ventricular response.

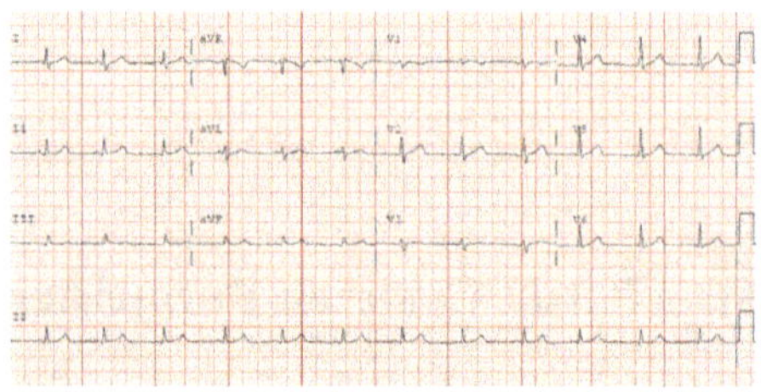

FIGURE 2: Post gag reflex-mediated cardioversion electrocardiogram showing normal sinus rhythm.

The following morning, the patient was scheduled for a transesophageal echocardiogram in anticipation of elective cardioversion as he remained in atrial fibrillation. Prior to the procedure, he received midazolam injection, topical butamben-tetracaine-benzocaine (CETACAINE) spray to the oropharynx, and propofol intravenously. Upon introduction of the TEE probe, the patient had several episodes of severe gagging following aggressive premedication. His rhythm then spontaneously reverted to sinus and no electrical cardioversion was necessary (Figure 2). TEE was completed and confirmed as having no valvular abnormalities or thrombus in the left atrial appendage. The patient maintained a normal sinus rhythm and was asymptomatic for the rest of his stay. The patient was discharged home in stable condition with follow-up in the cardiology clinic.

3. Discussion

Vagal maneuvers are relatively safe and easily performed techniques. Although mainly considered therapeutic for atrioventricular reentrant tachycardia (AVRT) and atrioventricular nodal reentry tachycardia (AVNRT), vagal techniques are recommended as an initial therapeutic option in patients with any form of SVT, although some studies have not shown sufficient evidence to support or refute their effectiveness [2–4]. In addition to slowing conduction through the AV node, vagal maneuvers have also been known to contribute to atrial fibrillation resolution by reducing P-wave dispersion. Several studies have concluded that large P-wave dispersion is associated with recurrences of atrial fibrillation after cardioversion [5].

In the setting of newly diagnosed atrial fibrillation and unknown thrombus burden, it is important to be aware of the potential risk of embolization from vagal-mediated cardioversion. Introduction of the TEE probe, despite aggressive premedication, can lead to a severe gag reflex and vagal stimulation. Although there are current guidelines in place for sedation and anesthesia during TEE, these guidelines do not address dosages [6]. Therefore, in order to minimize this risk, operators should be conscious, providing adequate pharyngeal anesthesia, sedation, and adequate time for the sedation to help decrease the gag reflex stimulation.

4. Conclusion

Vagal maneuvers are recommended as an initial therapeutic option for SVTs before medical or electrical intervention is performed. Believed to be relatively safe, vagal maneuvers are widely used. However, vagally induced cardioversion of SVT and in particular atrial fibrillation carries a risk of embolization; this is especially relevant in situations of inadequate anticoagulation and unknown thrombus burden.

Operators must be cautious regarding the risk of embolization of a potential thrombus from vagal-mediated cardioversion with unknown thrombus burden in patients with newly diagnosed atrial fibrillation.

References

[1] D. E. Becker, "Fundamentals of electrocardiography interpretation," *Anesthesia Progress*, vol. 53, no. 2, pp. 53–64, 2006.

[2] C. J. Kirchhof, A. P. Gorgels, and H. J. Wellens, "Carotid sinus massage as a diagnostic and therapeutic tool for atrial flutter-fibrillation," *Pacing and Clinical Electrophysiology*, vol. 21, no. 6, pp. 1319–1321, 1998.

[3] R. L. Page, J. A. Joglar, M. A. Caldwell et al., "2015 ACC/AHA/HRS guideline for the management of adult patients with supraventricular tachycardia: a report of the American College of Cardiology/American Heart Association task force on clinical practice guidelines and the Heart Rhythm Society," *Circulation*, vol. 133, no. 14, pp. e506–e574, 2016.

[4] G. D. Smith, M. M. Fry, D. Taylor, A. Morgans, K. Cantwell, and Cochrane Heart Group, "Effectiveness of the Valsalva manoeuvre for reversion of supraventricular tachycardia," *The Cochrane Database of Systematic Reviews*, no. 3, article Cd009502, 2015.

[5] S. Okutucu, K. Aytemir, and A. Oto, "P-wave dispersion: what we know till now?," *JRSM Cardiovascular Disease*, vol. 5, 2016.

[6] R. T. Hahn, T. Abraham, M. S. Adams et al., "Guidelines for performing a comprehensive transesophageal echocardiographic examination: recommendations from the American Society of Echocardiography and the Society of Cardiovascular Anesthesiologists," *Anesthesia and Analgesia*, vol. 118, no. 1, pp. 21–68, 2014.

10

Periaortic Abscess following DeBakey Type-1 Aortic Dissection Repair with Dacron Graft—Early Diagnosis and Management

Rishi Raj[1] **Dileep Unnikrishnan**[2] **Aasems Jacob**[1] **Kumar Ashish**[3] **Amulya Prakash**[2] **and Ajay Shah**[2]

[1]*University of Kentucky, Lexington, KY, USA*
[2]*Monmouth Medical Center, Long Branch, NJ, USA*
[3]*Crozer-Chester Medical Center, Upland, PA, USA*

Correspondence should be addressed to Rishi Raj; rishiraj91215@gmail.com

Academic Editor: Alfredo E. Rodriguez

A 71-year-old male with history of DeBakey type-1 aortic dissection and repair with dacron graft three months prior to presentation was brought to the emergency room with complaints of high-grade fevers, chills, and shortness of breath. Chest X-ray revealed right lower lobe infiltrates and widened superior mediastinum. A follow-up CT chest with contrast showed fluid collection around the aortic graft. He was started on intravenous broad-spectrum antibiotics, and a TEE was done for further evaluation of periaortic fluid collection which showed findings to suggest periaortic abscess. The patient underwent surgical drainage of the abscess and was found to have an abscess around the surgical aortic graft which was drained followed by two weeks of antibiotic treatment. The patient was discharged to a rehabilitation facility and remained asymptomatic at three-month follow-up appointment. Type-1 aortic dissection is a medical emergency requiring acute surgical intervention, and despite significant advancements in diagnosis and management, the immediate and long-term complications remain high leading to increased risk of mortality. Our patient developed spontaneous periaortic abscess three months postoperatively requiring intensive antibiotic therapy along with surgical drainage. Our case emphasizes the importance of early diagnosis and management of late complications of periaortic abscess in patients with aortic dissection repair.

1. Background

Graft and perigraft infections are dreaded complications following aortic repair surgeries with high mortality rates. Accurate and early detection and prompt surgical treatment are of paramount importance in reducing mortality in such cases. Although it has been widely accepted that surgical explantation with long-term antibiotics reduces mortality drastically compared to conservative measures, there is no consensus on the treatment approach for this entity. Recent studies have shown graft-sparing surgical therapy to be safe and effective for aortic graft infection which occur within 1 month postaortic dissection repair surgery. However, replacement of graft with biological conduits was showed to be better when aortic infection happens 3-6 months post-aortic dissection repair [1]. Here, we present a case of early-onset periaortic infection and abscess formation following aortic dissection repair who was successfully managed without graft explantation.

2. Case Presentation

A 71-year-old Caucasian hypertensive, diabetic male with past medical history significant for critical coronary artery disease, hyperlipidemia, carotid artery stenosis, and subclavian vein thrombosis presented to the emergency room with chief complaints of high-grade fever of one day duration associated with chills and shortness of breath. Three months prior to presentation, the patient developed acute aortic dissection DeBakey type-1 for which he underwent emergent cardiothoracic surgery and dacron graft repair of the ascending aorta. Few days following his discharge, he started having low-grade fevers which was associated with night sweats, dry cough, and exertional dyspnea for which the patient did not seek medical attention until one week from the visit date. Prior to presentation, he was treated at an urgent-care facility with a five-day course of doxycycline for the same complaints with a working diagnosis of community-acquired pneumonia with only partial improvement of his symptoms. One day prior to presentation, he developed high-grade fever. He denied any chest pain, rashes on his body, and painful nodules on his hands or feet. On admission, his blood pressure was 137/68 mmHg, pulse rate 113 beats per minute, and respiratory rate 18/minute, and he was saturating of 99% on room air. He was febrile with temperature of 102.6°F. Physical examination was remarkable for tachycardia and early diastolic murmur in the aortic area and a pansystolic murmur best heard in the apex with radiation to the axilla. The sternotomy scar on his chest was well-healed.

Initial laboratory investigation results are presented in Table 1, along with reference range values. Notably, his WBCs, lactic acid level, and procalcitonin levels were within normal range. A chest X-ray as part of the routine work-up was ordered from the emergency room and showed widening of the superior mediastinum compared to his prior film (Figure 1). Due to this concerning finding, a CT scan of the chest with contrast was ordered and showed a new fluid collection surrounding the ascending aorta and extending into the aortic arch measuring 5 cm in mediolateral dimension at the level of aortic arch (Figure 2). The patient was admitted to the medical floors with working diagnosis of aortic graft infection. Blood cultures were drawn and vancomycin 1 gm every 12 hours and piperacillin-tazobactam 4.5 g every 6 hours was started. Cardiothoracic surgeons were called in to evaluate the patient for possible surgical evacuation of the abscess and explantation of the graft. A transthoracic echocardiogram (TEE) was recommended by the surgical team for better visualization of the valves and their involvement. The TEE showed an echolucent area (Figure 3) consistent with fluid or blood around the ascending aorta conduit graft concerning for periconduit leak or abscess. It also revealed moderate-to-severe aortic regurgitation (Figure 4) with global left ventricular hypokinesis, but no valvular or perivalvular vegetations concerning for endocarditis. At this point, a decision was made to take the patient to the operating room for drainage of the abscess. On surgical exploration, purulent material was drained from the wall of the aorta around the graft and microbiological cultures were obtained. Intraoperatively, it was found that there was a clear demarcation between the graft and the abscess collection; and therefore, a decision was made not to explant the graft. Mediastinal drains were placed, and patient underwent continuous irrigation with betadine. Microbiological cultures from the abscess remained negative. Patient was continued on intravenous antibiotics for 2 weeks and was eventually discharge to rehabilitation after completion of two weeks of inpatient antibiotic treatment following sternotomy. He started to defervesce postoperatively and remained afebrile upon discharge. Interestingly, both his blood and pus cultures were negative, most likely because of early initiation of potent broad-spectrum antibiotics. The patient was advised to follow up with cardiology for aortic valve repair at a later date as an outpatient.

Table 1

Laboratory test	Levels	Reference range
White blood cells (WBCs)	4.1 K/CMM	4.5-11.0 K/CMM
Red blood cells (RBCs)	3.77 K/CMM	4.5-6.0 K/CMM
Hemoglobin	10.9 g/dL	13.5 to 17.5 g/dL
Lactic acid	0.9 mmol/L	0.5-2.2 mmol/L
Serum sodium	105 mEq/L	135–145 mEq/L
Serum chloride	74 mEq/L	99-109 mEq/L
Serum osmolality	234 mosm/kg	275–295 mosm/kg
Serum creatinine	0.69 mg/dL	0.40-1.10 mg/dL
Blood urea nitrogen (BUN)	10 mg/dL	5-21 mg/dL
Thyroid-stimulating hormone (TSH)	0.86 mcIU/mL	0.5-5.0 mcIU/mL
C-reactive protein (CRP)	60.5 mg/L	<7 mg/L
Erythrocyte sedimentation rate (ESR)	40 mm/hr	

3. Discussion

Infections of the aortic graft are rare postoperative complications of aortic surgeries such as repair of the aortic dissection and aneurysms. Although the incidence varies from based on center and expertise ranging anywhere from 1-3% to 0.2-5% in various studies, the condition can be catastrophic and is associated with very high mortality rate ranging from 25 to 75% [2, 3]. Due to its rarity, there are no large studies identifying the predisposing factors for aortic graft infection. Immediate postoperative infections are considered to be from direct inoculation of microbial flora, whereas delayed infection might be due to unevacuated thrombus, persistent leak around graft, nosocomial septicemia, and/or immunocompromised states. Although source of graft infection following open or endovascular procedure remains unrecognized, skin flora is considered to be most commonly encountered pathogen. There are reports of duodenal defects leading to graft infections in cases of abdominal aortic aneurysm; however, no such direct seeding of microbial flora has been reported following thoracic aorta dissection repair.

In cases where microbiological culture remains negative due to use of antibiotics, molecular testing (including qPCR or broad-range 16S rDNA) could be useful as they do not rely on the patient being antibiotic naïve and can help establish infectious etiology. In addition, it would also help in differentiating more aggressive organism (e.g., *Staphylococcus aureus*) from less virulent pathogen and potentially indicated the source of infection as low-grade infection tends to happen at time of surgery. Although broad -range 16S rDNA PCR is very specific and have high positive and negative predictive values, it can detect all bacterial DNA present in a sample, including the contaminants which are unavoidably present in reagents, thereby increasing false-

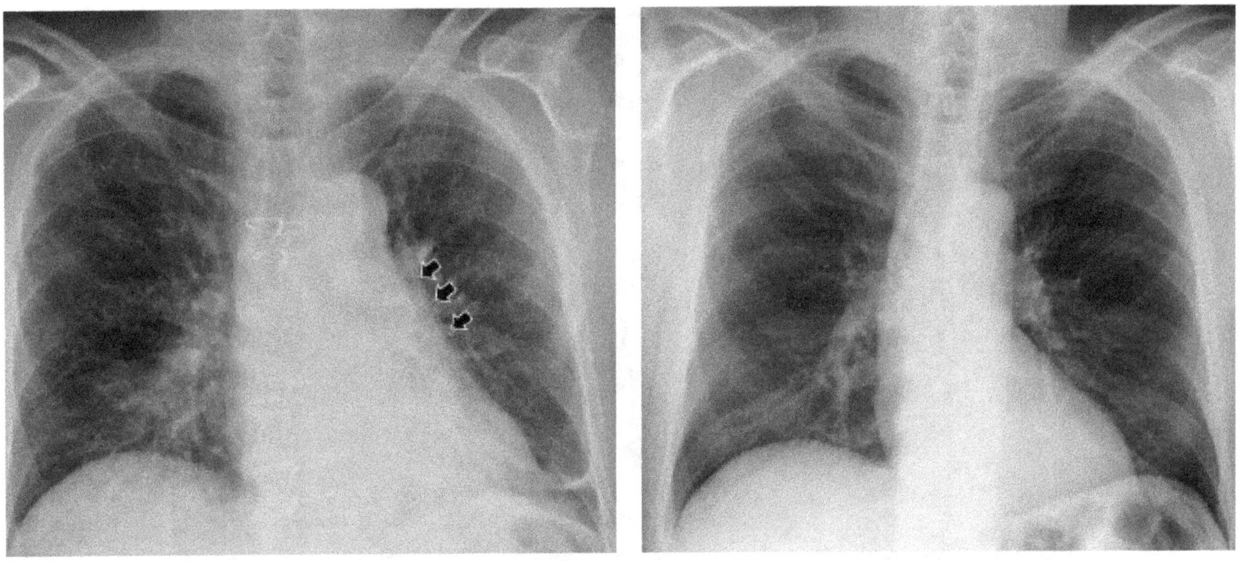

(a) (b)

FIGURE 1: Chest X-ray on admission (a) compared to the prior chest X-ray (b); black arrows show superior mediastinal fullness compared to the prior study.

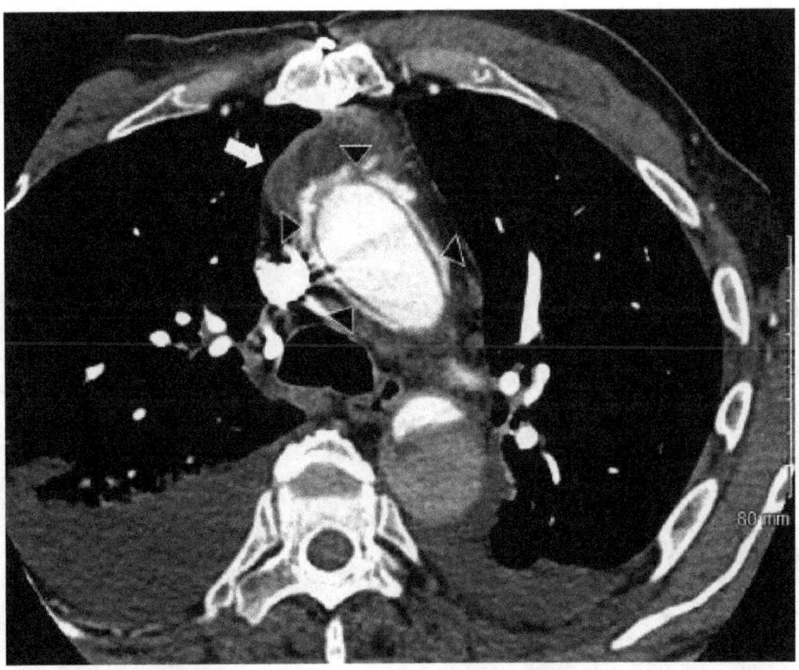

FIGURE 2: CT chest with contrast. White arrows show periaortic abscess in the ascending aorta.

positive rate and decreasing sensitivity. It is therefore important to use qPCR studies as the first line and only consider broad-range 16S rDNA PCR as an adjunct to microbiological diagnostics as a second line when infection of a sterile site is highly suspected, but culture and qPCR for the most likely pathogens have been proven negative [4].

Symptoms of aortic graft infection are often vague, and this requires a high degree of suspicion on the clinician's side while treating patients with aortic grafts. It could present as a constellation of symptoms that include fever, malaise, weight loss, back pain, leukocytosis, or abdominal pain. Severe fulminant sepsis can be seen in about one-third of cases of early graft infections. Computerized tomography (CT) with contrast enhancement is the diagnostic modality of choice in aortic graft infections [5]. CT angiography can be supplemented by indium-leucocyte scanning and sinography, which could illustrate whether a draining sinus extends to the graft [6]. Findings to look for in CT scan includes the following:

(a) Persistence of perigraft fluid after 3 months of procedure.

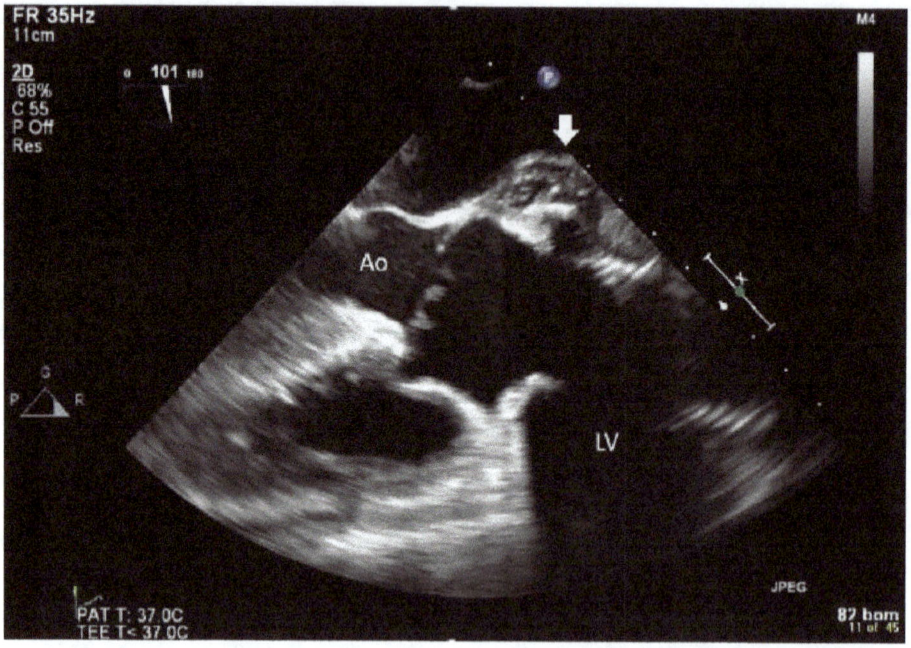

FIGURE 3: Mid-esophageal long-axis view of the heart with Doppler in the transesophageal echocardiogram showing severe aortic regurgitation.

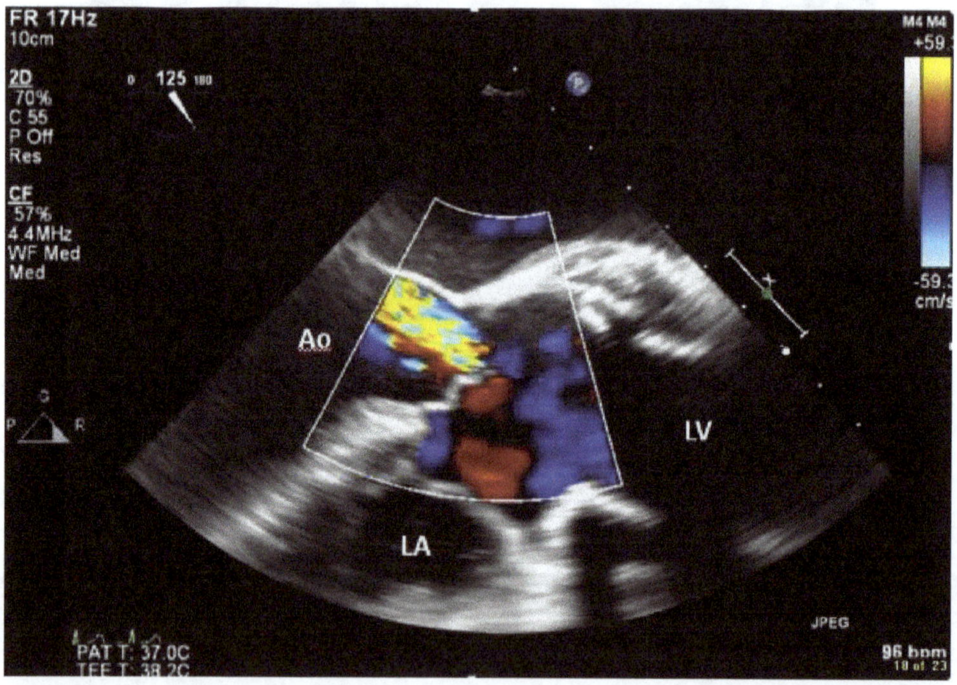

FIGURE 4: Mid-esophageal long-axis view of the heart in the transesophageal echocardiogram. White arrow shows periaortic abscess extending to the root of the aorta.

(b) Presence of ectopic gas in the aortic wall.

(c) Increased soft tissue and loss of normal tissue planes.

(d) Formation of pseudoaneurysm.

Transthoracic or transesophageal echocardiography can support a CT with contrast findings in cases where the thoracic aorta is involved. A 2016 study by Lyons et al. elucidated the diagnostic criteria to be used in suspected cases of aortic graft infection [7]. The management of aortic graft infection collaboration (MAGIC) criteria includes clinical, radiological, and laboratory findings and categorizes each into three major and two minor criteria. Although there are no established treatment guidelines for this clinical entity due to its rarity, most of the existing literature endorses surgical removal of graft over conservative management alone.

However, explantation of infected graft is not a good idea in very debilitated and patients with significant comorbidities. In case of conservative management, CT imaging-guided aspiration of the periaortic fluid can supplement antibiotic therapy. The choice of antibiotics is empirical until cultures are available and should have broad gram-positive coverage (both gram-positive and -negative in cases where aortoenteric fistula is suspected). There is no established consensus on the duration of treatment. Most published case reports opted for a minimum of 4-6 weeks of antibiotics with some cases resorting to lifelong antibiotic therapy [8]. Contraindication for conservative treatments are suture-line hemorrhage, graft-enteric fistula, and infected anastomotic aneurysm. High rate of mortality is the norm for aortic graft infection. As reported in an international enquiry with 62 reported cases from different international centers of vascular surgery, mortality among operative cases was 16.3% and that among conservative management was 36.4% [9]. With such high mortality rates, it is important to focus on prevention, early detection, and prompt treatment of this entity.

4. Conclusion

Aortic graft infection is a rare complication of postaortic repair surgeries with very high mortality. The presenting symptoms are often vague and depend on the time of presentation, part of the aorta that is infected, and the virulence of pathogen involved. Fever with new-onset murmur is red flag in patients with aortic grafts in situ and warrants further investigations. In addition, subtle findings such as widening of the mediastinum should not be neglected in such patients to ensure prompt diagnosis. CT chest with contrast enhancement is the diagnostic modality of choice which can reveal perigraft fluid, ectopic gas in the aortic wall, and loss of normal tissue. The criteria defined by MAGIC (Management of Aortic Graft Infection Collaboration) provides a handy tool to arrive at a diagnosis. Treatment with broad-spectrum antibiotics must be initiated at the earliest time after drawing blood cultures. Graft explantation with four to six weeks of antibiotics is the accepted practice in anyone who does not have contraindications for surgery. Conservative management has been resorted to in patients with debility with markedly higher mortality.

References

[1] J. Umminger, H. Krueger, E. Beckmann et al., "Management of early graft infections in the ascending aorta and aortic arch: a comparison between graft replacement and graft preservation techniques," *European Journal of Cardio-Thoracic Surgery*, vol. 50, no. 4, pp. 660–667, 2016.

[2] K. Laohapensang, S. Arworn, S. Orrapin, T. Reanpang, and S. Orrapin, "Management of the infected aortic endograft," *Seminars in Vascular Surgery*, vol. 30, no. 2-3, pp. 91–94, 2017.

[3] R. O. Darouiche, "Treatment of infections associated with surgical implants," *New England Journal of Medicine*, vol. 350, no. 14, pp. 1422–1429, 2004.

[4] A. Patel, K. A. Harris, and F. Fitzgerald, "What is broad-range 16S rDNA PCR?," *Archives of disease in childhood - Education & practice edition*, vol. 102, no. 5, pp. 261–264, 2017.

[5] P. Rossi, F. M. Arata, F. M. Salvatori et al., "Prosthetic graft infection: diagnostic and therapeutic role of interventional radiology," *Journal of Vascular and Interventional Radiology*, vol. 8, no. 2, pp. 271–277, 1997.

[6] P. F. Lawrence, "Conservative treatment of aortic graft infection," *Seminars in Vascular Surgery*, vol. 24, no. 4, pp. 199–204, 2011.

[7] O. T. A. Lyons, M. Baguneid, T. D. Barwick et al., "Diagnosis of aortic graft infection: a case definition by the Management of Aortic Graft Infection Collaboration (MAGIC)," *European Journal of Vascular and Endovascular Surgery*, vol. 52, no. 6, pp. 758–763, 2016.

[8] M. Blanch, J. Berjón, R. Vila et al., "The management of aortic stent-graft infection: endograft removal versus conservative treatment," *Annals of Vascular Surgery*, vol. 24, no. 4, pp. 554.e1–554.e5, 2010.

[9] P. Fiorani, F. Speziale, A. Calisti et al., "Endovascular graft infection: preliminary results of an international enquiry," *Journal of Endovascular Therapy*, vol. 10, no. 5, pp. 919–927, 2003.

11

Odynophagia after Cardiac Catheterization: A Rare Complication in the Presence of Aberrant Subclavian Artery

Moumita Naidu, Robby Singh, and Marcel Zughaib

Providence Hospital-Michigan State University, USA

Correspondence should be addressed to Moumita Naidu; monaidu7@gmail.com

Academic Editor: Christopher S. Snyder

Background. Vascular complications from transradial cardiac catheterization are uncommon. Mediastinal hematoma is a rare complication with life-threatening potential. We present a case of a patient who underwent cardiac catheterization and subsequently experienced odynophagia from injury to an aberrant subclavian artery that led to a mediastinal hematoma. *Case Report.* A 59-year-old female with past medical history of coronary artery disease presented with complaints of angina and underwent a transradial cardiac catheterization. Immediately after the procedure, the patient complained of chest pain and odynophagia. EKG and echocardiogram were unremarkable, and a CT scan of the chest demonstrated an ill-defined fluid collection present in the superior mediastinum and an aberrant right subclavian artery. The patient was closely monitored in the Intensive Care Unit, and the patient remained hemodynamically stable throughout the admission. The patient was subsequently discharged home in good condition and did well on outpatient follow-up. *Conclusion.* Vascular injuries associated with delivery of standard radial catheters in the subclavian artery are rare, with very few cases reported in the literature. We presented the case of a patient who had a previously unidentified right aberrant subclavian artery with a retroesophageal course which precipitated the hematoma and subsequently resulted in odynophagia despite an uncomplicated catheterization. This rare complication of a commonplace procedure necessitates prompt recognition, appropriate hemodynamic management, and possible repair of the injured vessel to appropriately manage a potentially life-threatening condition.

1. Introduction

Transradial cardiac catheterization is a commonplace procedure due to increased patient comfort and low rates of vascular complications. Radial artery occlusion is the most frequent complication (1.77%) though pseudoaneurysms (0.38%) and AV-fistulas (0.19%) can also be seen postprocedure [1, 4]. Potentially life-threatening vascular complications such as mediastinal hematoma are extremely rare and are usually due to trauma, laceration, or perforation of the thoracic arch vessels and can lead to significant morbidity [2, 3]. Previously unidentified anatomic variants, calcification, and rigid, large-bore catheters are some of the contributing factors which can predispose patients to vascular injuries.

Although patients with mediastinal hematoma typically present with chest pain, bleeding, or hemodynamic instability, this very rare albeit feared complication (.01% of cases) and carries a mortality rate is forty-nine percent within the first 24 hours [5]. Odynophagia is a rare presenting symptom for a patient with a mediastinal hematoma and should not be dismissed especially after a transradial catheterization. It is important for astute clinicians to familiarize themselves with not only the predisposing risk factors for vascular injuries but also the variety of symptoms which can lead to a diagnosis of mediastinal hematoma which is potentially fatal.

2. Case Report

A 59-year-old female with a past medical history of tobacco abuse, hypertension, and coronary artery disease and prior percutaneous coronary intervention presented with complaints of angina and subsequently underwent coronary angiography. The procedure was performed via the right radial artery approach. A 5 French Jacky catheter was used to engage the left coronary artery system, and a 6 French

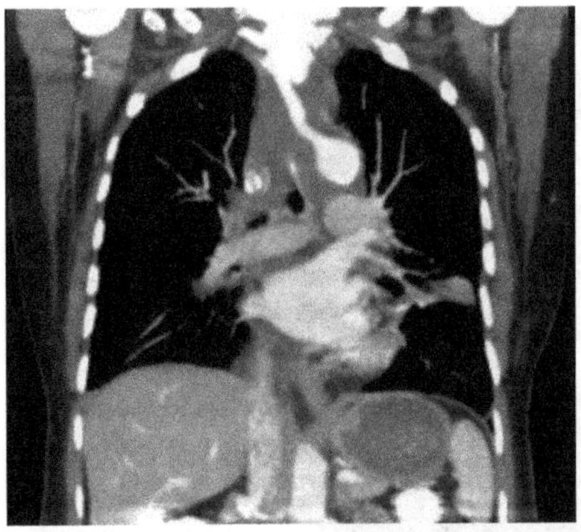

FIGURE 1: CT scan demonstrating ill-defined fluid collection in the superior mediastinum (arrow).

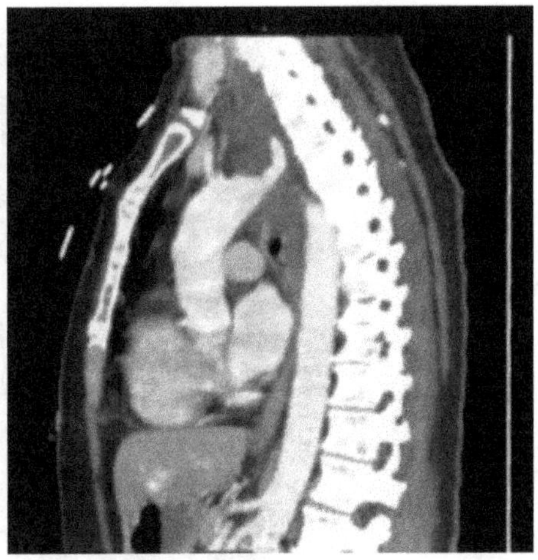

FIGURE 2: Aberrant right subclavian artery coursing posterior to the trachea and esophagus (arrow).

Judkins Right 4 catheter was used to engage the right coronary artery system. The procedure was completed without difficulty from the operator, and the patient was transferred to the postoperative holding area in stable condition.

However, immediately after the procedure, the patient began to experience chest pain and odynophagia. Stat electrocardiogram and bedside echocardiogram were unremarkable, and a CT scan demonstrated an ill-defined fluid collection present in the superior mediastinum (Figure 1).

While a hematoma and a mass were both considered to be in the differential diagnosis, the CT scan also made note of an aberrant right subclavian artery (ARSA) coursing posterior to the trachea and esophagus (Figure 2). Esophageal anomalies were otherwise ruled out with an esophagram, and the differential diagnosis was narrowed down to a mediastinal hematoma.

Consequently, the patient was admitted to the cardiac care unit but continued to complain of midsternal chest pain and odynophagia. The patient remained hemodynamically stable and without any airway compromise. The patient was managed expectantly with analgesia. A repeat CT scan a day later again demonstrated the ill-defined collection which had now extended into the inferior right paravertebral aspect near the gastroesophageal junction. This was deemed to be an extension of the same fluid collection with the size of the hematoma remaining stable. The patient was monitored closely and improved clinically over the course of four days and was subsequently discharged home in good condition. On outpatient follow-up, the patient reported her symptoms had completely resolved.

3. Discussion

Vascular injury can be the result of a routine cardiac catheterization, but the injury associated with the delivery of standard radial catheters in the subclavian artery is rare, with only a few cases reported in the literature [1]. Most vascular complications occur due to laceration or perforation of thoracic arch vessels due to the tension created on the ostium of the artery from catheter manipulation. These previously reported cases highlight the importance of careful catheter placement and the use of fluoroscopy to confirm the relative position of the equipment during the procedure. In addition, choosing the right catheter type plays a vital role in preventing injury since rigid guide catheters, curved catheters, and larger French sizes are all associated with increased risk of vessel trauma. Calcified vessels are a separate risk which predisposes patients to vascular injuries, but most experienced operators are keenly aware of such complications.

In addition to appropriate catheter choice, operators must be aware of anatomic variants which can predispose patients to vascular complications. Aberrant right subclavian artery (ARSA) is one such variant (Figure 3), and it can be encountered during a radial catheterization. Though rare, as it is only reported in 0.4-1.8% of the general population; this artery can arise directly from the aortic arch distal to the left subclavian artery [5], instead from the brachiocephalic artery. ARSA does pose an increased risk for vessel trauma especially since its presence is often unbeknownst to the operator.

One of the most feared consequences of vessel trauma is mediastinal hematoma, and most patients present with chest pain, bleeding, or hemodynamic instability immediately after cardiac catheterization. Odynophagia, however, as a chief complaint is extremely rare. In our case, a likely injury of an ARSA led to a mediastinal hematoma which was only discovered when the patient complained of odynophagia in recovery. This complication was not detected on initial electrocardiography or echocardiography. Despite this, the physicians involved in the procedure maintained a high index of suspicion for possible hematoma which was discovered on CT scan. The anatomic variant ARSA which was only discovered postprocedure likely placed this patient at an increased risk for this complication.

Although the patient was able to be managed with supportive care in this scenario, this may not always be possible. Prompt recognition and treatment are imperative in treating this complication. The aforementioned case highlights the fact that unusual complaints such as swallowing dysfunction following cardiac catheterization should not be ignored but rather alert operators to evaluate for potential rare complications such as mediastinal hematoma.

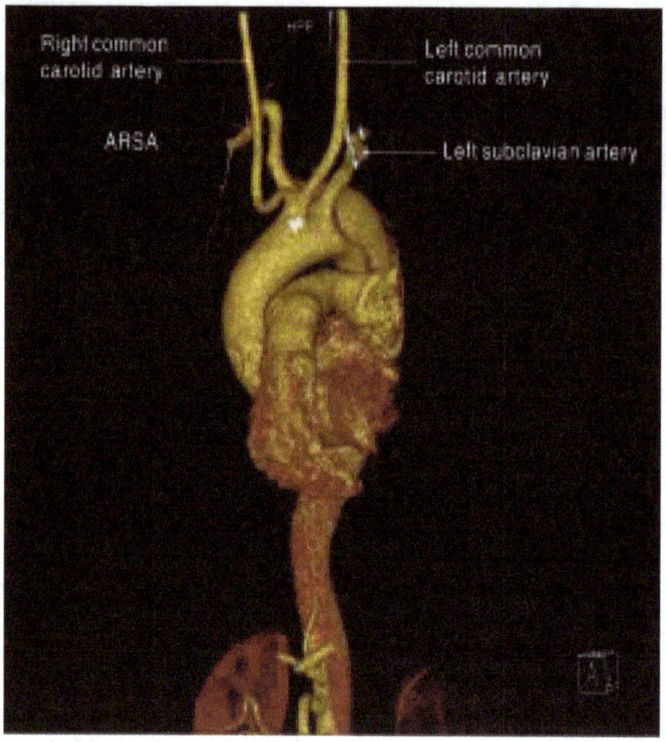

FIGURE 3: Adapted from "Repair of a type B aortic dissection with a re-vascularization of the aberrant right subclavian artery in an adult patient."

4. Conclusion

Mediastinal hematoma is a known but rare complication of transradial cardiac catheterization and is related to vessel trauma during instrumentation [3]. We presented a case where the routine use of 5 French and 6 French catheters led to an ARSA injury and subsequently a mediastinal hematoma. This raises the question of whether a transfemoral approach is better suited for these patients if this aberrancy is identified prior to the procedure.

This patient, however, had a previously unidentified vascular anomaly (ARSA), which likely predisposed her to this complication despite a seemingly uncomplicated transradial catheterization. Prompt recognition of unusual symptoms postprocedure, appropriate hemodynamic and airway management, and possible endovascular repair of the injured vessel are all components of successful management of this potentially life-threatening condition. In addition, a post catheterization angiography of the aberrancy may be helpful to assess for any injury to the vessel prior to sending the patient to recovery if it is recognized during the procedure.

In this case, ARSA was not identified during the catheterization and there was no reported difficulty in engaging the coronaries which would have otherwise alerted the operator. Because of this, operators must have the knowledge of this anatomic aberrancy even if undetected during the procedure. In addition, when vascular injury is suspected, there are a wide variety of symptoms which should raise concern post-procedure, and odynophagia is one such presentation which should not be ignored. This patient's complaint of odynophagia was the direct result of a mediastinal hematoma, and this association has not been previously reported in the literature to the best of our knowledge.

References

[1] M. Sanmartin, D. Cuevas, and J. Goicolea, "Vascular complications associated with radial artery access for cardiac catheterization," *Revista Española de Cardiología*, vol. 57, no. 6, pp. 581-584, 2004.

[2] T. Patel, S. Shah, K. Sanghavi, and S. Pancholy, "Management of radial and brachial artery perforations during transradial procedures–a practical approach," *Journal of Invasive Cardiology*, vol. 21, no. 10, pp. 544-547, 2009.

[3] N. Habib, A. Jerzewski, E. M. Koomen et al., "Subclavian artery perforation complicating coronary angiography," *Netherlands Heart Journal*, vol. 20, no. 6, pp. 288–290, 2012.

[4] F. Farooqi, J. Alexander, and A. Sarma, "Rare vascular perforation complicating radial approach to percutaneous coronary angioplasty," *Case Reports*, vol. 2013, no. jan28 1, p. bcr2012007732, 2013.

[5] J. Woodring and M. Dillon, "Radiographic manifestations of mediastinal hemorrhage from blunt chest trauma," *The Annals of Thoracic Surgery*, vol. 37, no. 2, pp. 171–178, 1984.

12

Hemangioma of the Atherosclerotic Changed Aortic Valve

A. van Broekhoven[1,2,3] **P. A. J. Krijnen,**[1,2] **H. W. M. Niessen,**[1,2,3] **and A. B. A. Vonk**[2,3]

[1] *Department of Pathology, Amsterdam UMC, Vrije Universiteit, Amsterdam, Netherlands*
[2] *Amsterdam Cardiovascular Sciences, Amsterdam, Netherlands*
[3] *Department of Cardiac Surgery, Amsterdam UMC, Vrije Universiteit, Amsterdam, Netherlands*

Correspondence should be addressed to A. van Broekhoven; a.vanbroekhoven@vumc.nl

Academic Editor: Aiden Abidov

The incidence of heart valve hemangioma is very low and is mostly observed in the mitral and tricuspid valve. In 2006, two cases of aortic valve hemangioma were reported for the first time, including one with calcifying aortic valve stenosis. We now present a case of aortic valve hemangioma in a patient suffering from aortic valve insufficiency combined with atherosclerotic thickening.

1. Introduction

Primary benign tumors of the heart are rare, accounting for 72% of all primary cardiac tumors [1]. Of these benign tumors, only 5-10% consist of hemangiomas. Valvular hemangiomas are even less frequent [2, 3]. Most previous case reports described valve hemangiomas observed in the mitral or tricuspid valve [4–14]. To the best of our knowledge, only two aortic valve hemangiomas have been reported to date, including one hemangioma observed in a calcified stenotic aortic valve [15, 16]. In this report, we present a new case of hemangioma which was unexpectedly detected in an aortic valve with atherosclerotic changes after pathological examination.

2. Case Presentation

A 74-year-old man was referred to our hospital with severe aortic valve insufficiency and left ventricle dilatation. His past medical history showed hypercholesterolemia and a recent episode of de novo atrial flutter which was treated with electrical cardioversion. His medication included atorvastatin, nebivolol, and dabigatran. He stopped smoking 40 years ago and uses 14 units of alcohol per week.

The patient's vital signs were normal. Physical examination revealed normal pulmonary, abdominal, and neurological functions. Except for a diastolic murmur at the right lower sternal border, cardiovascular examination revealed normal heart sounds. Coronary angiography did not show significant coronary artery disease. Transthoracic echocardiography revealed a severe aortic valve insufficiency with a somewhat impaired function of the left ventricle. Cardiac MRI showed severe aortic valve insufficiency combined with a dilated aortic root (46 mm) and a severely dilated left ventricle with an ejection fraction of 50%. Aortic valve replacement with a biological device (Edwards Lifesciences Perimount 27 mm) was performed. No complications occurred during surgery. Except for a ventral pneumothorax, the patient's recovery was uneventful. He was discharged in good condition to the cardiology nursing ward of a peripheral hospital on postoperative day 4. At two weeks follow-up, the patient was doing well. He did not experience any cardiac complaints. For further recovery, the patient was referred back to the referring cardiology department. After 6 weeks, the patient was reevaluated for his recovery at the policlinic of cardiothoracic surgery, where no abnormal findings were observed during physical examination.

The excised aortic valve was tricuspid and measured $3.5 \times 1.3 \times 0.3$ cm. The cusps were partially calcified. Microscopic examination of cross-sections of the aortic valve leaflets showed areas of calcification with focal ceroid, as can be found in the atherosclerotic valves [17, 18]. In between the calcification areas, a few reactive small thin-walled

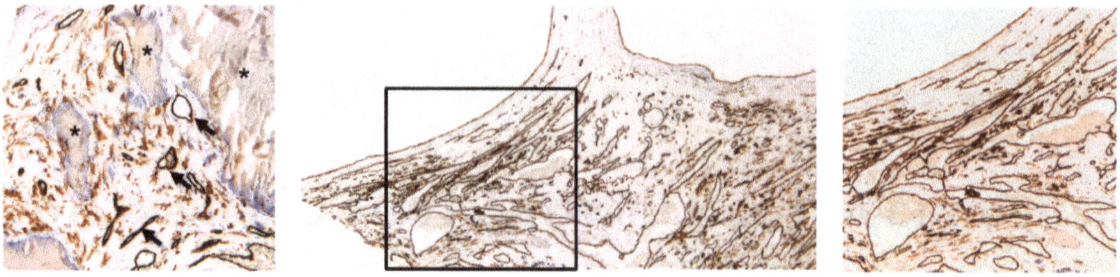

FIGURE 1: Reactive proliferation of blood vessels. (a) Reactive proliferation of dense blood vessels (arrows) surrounding calcified areas (asterisk) visualised by CD31 staining. Magnification 50x. (b) Overview of aortic valve hemangioma stained for CD31, showing an agglomerate of thin-walled vessels. Magnification 25x. (c) Detailed view of aortic valve hemangioma stained for CD31. Magnification 50x.

blood vessels were found (Figure 1(a)). Next to calcification, fibrosis and mucoid degeneration was also observed (not shown). In the periphery of the valve, an agglomerate of thin walled, often dilated, blood vessels was observed (Figures 1(b) and 1(c)). These vessels stained positive for CD31 and were negative for D2-40 (staining lymphatic vessels). The vessels were predominantly negative for SMA (not shown). These findings supported the diagnosis of hemangioma of the aortic valve. In retrospect, no clear abnormalities indicative for a hemangioma in the aortic valve were seen in preoperative TTE. The aortic valve did appear slightly thickened, which was assumed to be due to atherosclerotic changes (Figure 2).

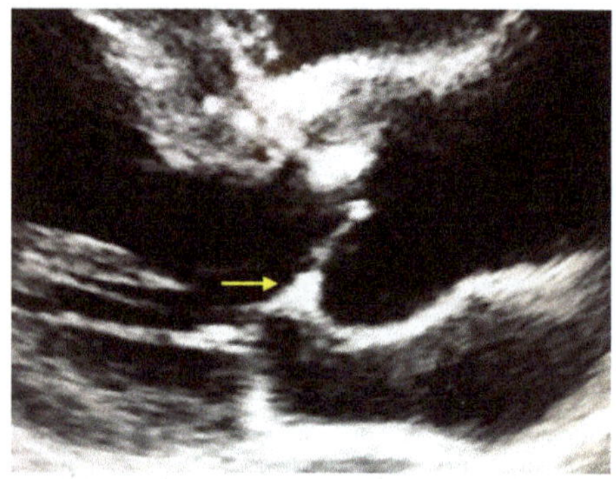

FIGURE 2: Preoperative transthoracic echocardiography. Apart from a slightly thickened aortic valve (arrow), no clear abnormalities indicative for a hemangioma could be observed.

3. Discussion

Hemangiomas of the cardiac valves are exceptional, especially in the aortic valves [15, 16].

We now describe the finding of a hemangioma in the atherosclerotic aortic valve. Previously, Val-Bernal et al. also described a hemangioma in a calcified aortic valve [16], while Vivirito et al. described a hemangioma in a nondegenerated valve, indicating that hemangiomas also occur independent of atherosclerosis. It is known that in atherosclerotic aortic valves, reactive vessel wall proliferation occurs. Normally, these are small solitary vessels. In contrast, in hemangioma, an agglomerate of multiple thin-walled and mostly dilated vessels occurs, excluding a reactive vessel wall proliferation as demonstrated in our case.

The clinical presentation of cardiac hemangiomas is variable and depends on multiple factors including location, size, growth rate, sex, and patient's age. Heart valve hemangiomas may present with palpitations and syncope, exertional dyspnea, heart failure due to hemodynamic instability, and atypical chest pain [2, 6, 8, 10, 14, 19–21]. In our patient, it is likely that the hemangioma of the aortic valve contributed to the development of aortic valve regurgitation. As most patients with heart valve hemangiomas remain asymptomatic (Edwards [2]), it cannot be precluded that aortic valve hemangiomas are more common than observed, since they may not cause clinically relevant valve dysfunction.

Cardiac hemangiomas can be detected by transthoracic echocardiography (TTE), transesophageal echocardiography (TEE), and cardiac CT or MRI scan [22]. To differentiate hemangiomas from other cardiac tumors, a three-dimensional TTE (3D TTE) may be more precisely related to so-called echolucencies [8, 9]. However, the golden standard for diagnosis of most cardiac hemangiomas is histological examination upon surgical excision [8, 9]. In our case, no signs indicative for the presence of an aortic valve hemangioma on preoperative TTE and cardiac MRI were seen, even in retrospect. The thickening of the aortic valve that was observed was assumed to be due to atherosclerosis. However, we did not perform 3D TTE in our patient. Previous case reports regarding aortic valve hemangioma also did not detect the hemangioma using TTE [15, 16].

In general, cardiac hemangiomas are classified as benign tumors and lack the ability to metastasize. Their growth patterns are unpredictable and range from dormancy to accelerated growth or to spontaneous regression [3, 8, 23–25]. To the best of our knowledge, the growth pattern of valvular hemangiomas specifically is unknown, since all the previous documented cases were obtained from excised heart valves and therefore the natural course of these hemangiomas was not studied. In one case of a surgically excised histiocytoid hemangioma of the left atrium, an angiosarcoma was found 7 years after surgery, which supports the recommendation of regular follow-up by echocardiography of cardiac hemangiomas [8, 11, 26]. Though, as far as we are aware, in all patients with heart valve hemangiomas described so far, no signs of recurrence of the hemangioma have been observed [27] nor malignant degeneration of heart valve hemangiomas or any other complications have been described upon excision [6, 27].

In our case, the patient was reevaluated six weeks after aortic valve replacement by the cardiothoracic surgeon. No abnormal findings were observed during the physical examination. Therefore, upon en bloc removal of the aortic valve containing the hemangioma, there are no specific consequences regarding surgical follow-up for our patient. Instead, regular check-ups need to be aimed at evaluating the prosthetic valve and the patient's status after severe aortic valve insufficiency.

In conclusion, we present a hemangioma localized in an atherosclerotic aortic valve [15, 16]. Several imaging techniques, including TTE and cardiac MRI, did not reveal the existence of a tumor mass in our patient, indicating the importance of pathological examination of excised heart valves.

References

[1] A. Burke and R. Virmani, *Tumors of the Heart and Great Vessels*, Armed Forces Institute of Pathology, Washington, DC, USA, 1996.

[2] F. H. Edwards, D. Hale, A. Cohen, L. Thompson, A. T. Pezzella, and R. Virmani, "Primary cardiac valve tumors," *The Annals of Thoracic Surgery*, vol. 52, no. 5, pp. 1127–1131, 1991.

[3] W. Li, P. Teng, H. Xu, L. Ma, and Y. Ni, "Cardiac hemangioma: a comprehensive analysis of 200 cases," *The Annals of Thoracic Surgery*, vol. 99, no. 6, pp. 2246–2252, 2015.

[4] G. H. Luo, W. G. Ma, H. S. Sun et al., "Surgical treatment for primary mitral valve tumor: a 25-year single-center experience," *Cardiology*, vol. 119, no. 2, pp. 81–87, 2011.

[5] A. L. Cook, D. A. Williams, S. Bergman, and M. H. Hines, "Atypically located cardiac haemangioma of the mitral valve," *Cardiology in the Young*, vol. 21, no. 5, pp. 598–600, 2011.

[6] M. Floria, A. Guedes, M. Buche, R. Deperon, and B. Marchandise, "A rare primary cardiac tumour: cavernous hemangioma of the tricuspid valve," *European Journal of Echocardiography*, vol. 12, no. 6, p. 477, 2011.

[7] A. Cannata, C. F. Russo, B. Merlanti et al., "Cavernous hemangioma replacing the septal leaflet of the tricuspid valve," *Journal of Cardiac Surgery*, vol. 25, no. 5, pp. 524–527, 2010.

[8] V. Yaganti, S. Patel, S. Yaganti, and M. Victor, "Cavernous hemangioma of the mitral valve: a case report and review of literature," *Journal of Cardiovascular Medicine*, vol. 10, no. 5, pp. 420–422, 2009.

[9] H. S. Dod, M. V. Burri, D. Hooda et al., "Two- and three-dimensional transthoracic and transesophageal echocardiographic findings in epithelioid hemangioma involving the mitral valve," *Echocardiography*, vol. 25, no. 4, pp. 443–445, 2008.

[10] L. Muzzi, G. Davoli, L. Specchia, and M. Chiavarelli, "Primary hemangioma of the mitral valve: an unusual presentation," *The Journal of Heart Valve Disease*, vol. 16, no. 2, pp. 209–211, 2007.

[11] S. Ugras and I. Bayram, "Cavernous haemangioma of the mitral valve in a child: report of a case and review of the literature," *Pathology*, vol. 37, no. 5, pp. 396–398, 2005.

[12] K. K. Wong, G. G. S. Sandor, and S. S. Sett, "Isolated haemangioma of the tricuspid valve," *Cardiology in the Young*, vol. 14, no. 3, p. 324, 1999.

[13] E. Lapenna, M. de Bonis, L. Torracca, G. la Canna, G. Dell'Antonio, and O. Alfieri, "Cavernous hemangioma of the tricuspid valve: minimally invasive surgical resection," *The Annals of Thoracic Surgery*, vol. 76, no. 6, pp. 2097–2099, 2003.

[14] S. W. Nye, D. A. Orsinelli, P. B. Baker, and D. A. Brown, "Surgical treatment of a hemangioma of the mitral valve," *The Annals of Thoracic Surgery*, vol. 71, no. 1, pp. 345–347, 2001.

[15] M. Vivirito, R. Boldorini, L. Rossi, P. P. Caimmi, M. Bernardi, and G. Teodori, "Capillary hemangioma of the aortic valve: false preoperative diagnosis of endocarditis," *The Journal of Thoracic and Cardiovascular Surgery*, vol. 132, no. 3, pp. 690-691, 2006.

[16] J. F. Val-Bernal, M. Cuadrado, M. F. Garijo, and J. M. Revuelta, "Incidental in vivo detection of an isolated hemangioma of the aortic valve in a man with a history of renal transplantation," *Virchows Archiv*, vol. 449, no. 1, pp. 121–123, 2006.

[17] C. M. Otto, J. Kuusisto, D. D. Reichenbach, A. M. Gown, and K. D. O'Brien, "Characterization of the early lesion of 'degenerative' valvular aortic stenosis. Histological and immunohistochemical studies," *Circulation*, vol. 90, no. 2, pp. 844–853, 1994.

[18] K. Kupreishvili, A. Baidoshvili, M. ter Weeme et al., "Degeneration and atherosclerosis inducing increased deposition of type IIA secretory phospholipase A2, C-reactive protein and complement in aortic valves cause neutrophilic granulocyte influx," *The Journal of Heart Valve Disease*, vol. 20, no. 1, pp. 29–36, 2011.

[19] R. Ray, A. Rishi, P. Venugopal, and P. Chopra, "Hemangioma of the tricuspid valve: a report of two cases with review of literature," *Cardiovascular Pathology*, vol. 13, no. 2, pp. 120–122, 2004.

[20] C. Abad, S. de Varona, M. A. Limeres, J. Morales, and J. Marrero, "Resection of a left atrial hemangioma. Report of a case and overview of the literature on resected cardiac hemangiomas," *Texas Heart Institute Journal*, vol. 35, no. 1, pp. 69–72, 2008.

[21] I. Juric, I. Hadzibegovic, P. Kes, B. Biocina, D. Milicic, and N. Basic-Jukic, "An exceptional cause of progressive dyspnoea in a renal transplant recipient: hemangioma of the mitral valve," *Kidney & Blood Pressure Research*, vol. 37, no. 1, pp. 9–14, 2013.

[22] P. A. Araoz, S. L. Mulvagh, H. D. Tazelaar, P. R. Julsrud, and J. F. Breen, "CT and MR imaging of benign primary cardiac neoplasms with echocardiographic correlation," *RadioGraphics*, vol. 20, no. 5, pp. 1303–1319, 2000.

[23] K. Nakamura, N. Funabashi, H. Miyauchi et al., "Hemangioma located just above the left main coronary artery, in a subject who had cardiac arrest due to ventricular fibrillation, led to a diagnosis of Brugada syndrome," *International Journal of Cardiology*, vol. 127, no. 3, pp. 437–441, 2008.

[24] T. E. Palmer, D. D. Tresch, and L. I. Bonchek, "Spontaneous resolution of a large, cavernous hemangioma of the heart," *The American Journal of Cardiology*, vol. 58, no. 1, pp. 184-185, 1986.

[25] J. S. Chang, M. L. Young, W. M. Chuu, and H. C. Lue, "Infantile cardiac hemangioendothelioma," *Pediatric Cardiology*, vol. 13, no. 1, pp. 52 55, 1992.

[26] Y. Chalet, L. Mace, B. Franc, J. Y. Neveux, and B. Lancelin, "Angiosarcoma 7 years after surgical excision of histiocytoid haemangioma in left atrium," *The Lancet*, vol. 341, no. 8854, p. 1217, 1993.

[27] T. Eichler, T. Paul, and H. E. Schneider, "Hemangioma as a rare cause of a neonatal cardiac tumor resulting in inflow obstruction of the tricuspid valve," *Clinical Research in Cardiology*, vol. 100, no. 5, pp. 469-470, 2011.

13

Surgical Repair of a Giant Sinus of Valsalva Aneurysm with an Anomalous Left Circumflex Artery in a Patient with Bicuspid Aortic Valve

Kristin Stawiarski, Asiya Mamhut, Elenita Kanin, and Stuart Zarich

Yale New Haven Health Heart and Vascular Center, Bridgeport Hospital, Bridgeport, CT, USA

Correspondence should be addressed to Kristin Stawiarski; kristin.stawiarski@bpthosp.org

Academic Editor: Kathleen Ngu

Congenital cardiac abnormalities are not always found in isolation. We describe a case of a giant right coronary sinus of Valsalva aneurysm with anomalous left circumflex artery in a 46-year-old male with bicuspid aortic valve and prior ventricular septal defect repair.

1. Introduction

Sinus of Valsalva aneurysms (SOVAs) account for only 0.09% of congenital or acquired cardiac defects [1]. However, when present, they may be associated with other cardiac anomalies [1].

2. Clinical Summary

A 46-year-old male with ventricular septal defect repair at age 3, bicuspid aortic valve, diabetes mellitus, hypertension, and previous tobacco use presented to clinic for routine follow-up. He was first diagnosed with an ascending aortic aneurysm 13 years prior and remained asymptomatic with a stable echocardiographic measurement of 5 cm. There was only mild aortic and mitral regurgitation with no residual shunt post-VSD repair. Electrocardiogram revealed normal sinus rhythm with incomplete right bundle branch block, right axis deviation, and poor R wave progression.

Computed tomography angiography (CTA) was obtained for further assessment. A SOVA was identified measuring $3.5 \times 4.7 \times 6.9$ cm at the level of the sinotubular junction (Figures 1 and 2). Immediately to the aneurysm, the ascending aorta measured 4.5×3.7 cm. The aortic arch was markedly tortuous (Figure 3). Suspicion was raised for possible anomalous coronary artery origin; however, gated acquisition was not performed.

Surgery was planned, and preoperative angiography was completed. Aortography demonstrated a giant SOVA with a fused right and noncoronary cusp and a small appearing left coronary sinus (Video 1). The coronary system was right dominant with the right coronary and left main arteries originating from their respective cusps. The left main artery gave rise to a left anterior descending and a left circumflex artery. An ectopic duplicate left circumflex artery was also seen coming off the right coronary sinus (Video 2). All vessels were free from significant disease.

The patient underwent redo sternotomy with SOVA and ascending aorta resection. A 27 mm Hemashield valved conduit, with St. Jude mechanical valve, was sewn in place along with correct reimplantation of coronaries including the anomalous left circumflex artery.

3. Discussion

SOVA can manifest at any age usually with a male predisposition. These aneurysms can coexist with other congenital abnormalities such as VSD (30-60%), bicuspid aortic valves (10%), and coronary anomalies [1]. The anomalous origin of the circumflex artery from the right coronary sinus was first described in 1933 and has since had a reported incidence

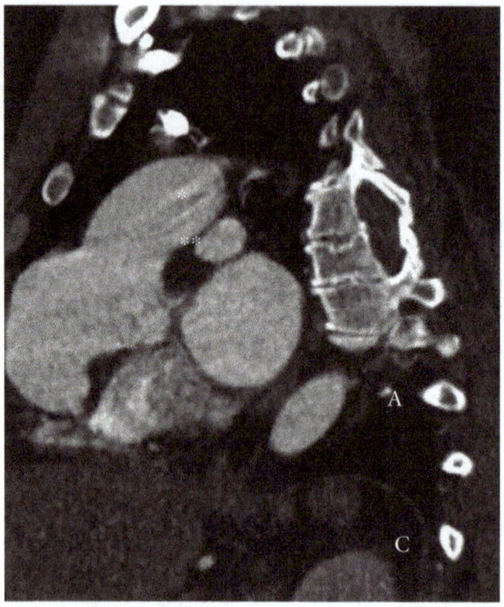

Figure 1: Transverse computed tomography angiography view of the aneurysm with a 2-dimensional diameter of 4.7 cm at the level of sinotubular junction.

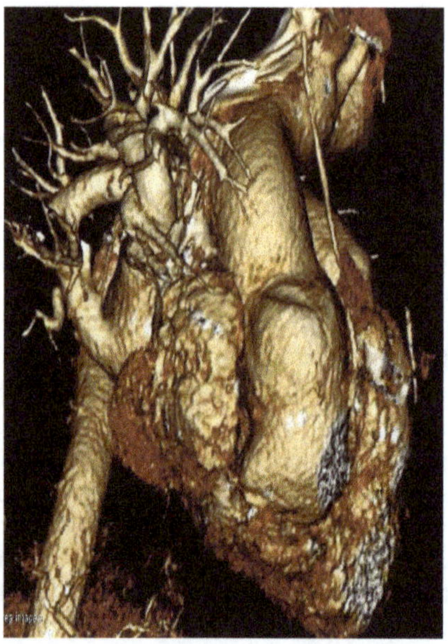

Figure 2: Computed tomography angiography of the sinus of Valsalva aneurysm, sagittal view. The right and noncoronary cusps are fused, separated by a raphe.

of 0.35% [2]. This variant carries a low risk of sudden cardiac death albeit the risk of coronary artery disease remains debatable [2].

Coronary angiography is considered the gold standard for diagnosing a SOVA [1]. However, up to 90% of cases published in the past 10 years have been diagnosed via echocardiography [1]. This diagnostic method proves to be suboptimal in evaluating rare concomitant coronary anomalies as seen with our patient [3]. The American College of Cardiology/American Heart Association (ACC/AHA) 2008 recommendations for the management of adult congenital heart disease recommend the use of CTA or magnetic reso-

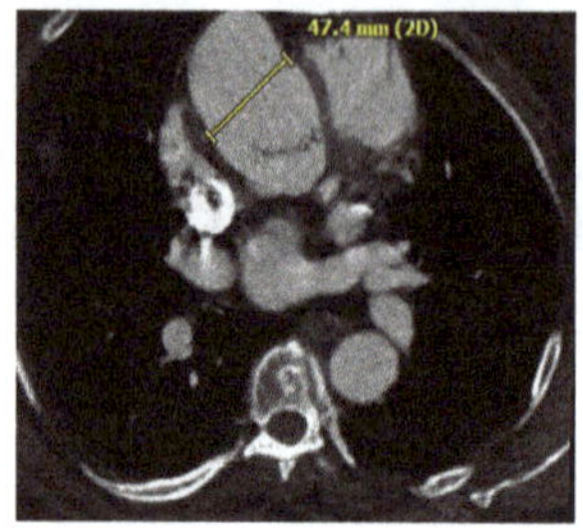

Figure 3: 3-dimensional reconstructed view of the sinus of Valsalva aneurysm and tortuous aortic arch.

nance imaging (MRI) for initial congenital coronary anomaly screening in patients who *survived unexplained cardiac death, life-threatening arrhythmia, coronary ischemic symptoms, or left ventricular dysfunction* (*class I, level of evidence* (*LOE*) *B*) [4]. However, the more recent ACC/AHA 2018 guidelines have removed this recommendation as the data supporting a surgical approach for secondary prevention of sudden cardiac death are limited [5]. These guidelines offer coronary angiography, CTA or, MRI as the choice image modalities for the evaluation of coronary anomalies (class I, LOE C-limited) [5].

It is generally accepted to apply aortic root aneurysm repair guidelines to SOVA repair as was done in our patient. Surgical repair of the aneurysm is usually considered if the aortic diameter is ≥5.5 cm in asymptomatic patients with a bicuspid aortic valve. Exceptional consideration is given to patients who have diameter of ≥5.0 cm with either additional risk factors for dissection or an expansion rate of ≥0.5 cm per year. Likewise, aneurysm repair is reasonable in patients undergoing aortic valve replacement due to severe bicuspid valve stenosis/regurgitation [6].

A thorough evaluation of the coronary anatomy is vital prior to any cardiac surgery. Failure to recognize coronary anomalies can result in intraoperative complications such as accidental vessel laceration or compression. However, primary surgery for anomalous coronary arteries is usually reserved for cases of ischemia (class I, LOE B nonrandomized) or ventricular arrthymias (class IIA, LOE C—expert opinion), both of which are lacking in our patient [5]. Surgery would also be reasonable if the left coronary artery arises from the right coronary sinus in the absence of symptoms (class IIA, LOE C—limited data) [5]. In our case, decision was made to relocate the anomalous artery to its usual course to reduce the potential risk of coronary artery disease from angular vessel insertion.

For patients with an identified congenital cardiac abnormality, it is prudent to comprehensively evaluate the entire cardiac anatomy for other clustered anomalies as seen in this case. The risk of ischemic events and sudden cardiac death from ectopic coronary arteries remains unclear but can pose a surgical risk for patients undergoing other cardiac surgery.

References

[1] A. O. Bricker, B. Avutu, E. E. Mohammed et al., "Valsalva sinus aneurysms: findings at CT and MR imaging," *Radiographics*, vol. 30, no. 1, pp. 99–110, 2010.

[2] G. Mohsen, K. G. Mohsin, M. Forsberg, E. Miller, M. Taniuchi, and A. J. Klein, "Anomalous left circumflex artery from the right coronary cusp: a benign variant?," *The Journal of Invasive Cardiology*, vol. 25, no. 6, pp. 284–287, 2013.

[3] P. Angelini, "Novel imaging of coronary artery anomalies to assess their prevalence, the causes of clinical symptoms, and the risk of sudden cardiac death," *Circulation. Cardiovascular Imaging*, vol. 7, no. 4, pp. 747–754, 2014.

[4] C. A. Warnes, R. G. Williams, T. M. Bashore et al., "ACC/AHA 2008 Guidelines for the Management of Adults With Congenital Heart Disease: A Report of the American College of Cardiology/American Heart Association Task Force on Practice Guidelines (Writing Committee to Develop Guidelines on the Management of Adults With Congenital Heart Disease)," *Journal of the American College of Cardiology*, vol. 52, no. 23, pp. e143–e263, 2008.

[5] K. K. Stout, C. J. Daniels, J. A. Aboulhosn et al., "2018 AHA/ACC guideline for the management of adults with congenital heart disease: executive summary: a report of the American College of Cardiology/American Heart Association Task Force on Clinical Practice Guidelines," *Journal of the American College of Cardiology*, vol. 73, no. 12, pp. 1494–1563, 2019.

[6] 2010 ACCF/AHA/AATS/ACR/ASA/SCA/SCAI/SIR/STS/SVM Guidelines for the Diagnosis and Management of Patients With Thoracic Aortic Disease Representative Members, L. F. Hiratzka, M. A. Creager et al., "Surgery for aortic dilatation in patients with bicuspid aortic valves: a statement of clarification from the American College of Cardiology/American Heart Association Task Force on Clinical Practice Guidelines," *The Journal of Thoracic and Cardiovascular Surgery*, vol. 151, no. 4, pp. 959–966, 2016.

14

Percutaneous Coronary Intervention Strategy for Spontaneous Coronary Artery Dissection of Left Main Coronary Artery with Extensive Intramural Hematoma in the Main Side Branch

Makio Muraishi,[1] **Kosuke Maeda**,[2] **Takuya Okada**,[2] **and Masahiko Noguchi**[1]

[1]*Department of Cardiology, Tokyo Bay Urayasu Ichikawa Medical Center, Urayasu, Japan*
[2]*Department of Cardiology, Yokosuka General Hospital Uwamachi, Yokosuka, Japan*

Correspondence should be addressed to Masahiko Noguchi; m.noguchi.0918@gmail.com

Academic Editor: Dirk Bandorski

A 46-year-old pregnant woman, presented with worsening episodes of intermittent chest pain. The patient was diagnosed with a non-ST-elevation myocardial infarction. On arrival, she had a stable hemodynamic status without chest pain. She was initially treated with conservative medical therapy. One day later, she complained of severe chest pain, and an electrocardiogram showed ST elevation in leads I, aVL, and V2-5. Emergency coronary angiography showed total occlusion of the left anterior descending artery (LAD) and intermediate stenosis of the left main coronary artery (LMCA). The intravascular ultrasound (IVUS) revealed an intramural hematoma (IMH) from the LMCA to the LAD, extending to the left circumflex artery (LCX) ostium. This finding was consistent with spontaneous coronary artery dissection (SCAD). After stent implantation from the LMCA to the LAD, severe stenosis was noted at the proximal site of the LCX. IVUS showed that the IMH extended to the LCX. The provisional crush stent technique was performed, and the final angiography revealed satisfactory results with thrombolysis in myocardial infarction flow grade 3 in the LAD and LCX. This case report highlighted that stent implantation in the SCAD lesions facilitated the extension of the IMH longitudinally and laterally into the side branch, resulting in stenosis or occlusion. Therefore, the side branch should be evaluated using IVUS before stent implantation. In cases where the IMH extends to the ostium of the side branch, two-stent techniques that do not require guidewire recrossing, such as crush stents, should be considered to avoid side branch occlusion.

1. Introduction

Spontaneous coronary artery dissection (SCAD) is defined as epicardial coronary artery dissection. It has been recognized as a significant cause of myocardial infarction, especially in younger women [1, 2]. Observational data have reported spontaneous angiographic healing in most patients (70-97%) [3, 4]. Meanwhile, percutaneous coronary intervention (PCI) for SCAD has been associated with high technical failure (36-53%) [3, 5]. In this procedure, the coronary guidewire may enter the false lumen and occlude the true lumen. Alternatively, balloon dilation and stent placement can result in extended intimal dissection, leading to intramural hematoma (IMH) formation, which propagates upstream and downstream. Thus, PCI for SCAD was recommended for patients, who have ongoing ischemia, cardiogenic shock, sustained ventricular arrhythmias, or left main coronary artery (LMCA) dissection, with a favorable anatomy for PCI [1]. However, the PCI strategy for SCAD has not been established. In this study, we describe a case of a 46-year-old woman, who presented with ST-elevation myocardial infarction (STEMI), caused by SCAD in the LMCA, treated with PCI. Furthermore, we discuss SCAD, including LMCA, focusing on the PCI strategy.

2. Case Series

A 46-year-old, five-week pregnant woman with hypertension and hyperlipidemia was transferred to our hospital with worsening episodes of intermittent chest pain. She experienced non-ST-elevation myocardial infarction (NSTEMI)

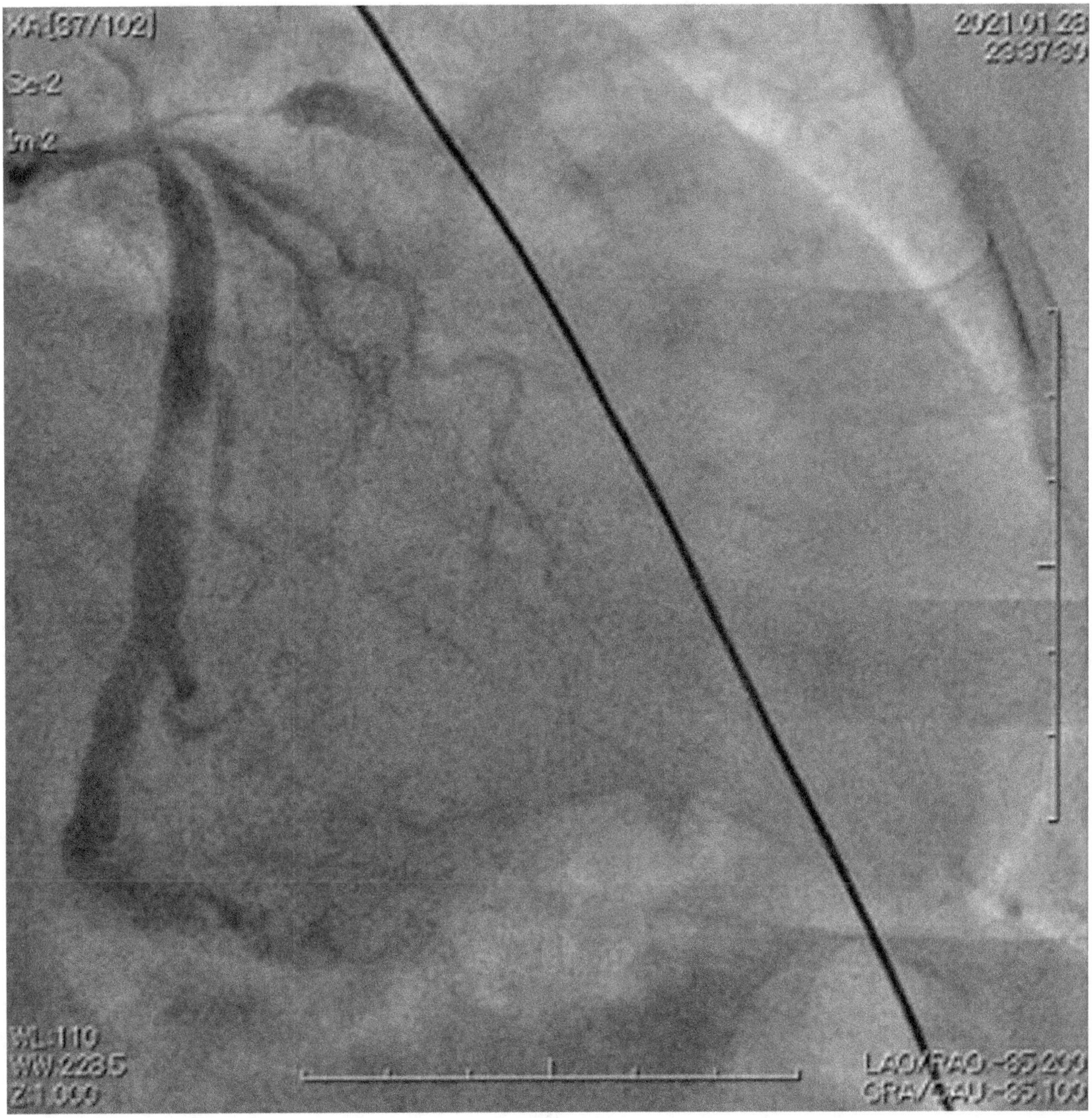

(a)

Figure 1: Continued.

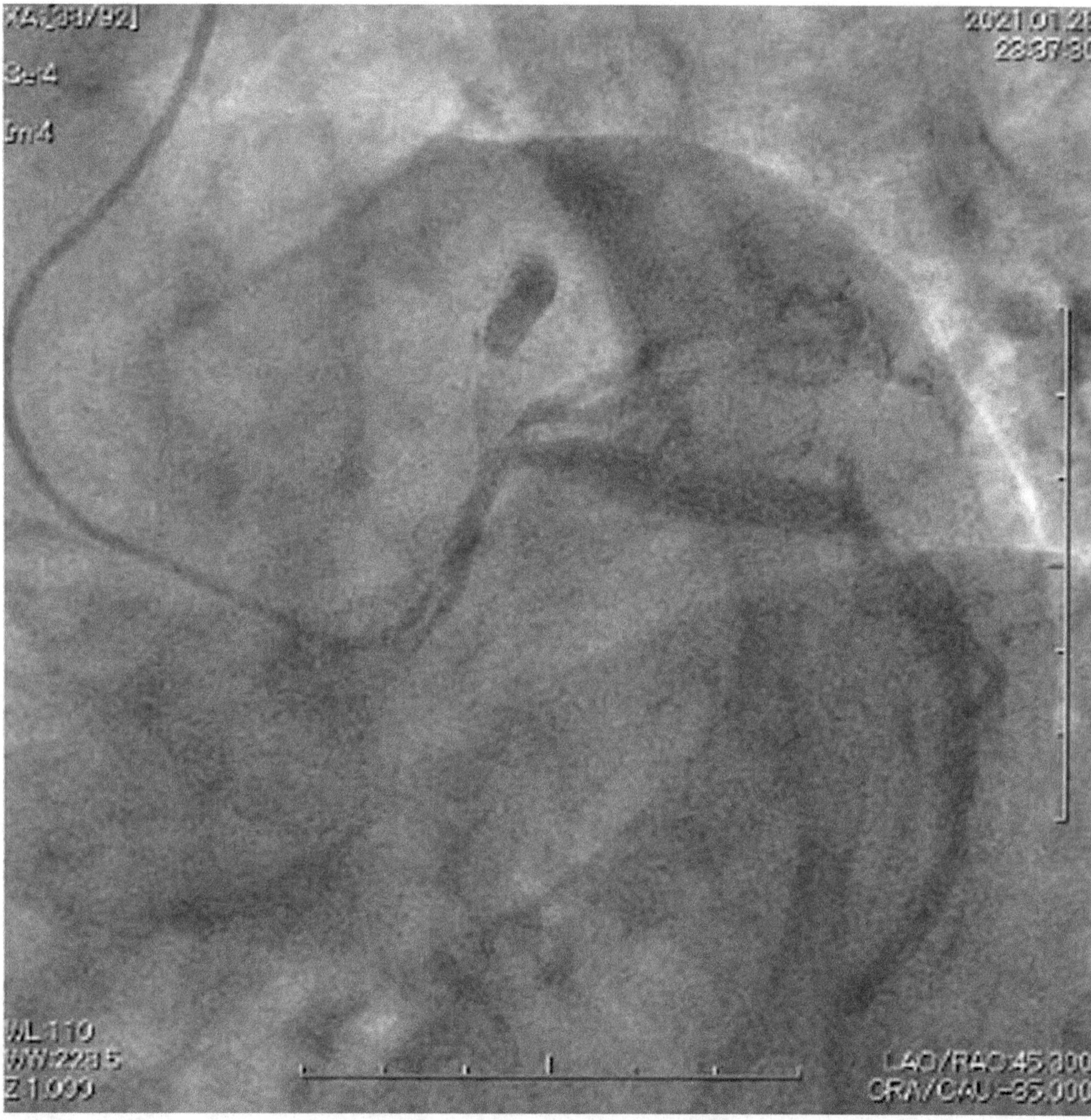

(b)

Figure 1: Emergency coronary angiography. (a) Right anterior oblique caudal projection and (b) left anterior oblique caudal projection showing TIMI flow 0 in the left anterior descending artery. Significant stenosis in the left main coronary artery and intermediate stenosis in the left circumflex artery were observed. In this case, the patient's abdomen and back were protected because she was pregnant, and the working view was limited to the right anterior oblique caudal projection and left anterior oblique caudal projection. TIMI: thrombolysis in myocardial infarction.

due to type 2 SCAD, treated conservatively two years ago. Subsequently, she was maintained on antiplatelet therapy (aspirin 100 mg daily) and a beta blocker (bisoprolol 2.5 mg daily). On arrival, her chest pain disappeared, and she had stable vital signs. The physical examination was unremarkable, with no noted murmur, rub, gallop, or signs of cardiac enlargement. The initial electrocardiogram showed T-wave inversion in leads I, aVL, and V2-V4, but ST elevation or Q wave was not observed. Laboratory testing showed elevated cardiac enzymes, such as positive troponin T, creatinine phosphokinase (CK) (646 U/L), and CK-MB (54 U/L). Bedside transthoracic echocardiography revealed impaired contractility in the anterior and septal segments of the left ventricle. Since she was pregnant and hemodynamically stable without chest pain, she was treated conservatively with aspirin, nitroglycerin, heparin, and bisoprolol.

One day later, she complained of severe chest pain, and an electrocardiogram showed ST elevation in leads I, aVL,

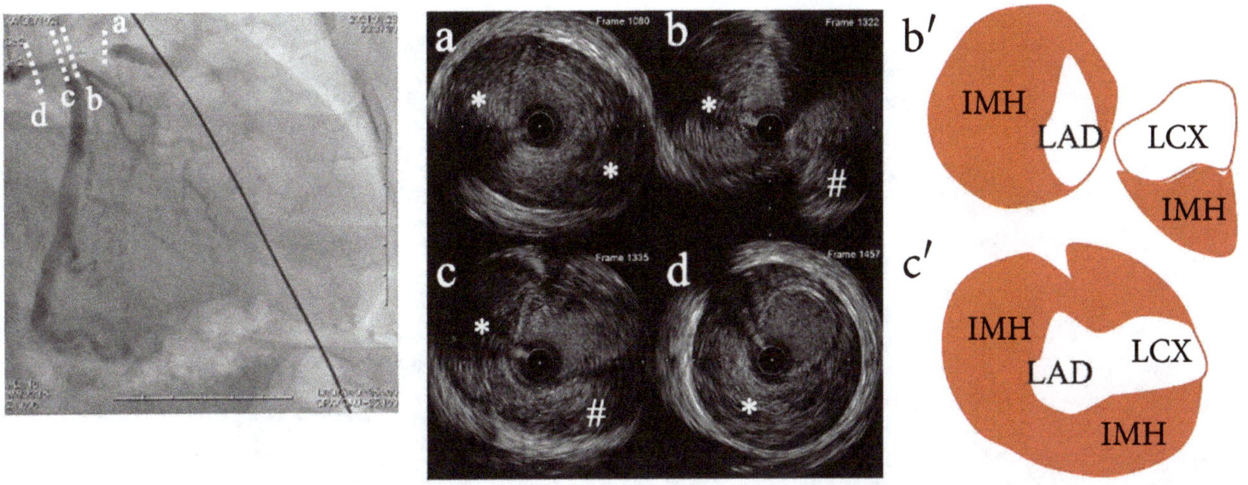

Figure 2: IVUS images of the left main coronary artery to left anterior descending artery and scheme of IVUS images. (a) IVUS image of the left anterior descending artery showing intramural hematoma (asterisk) compressing the true lumen. (b, b′) IVUS images of left anterior descending artery ostium showing intramural hematoma (asterisk). The left circumflex artery and intramural hematoma (sharp) extending to the left circumflex artery can also be observed. (c, c′) IVUS image of left main coronary artery bifurcation showing intramural hematoma extension to the left anterior descending artery (asterisk) and left circumflex artery (sharp). (d) IVUS image of left main coronary artery showing intramural hematoma (asterisk) compressing the true lumen. IVUS: intravascular ultrasound; LAD: left anterior descending artery; LCX: left circumflex artery; IMH: intramural hematoma.

and V2-5. Emergency coronary angiography revealed total occlusion of the left anterior descending artery (LAD) with thrombolysis in myocardial infarction (TIMI) flow grade 0 and intermediate stenosis of the LMCA (Figure 1). After the guidewire had been advanced into the LAD, the occluded lesion was dilated using a 2.0 mm coronary balloon, and the cause of the occlusion was determined via intravascular ultrasound (IVUS). IVUS revealed an intramural hematoma (IMH) from the LMCA to the LAD. The IMH extended to the left circumflex artery (LCX) ostium (Figure 2). Then, a 4.0 mm drug-eluting stent was implanted from the LMCA to the LAD to cover all IMHs. After stent implantation, a TIMI flow grade 3 was obtained in the LAD. However, the stenosis at the proximal segment of the left circumflex artery (LCX) progressed severely, and the LCX blood flow worsened to TIMI flow grade 2 (Figure 3). The guidewire was rewired through the stent struts. IVUS for LCX revealed a large IMH compressing the true lumen (Figure 4). Then, an additional drug-eluting stent (4.0 mm) was implanted into the LCX, using the provisional crush stent technique. The final angiography yielded satisfactory results with a TIMI grade 3 flow in both the LAD and LCX (Figure 5).

The postprocedural course was uneventful, and no major adverse cardiovascular events were observed. ECG before discharge revealed ST-segment resolution in the anterolateral leads. The patient's clinical course was uneventful during follow-up at the outpatient clinic.

3. Discussion

This case report highlighted that IMH can extend to the side branch. The PCI strategy for SCAD, including bifurcating lesions, should be carefully considered to avoid side branch occlusion. PCI has achieved a low success rate and high complication rate for SCAD due to difficulties in guidewire manipulation and the development of dissection and IMH [3, 5]. These challenging aspects are crucial, especially in bifurcation lesions, such as LMCA bifurcation. The present case illustrated two important lessons regarding the PCI strategy for SCAD.

First, intracoronary imaging was important in establishing the correct diagnosis and successfully performing PCI. It was difficult to distinguish between the true and false lumens using coronary angiography alone [6]. However, intracoronary imaging identified intimal tear, false lumen, IMH, and intraluminal thrombi [7]. Moreover, it confirmed the passage of the guidewire through the distal true lumen. Detecting the partial passage of the guidewire through the false lumen, including the bifurcation, allows manipulation of the guidewire into the true lumen under IVUS guidance. Numasawa et al. reported an IVUS-guided rewiring technique, which confirmed the passage of the guidewire through the true lumen of the LMCA and the false lumen of the LAD from the bifurcation. The second wire was inserted into the true lumen using a double-lumen catheter, placed in the true lumen of the LCX [8]. Intracoronary imaging can also be used to evaluate IMH expansion. In this case, severe stenosis was observed in the LAD, and the IMH was expected to extend mainly from the LMCA to the LAD. IVUS documented the expansion of the IMH from the LMCA to the LAD, and the extension of the IMH to the LCX ostium. This finding was a significant predictor of IMH propagation into the LCX after stent implantation in the LAD.

Second, the one-stent strategy should be avoided in cases wherein the IMH of the main vessel extends into the side branch, because stent implantation in the main vessel can result in side branch occlusion secondary to IMH propagation, as seen in this case. When managing PCI for true LMCA bifurcation lesions due to atherosclerotic coronary

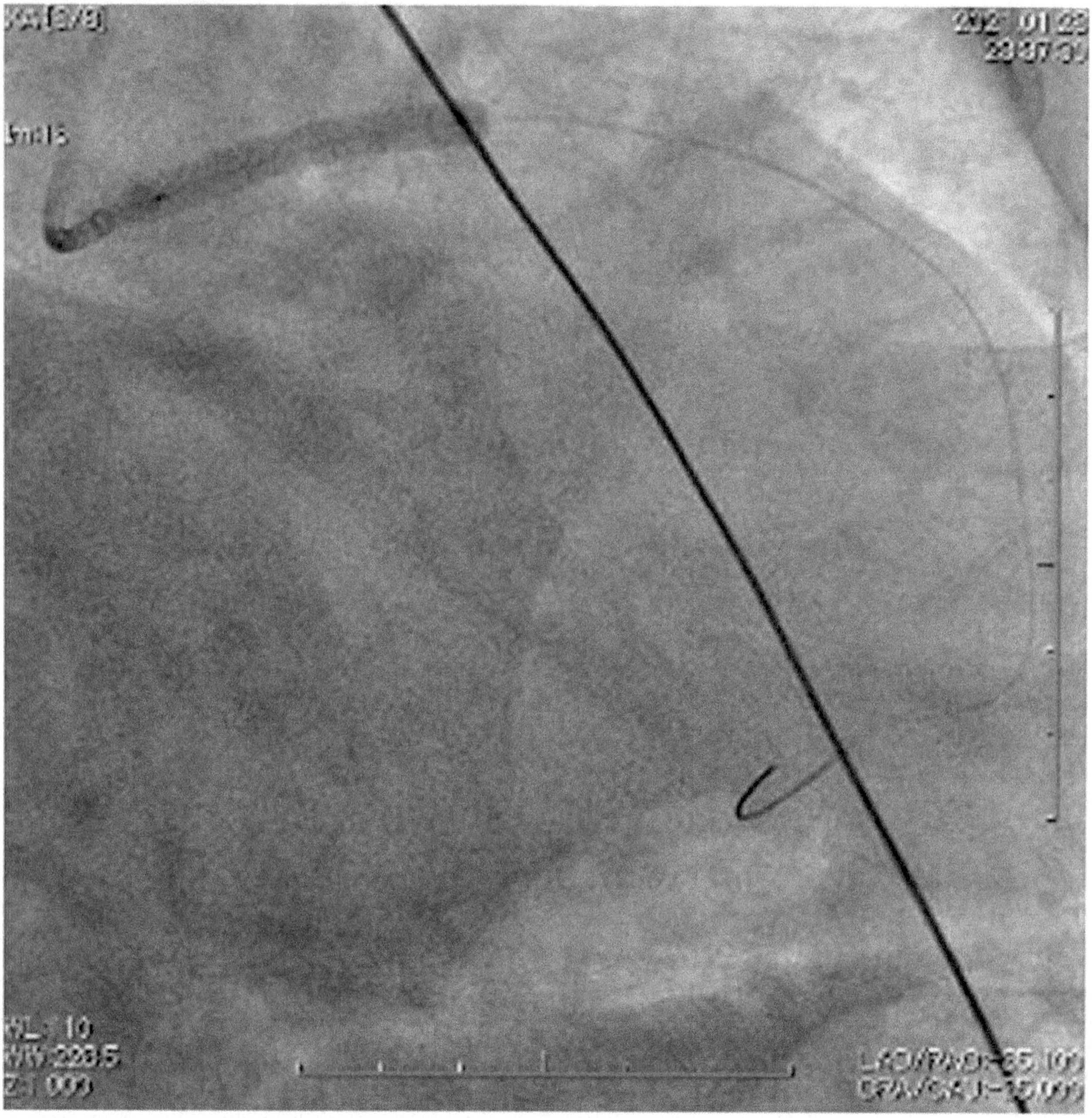

(a)

FIGURE 3: Continued.

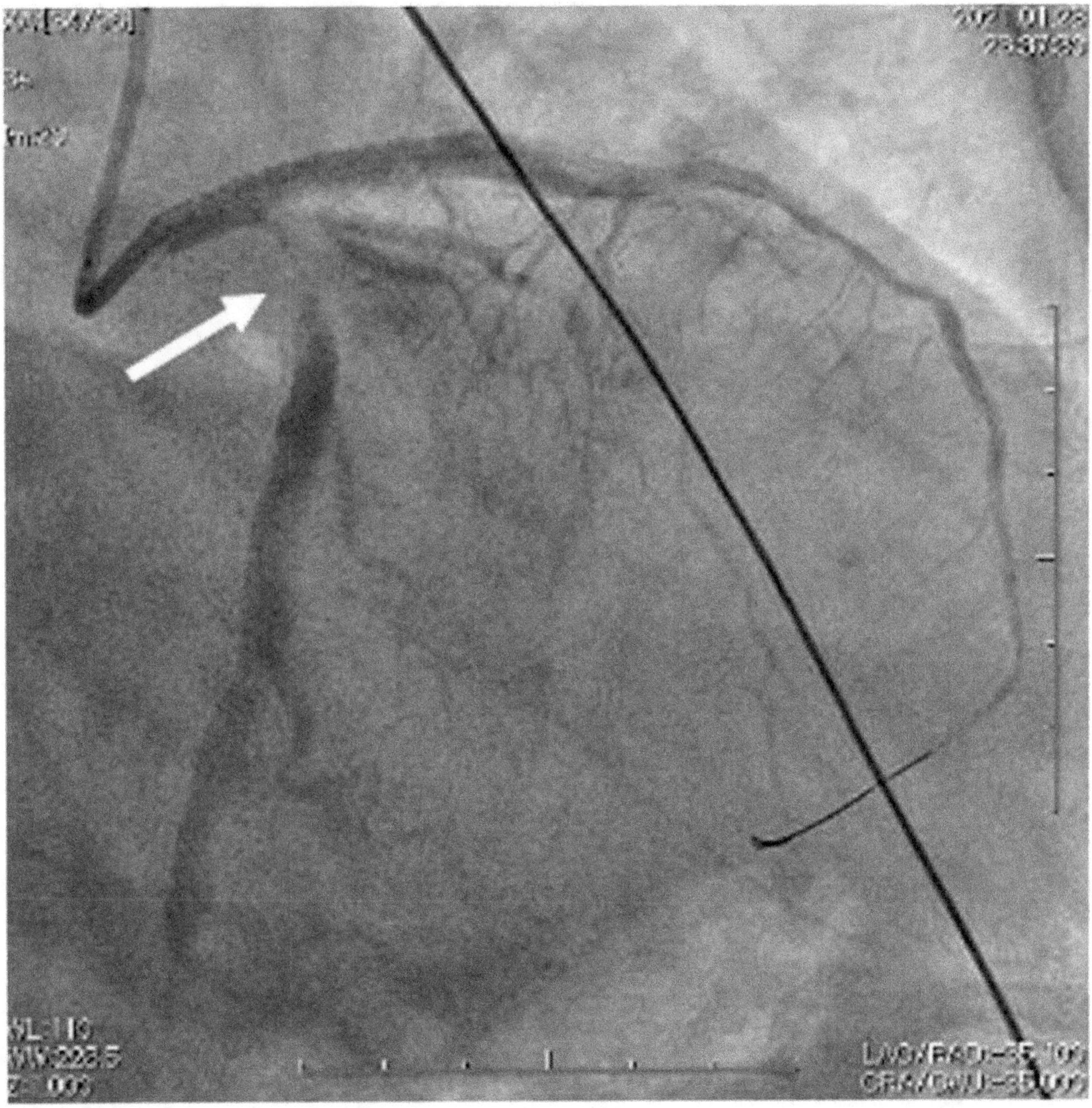

(b)

FIGURE 3: (a) The angiogram showing stent implantation from the left main coronary artery to the left anterior descending artery. (b) The angiogram after stent implantation. Significant stenosis appeared at the proximal site of the left circumflex artery (white arrow) which was not observed before stent implantation.

artery disease, the stepwise provisional strategy can serve as the default intervention for distal LMCA bifurcation, rather than the two-stent strategy [9, 10]. However, for true LMCA bifurcation lesions due to SCAD, the provisional strategy harbors the risk of side branch occlusion due to IMH extension after stent implantation. Side branch occlusion secondary to IMH extension hinders the recrossing of another guidewire into the true lumen of the side branch through stent struts. In this situation, a two-stent strategy, such as a crush stent, is preferred because this technique does not require guidewire recrossing. This case, which involved a lesion crossing over the major side branch, documented the proposed PCI algorithm for SCAD (Figure 6).

SCAD is a common cause of myocardial infarction in pregnant or postpartum women [2]. Therefore, postoperative antiplatelet therapy is crucial when PCI is performed for SCAD in pregnant patients. Although there are few data on dual antiplatelet therapy (DAPT) during pregnancy, the European Society of Cardiology guideline states that no complications have been reported in stented pregnant patients treated with aspirin and clopidogrel and that the duration of DAPT can be shortened with second-/third-

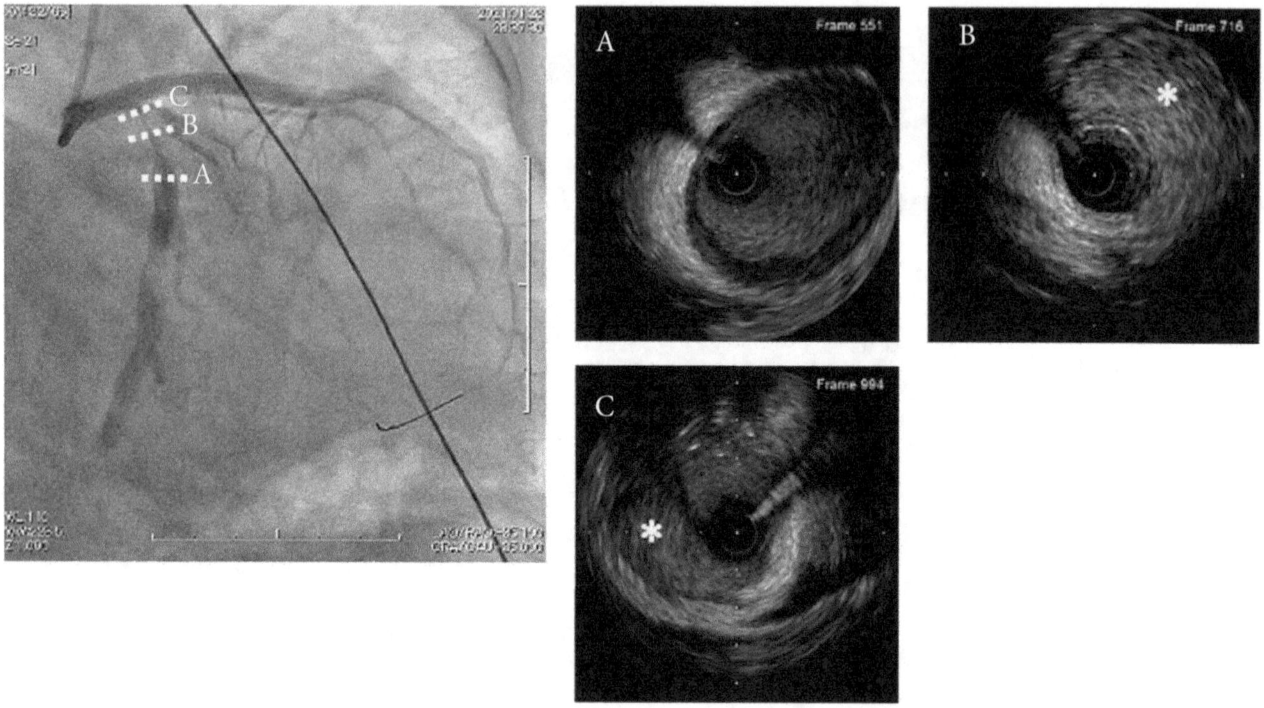

(a)

FIGURE 4: Continued.

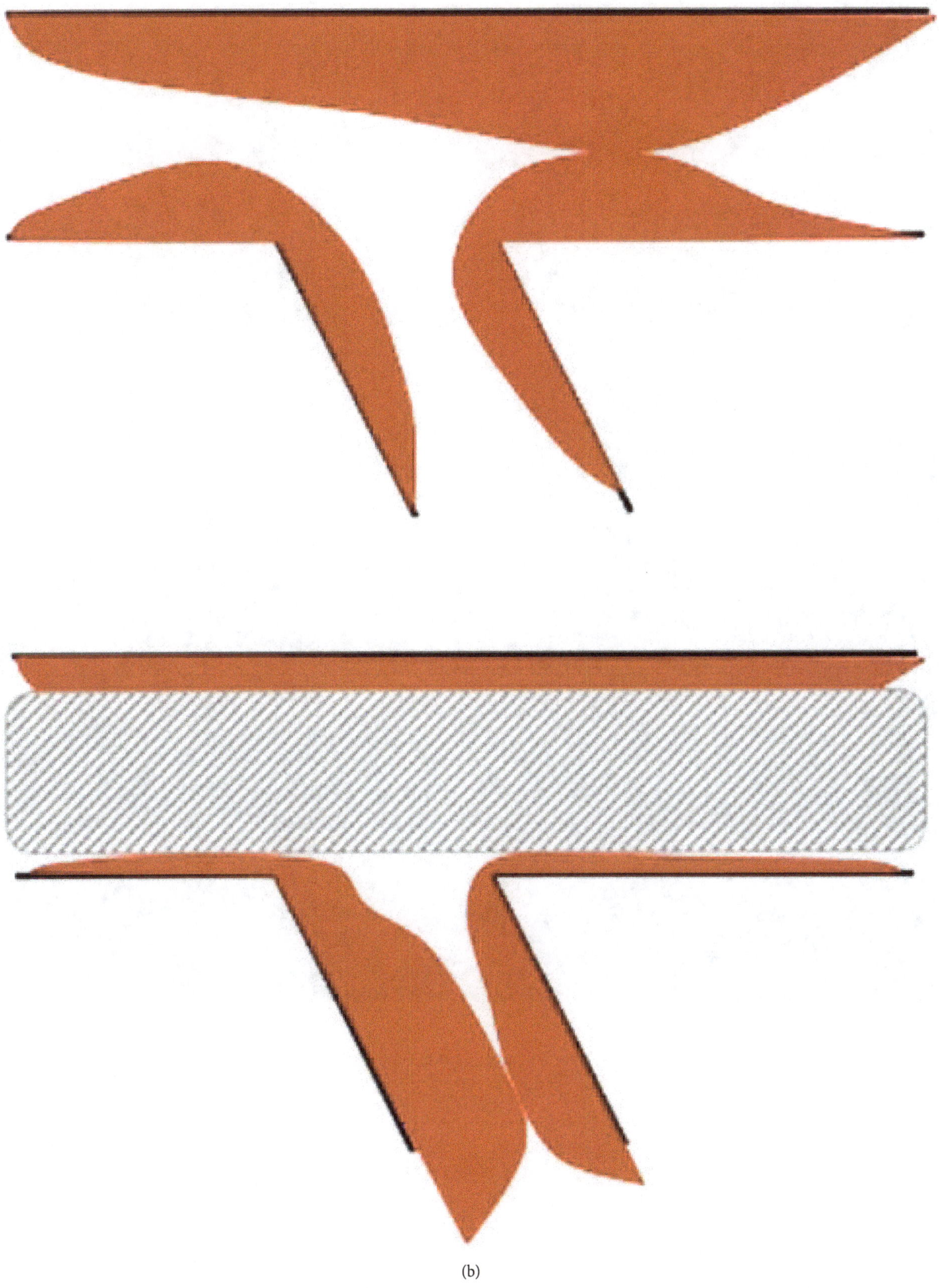

(b)

FIGURE 4: (a) The angiogram and IVUS images after stent implantation from the left main coronary artery to left anterior descending artery. (A) IVUS image of the midsite of left circumflex artery showing health vessel at this site. (B, C) IVUS image of the proximal site of left circumflex with significant stenosis showing huge intramural hematoma compressing the true lumen. (b) The scheme of extension of intramural hematoma to left circumflex after stent implantation from the left main coronary artery to left anterior descending artery.

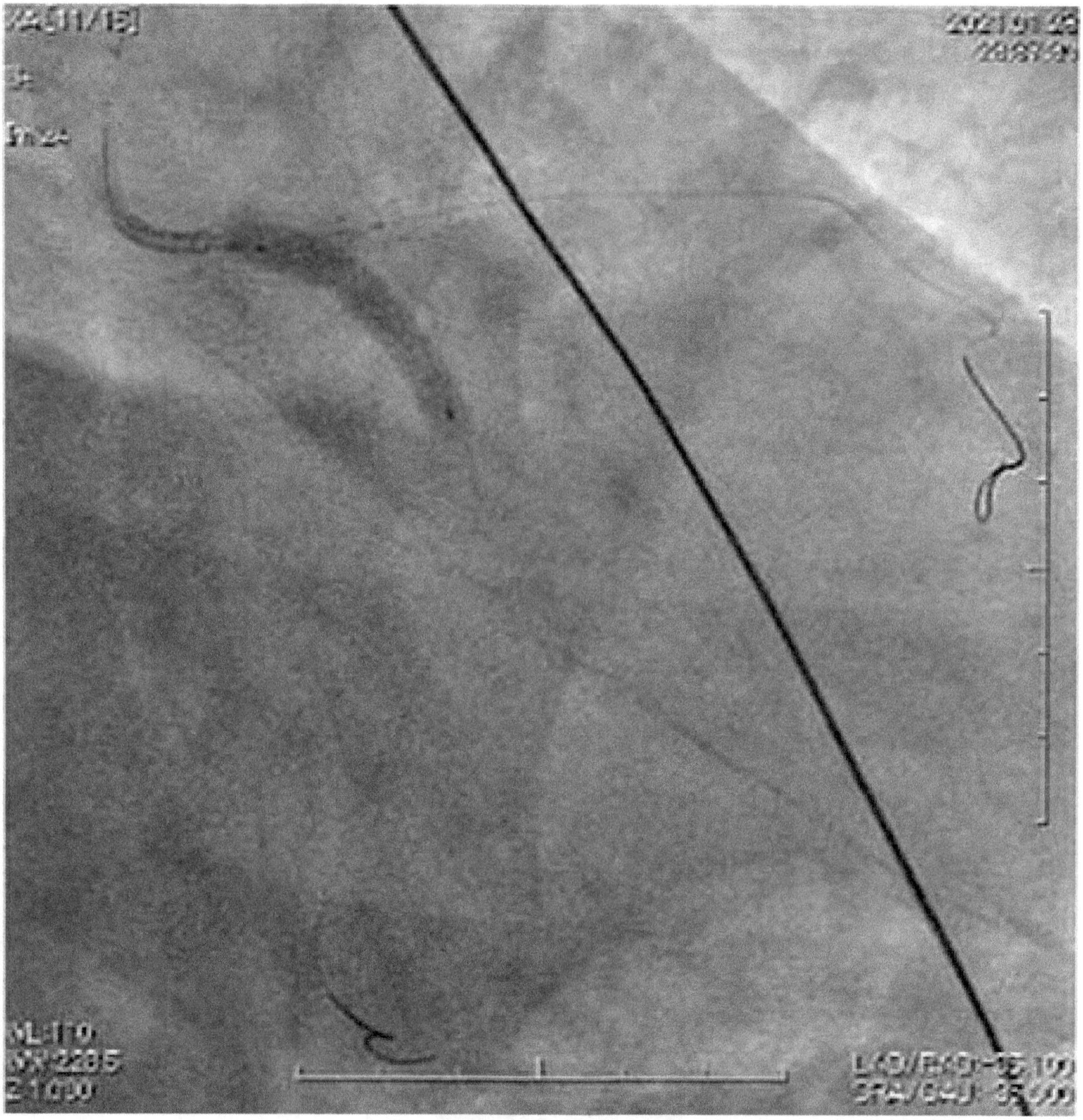

(a)

FIGURE 5: Continued.

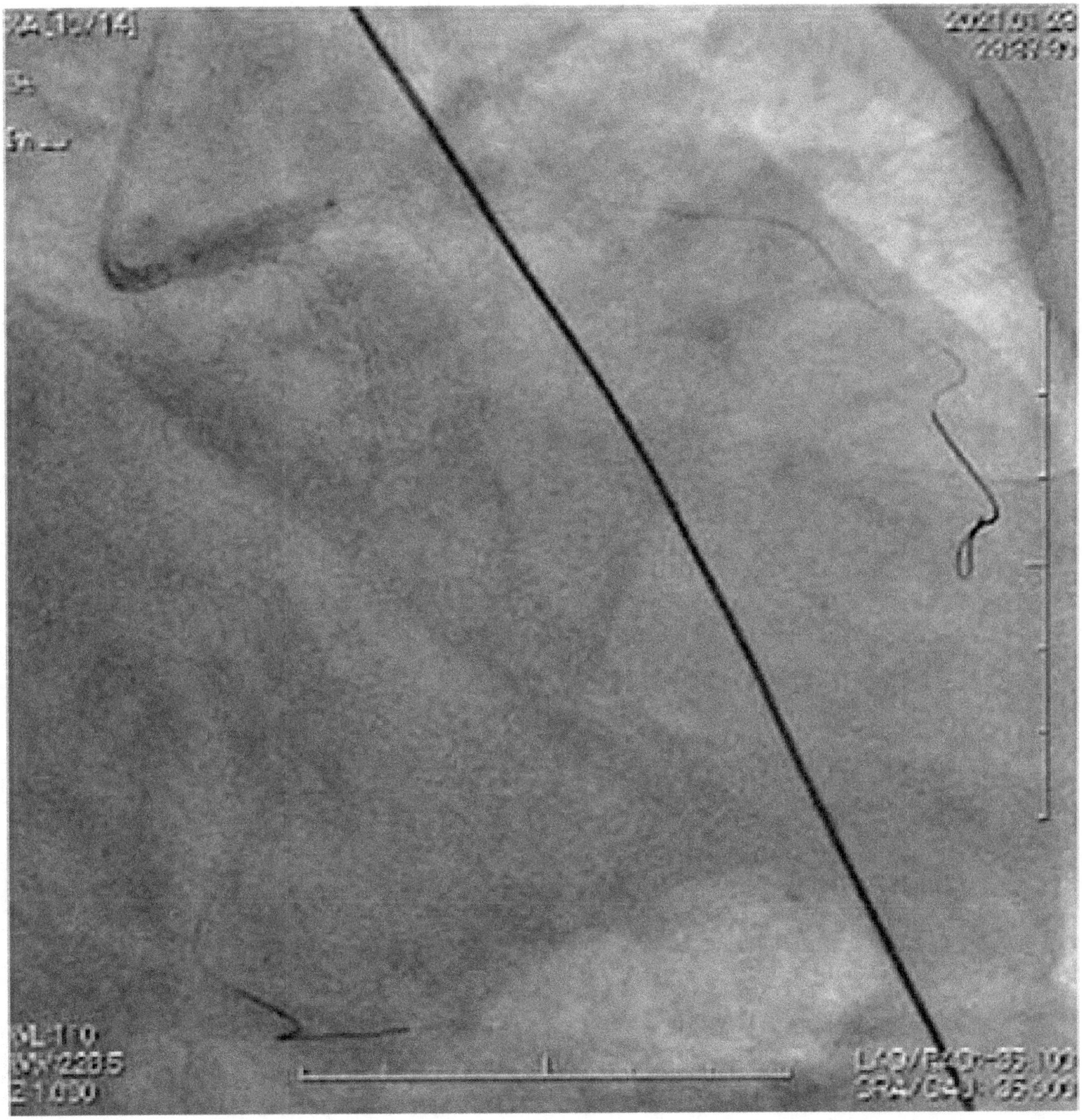

(b)

FIGURE 5: Continued.

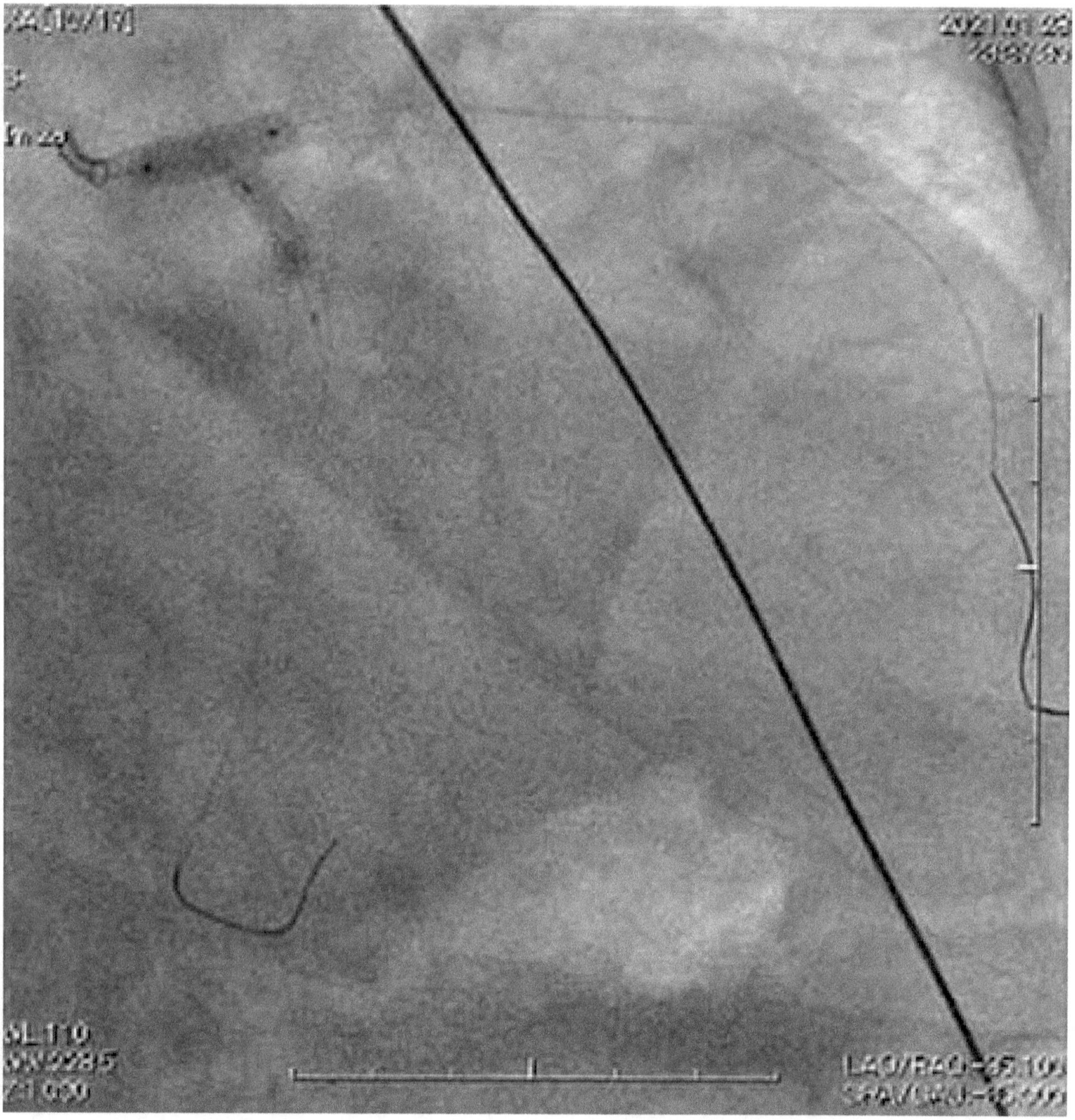

(c)

Figure 5: Continued.

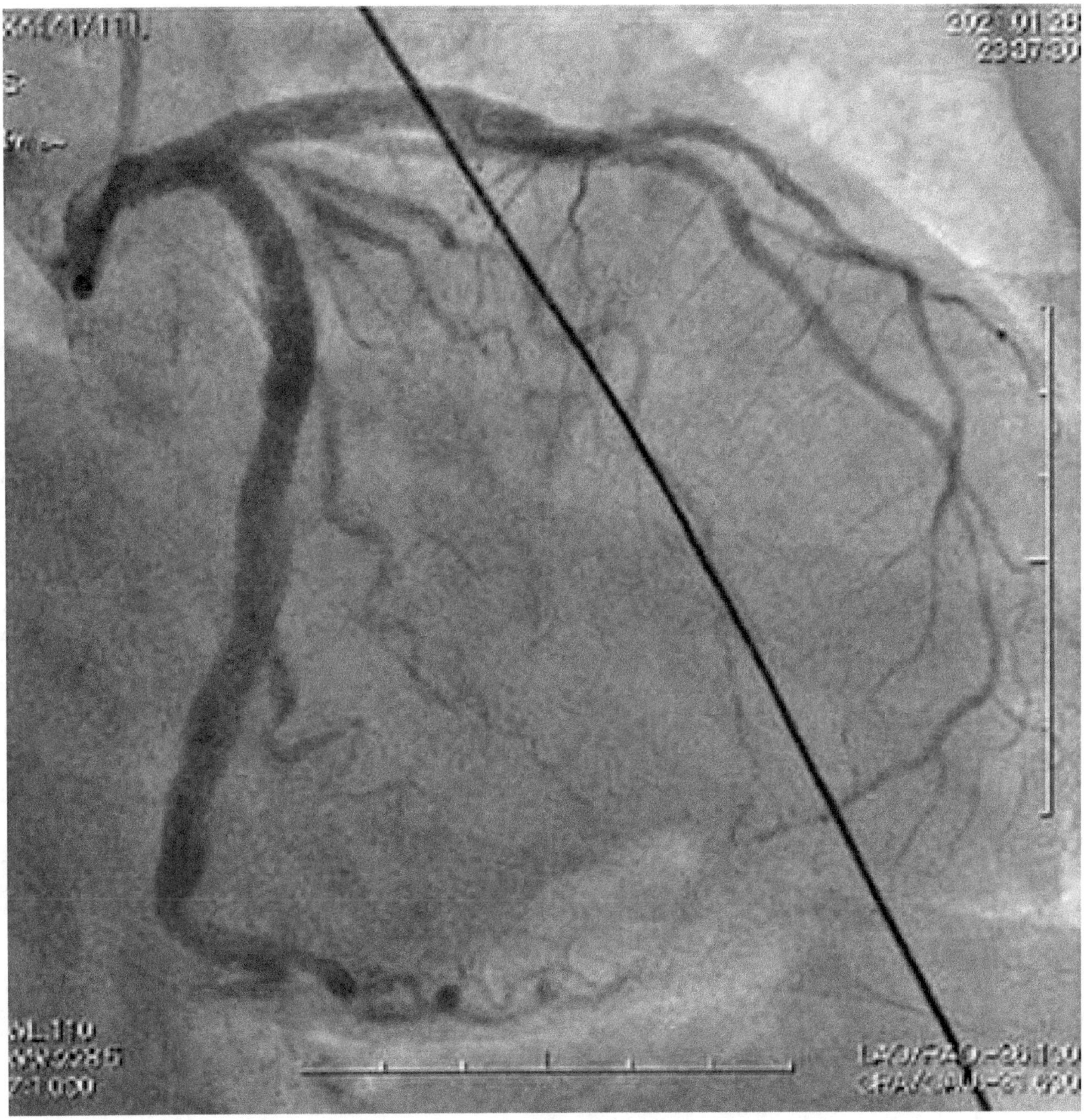

(d)

FIGURE 5: (a) The angiogram showing stent implantation from the left main coronary artery to the left circumflex artery through stent strut of the first stent. (b) The angiogram shows an inflated balloon at the left main coronary artery and a crushed stent. (c) The angiogram showing the kissing balloon technique after guidewire recrossing. (d) The final angiogram shows TIMI grade 3 flow in the left anterior descending artery and left circumflex artery.

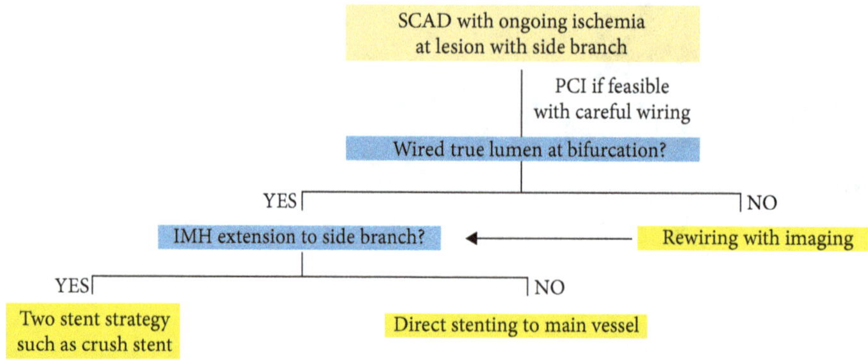

Figure 6: Proposed algorithm for management of SCAD with ongoing ischemia, which has the lesion crossing over the major side branch. SCAD: spontaneous coronary artery dissection; PCI: percutaneous coronary intervention; IMH: intramural hematoma.

generation drug-eluting stents [11]. In this patient, DAPT (aspirin and clopidogrel) was introduced at the time of PCI since she was undergoing complex stenting of an LM bifurcation lesion. The P2Y12 inhibitor was planned for discontinuation before delivery with closed monitoring.

4. Conclusion

SCAD is an uncommon but important cause of acute coronary syndrome. Emergent PCI for SCAD remains challenging because of the difficulty of manipulating the guidewire into the true lumen and extensive IMH. When performing PCI for SCAD with an IMH, crossing over the major side branch, the extension of the IMH to the side branch should be evaluated using intracoronary imaging. In cases wherein the IMH extends to the side branch, a two-stent strategy that does not require guidewire recrossing should be considered to avoid side branch occlusion.

Consent

Additional informed consent was obtained from all patients, for which identifying information was included in this article.

References

[1] A. Main and J. Saw, "Percutaneous coronary intervention for the treatment of spontaneous coronary artery dissection," *Interventional Cardiology Clinics*, vol. 8, no. 2, pp. 199–208, 2019.

[2] S. N. Hayes, E. S. Kim, J. Saw et al., "Spontaneous coronary artery dissection: current state of the science: a scientific statement from the American Heart Association," *Circulation*, vol. 137, no. 19, pp. e523–e557, 2018.

[3] M. S. Tweet, M. F. Eleid, P. J. Best et al., "Spontaneous coronary artery Dissection," *Circulation. Cardiovascular Interventions*, vol. 7, no. 6, pp. 777–786, 2014.

[4] S. Rogowski, M. T. Maeder, D. Weilenmann et al., "Spontaneous coronary artery Dissection," *Catheterization and Cardiovascular Interventions*, vol. 89, no. 1, pp. 59–68, 2017.

[5] J. Saw, E. Aymong, T. Sedlak et al., "Spontaneous coronary artery Dissection," *Circulation. Cardiovascular Interventions*, vol. 7, no. 5, pp. 645–655, 2014.

[6] F. Alfonso, M. Paulo, N. Gonzalo et al., "Diagnosis of spontaneous coronary artery dissection by optical coherence tomography," *Journal of the American College of Cardiology*, vol. 59, no. 12, pp. 1073–1079, 2012.

[7] M. Paulo, J. Sandoval, V. Lennie et al., "Combined use of OCT and IVUS in spontaneous coronary artery dissection," *JACC: Cardiovascular Imaging*, vol. 6, no. 7, pp. 830–832, 2013.

[8] Y. Numasawa, S. Yokokura, Y. Hitomi et al., "Successful Percutaneous Coronary Intervention Using Intravascular Ultrasound- Guided Rewiring Technique in a Case of Spontaneous Coronary Artery Dissection Involving Left Main Bifurcation," *Case Reports in Cardiology*, vol. 2020, 8890537 pages, 2020.

[9] T. K. Steigen, M. Maeng, R. Wiseth et al., "Randomized study on simple versus complex stenting of coronary artery bifurcation lesions: the Nordic bifurcation study," *Circulation*, vol. 114, no. 18, pp. 1955–1961, 2006.

[10] D. Hildick-Smith, M. Egred, A. Banning et al., "The European bifurcation club left main coronary stent study: a randomized comparison of stepwise provisional vs. systematic dual stenting strategies (EBC MAIN)," *European Heart Journal*, vol. 42, no. 37, pp. 3829–3839, 2021.

[11] V. Regitz-Zagrosek, J. W. Roos-Hesselink, J. Bauersachs et al., "2018 ESC guidelines for the management of cardiovascular diseases during pregnancy," *European Heart Journal*, vol. 39, no. 34, pp. 3165–3241, 2018.

15

Unique Findings and Novel Treatment Strategy of a Giant Coronary Artery Aneurysm Associated with a Significant Pericardial Effusion

Osayi Lawani[1] **and Rick Ganim**[2]

[1]*HCA Houston Healthcare, Kingwood, USA*
[2]*Vital Heart & Vein, HCA Houston Healthcare, Kingwood, USA*

Correspondence should be addressed to Osayi Lawani; osayi.lawani@hcahealthcare.com

Academic Editor: Konstantinos P. Letsas

Giant coronary artery aneurysms are a rare, asymptomatic occurrence. Presently, there is a lack of substantial research performed in the U.S., likely due to its low prevalence. As we are increasingly becoming a global community, strengthening data for seemingly rare disease processes such as this need to be addressed, particularly when they can progress to involve complications such as pericardial effusion caused by aneurysmal rupture or infection. A popular treatment option for these aneurysms is polytetrafluoroethylene-covered stents; they have been favorable with obtaining a high percentage of procedural success rates in aneurysms not associated with myocardial infarctions. In this paper, we present a case of a giant coronary artery aneurysm located in the left circumflex coronary artery that was complicated by a pericardial effusion. We will also present its unusual repair using a long drug-eluting stent as a scaffold to overlap covered coronary stents used to help exclude the aneurysm.

1. Introduction

Coronary artery aneurysms (CAAs) or ectasias are an unusual cardiac finding. As it is seen more often in males, the incidence for patients undergoing diagnostic imaging with incidental findings is currently between 0.3 to 5.3% [1]. Occurrence may increase due to the widespread use of computed tomography angiography in clinical practice. CAAs are described as a 1.5-fold dilation in a localized segment of a coronary artery in correlation to adjacent segments of the same vessel, although dilations can also be diffused [1]. Additionally, its morphology can be classified as either saccular, fusiform, or mixed (Figure 1) [2].

Italian physician Giovanni Battista Morgagni first described a giant CAA in 1761, where he relays the discovery of "an aneurysm the size of a walnut that had ruptured into the pericardium," during a postmortem evaluation [3]. CAAs are classified as "giant" when their diameter is greater than 8 mm or 4 times the reference vessel diameter [4]. Options for treatment consist of either percutaneous intervention, surgical excision, coronary artery bypass grafting, or conservative medical management. The aim of this paper is to describe challenges associated with providing intervention for giant CAAs. In this report, we present a case of a middle-aged male with multiple CAAs, which was also complicated with the development of a giant aneurysm and an associated pericardial effusion.

2. Case History

A 56-year-old male with a past medical history of coronary artery disease with stents, hypertension, hyperlipidemia, end-stage renal disease on hemodialysis, renal transplant, and prostate cancer with radiation presented with substernal chest pain and shortness of breath during an outpatient appointment.

Seven years earlier, the patient presented to the emergency department with similar symptoms. Electrocardiogram showed normal sinus rhythm with ST abnormalities, and he was diagnosed with unstable angina. An echocardiogram

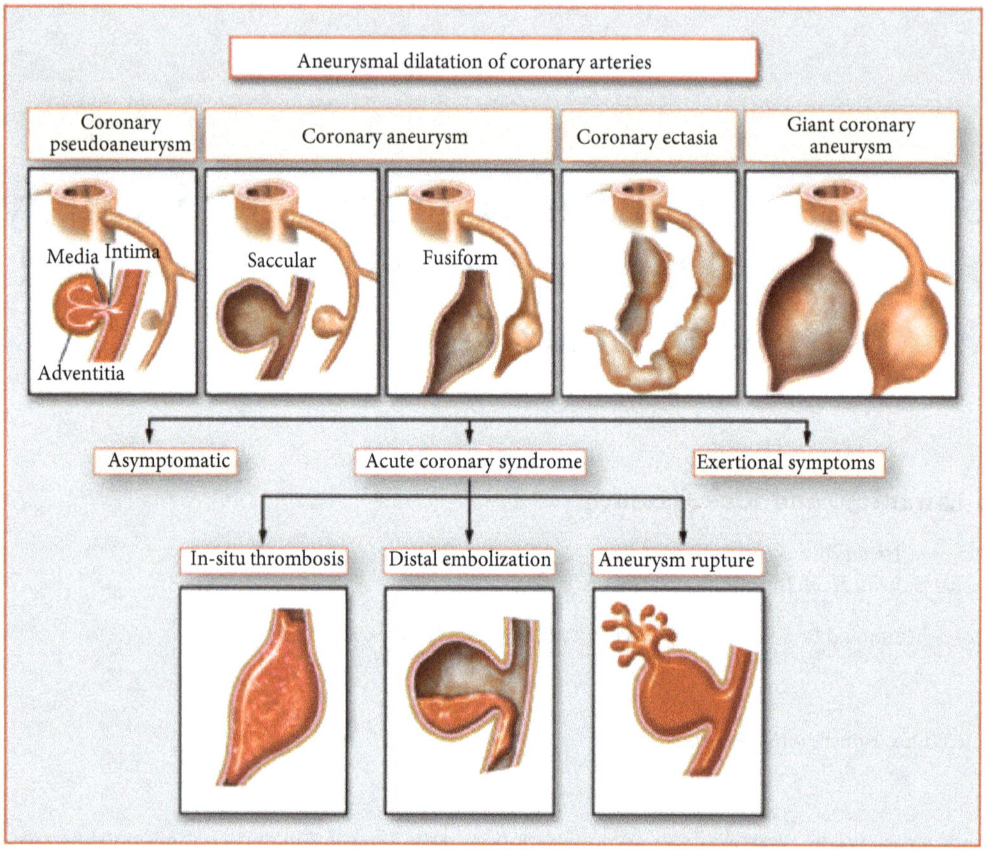

FIGURE 1: Morphologies of coronary artery aneurysms [2].

showed an ejection fraction of 45-50%, left ventricular hypertrophy, and left ventricle septal apical wall hypokinesis. Nuclear perfusion testing revealed moderate anteroseptal ischemia and decreased left ventricular systolic function, with an ejection fraction of 40%. A left heart catheterization was performed and showed diffuse ectasia of all three major coronary arteries. The left main had mild plaquing without any significant stenosis. The left anterior descending was large-caliber, and the mid-segment had eccentric 95-99% stenosis. The mid-to-distal left anterior descending had diffuse ectasia, as well as approximately 40% stenosis in its distal segment. The left circumflex artery was diffusely ectatic throughout. The right coronary artery was moderate in caliber, and the proximal segment and the posterolateral branch were diffusely ectatic without any critical stenosis. A percutaneous transluminal coronary angioplasty was performed with stent placement in the mid-left anterior descending with a 4.0 x 15 mm bare-metal integrity stent. Electrocardiogram following the procedure showed a normal sinus rhythm. The patient was discharged home on dual antiplatelet therapy and aggressive blood pressure and lipid control therapy.

Five years later, the patient presented to the emergency department after experiencing progressive shortness of breath, chest pressure, and lightheadedness for one week. Due to his history of unstable angina, a left heart catheterization was performed, and it was found that the left main coronary artery had no critical stenosis. Stent patency persisted in the mid-left anterior descending, and 40% stenosis in its mid-segment was consistent with the previous left heart catheterization. Within the left circumflex artery, the first obtuse marginal branch had a small aneurysm in its distal segment, and distal to the first take off, a very large CAA with sluggish flow was appreciated (Figure 2). An echocardiogram also revealed a large pericardial effusion with early tamponade physiology. Cardiovascular surgery was consulted, and the patient underwent urgent removal via a pericardial window. 1,100 ml of pericardial fluid was removed and was surmised to have originated from a rupture of the giant CAA.

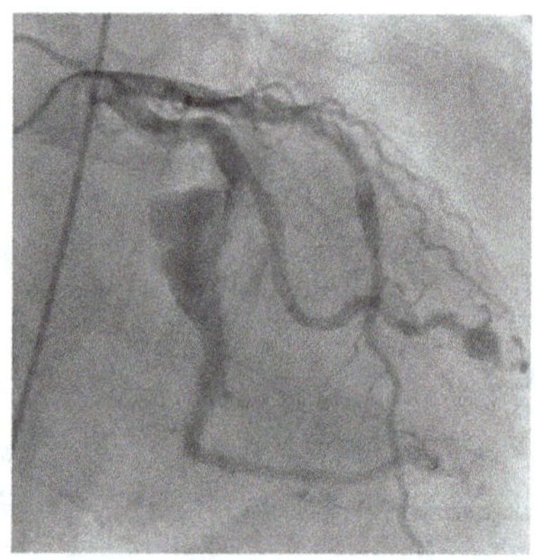

FIGURE 2: Giant coronary artery aneurysm in left circumflex coronary artery.

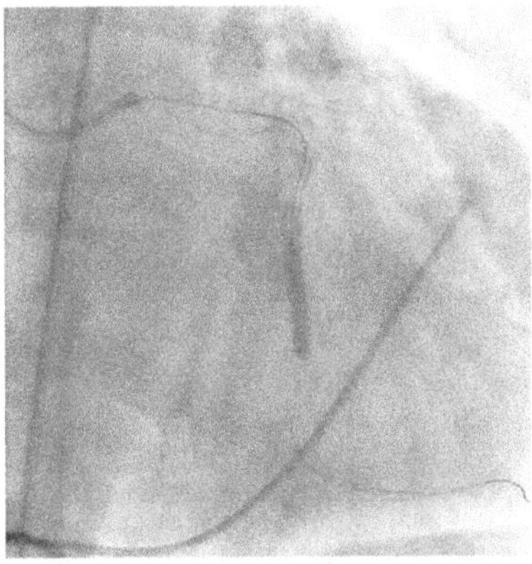

FIGURE 3: Synergy stent placement proximal and distal to a giant coronary artery aneurysm for support.

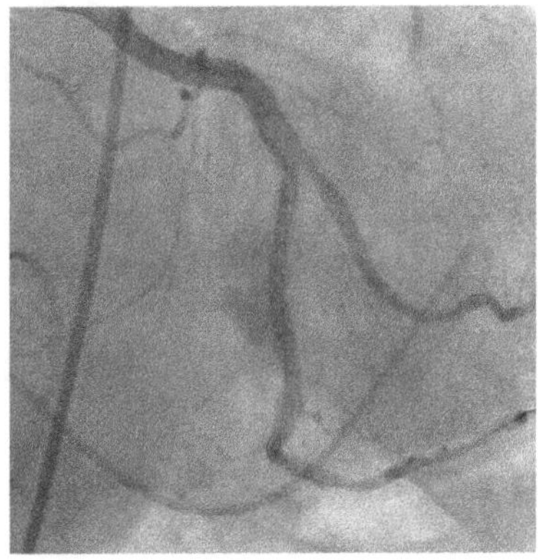

FIGURE 4: Resolution of a giant coronary artery aneurysm following repair with GraftMaster covered stents.

The following day the patient underwent a left heart catheterization of the left circumflex artery with plans to place a JOSTENT GraftMaster stent after receiving IRB and Abbott Vascular approval, due to its off-label use. The patient also consented to undergo covered stent placement for the aneurysm. A 7-french sheath was placed in the left femoral artery. A 7-french XB 3.5 guide catheter was used to engage the left main coronary artery, and a Luge wire was advanced into the distal obtuse marginal branch. Following intravenous anticoagulation, intravenous ultrasound was then advanced over the Luge wire and utilized to identify the size and length of the segment of the artery proximal and distal to the large aneurysm. Unexpectedly, the length of the aneurysm was longer than the longest GraftMaster covered stent (26 mm); intravenous ultrasound measured the length of the aneurysm at 32 mm. A 3.0 x 38 mm Synergy stent was then positioned proximal and distal to the aneurysm to provide support for placement of the covered stents. Next, the stent was postdilated with a 3.5 x 12 mm NC Emerge balloon and a 4.0 x 26 mm GraftMaster covered stent was positioned in the mid-to-distal segment of the aneurysm and was deployed at 15 atmospheres. A 2.8 x 16 mm GraftMaster covered stent was positioned in the proximal segment of the aneurysm and just proximal to the segment to the native coronary artery and was deployed at 16 atmospheres (Figure 3). The mid-to-distal segment was postdilated with a 4.0 x 20 mm NC Emerge balloon up to 16 atmospheres. Finally, the very proximal segment of the stent was postdilated with a 3.0 x 12 mm NC Emerge balloon.

Postintervention angiography revealed a resolution and complete sealing of the giant aneurysm with a Thrombolysis in Myocardial Infarction blood flow score of 3 (Figure 4). An echocardiogram showed an ejection fraction of 55-59% with no evidence of pericardial effusion. Electrocardiogram post-procedure displayed normal sinus rhythm with left axis deviation and left ventricular hypertrophy. The patient recovered well, and he was discharged a few days later on dual antiplatelet therapy.

Two years later, the patient presented with complaints of chest pain and shortness of breath during an outpatient visit. Following an abnormal stress test, a left heart catheterization was performed. It was found that the previously treated left circumflex artery stent was widely patent with continued resolution of the giant aneurysm (Figure 5). Previous stents in the midsegment of the left anterior descending also remained patent. New findings included 95% stenosis and ectasia of the mid posterolateral branch of the right coronary artery, and 75-80% stenosis in the left circumflex artery distal to the repaired aneurysmal lesion. Percutaneous intervention was performed, and a 3.0 x 16 mm Synergy stent was placed distal to the previously treated aneurysm. Also, a 3.5 x 16 mm Synergy stent was placed in the mid posterolateral branch. Following the procedure, he was discharged home to continue long-term dual antiplatelet therapy.

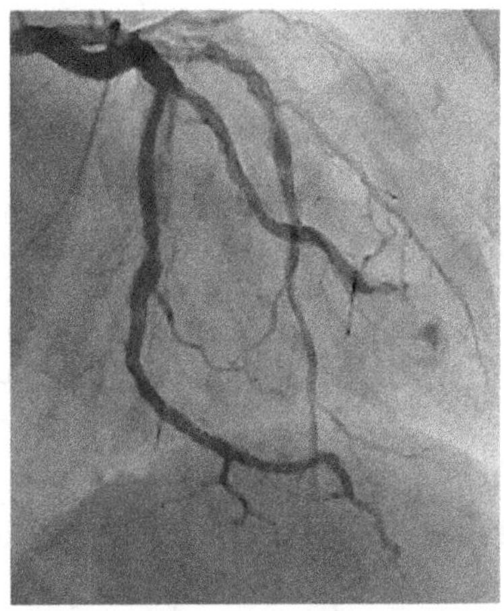

FIGURE 5: Continued resolution of a giant coronary artery aneurysm two years later.

3. Discussion

Since Dr. Charles Bougon published the first clinical description of CAAs in 1812 following a postmortem discovery, findings from autopsies are the basis for most of the knowledge on CAAs due to often treating them with percutaneous intervention or by minimal tissue excision [5]. CAAs are usually found in the right coronary artery, followed by the left anterior descending, left circumflex artery, and the left main.

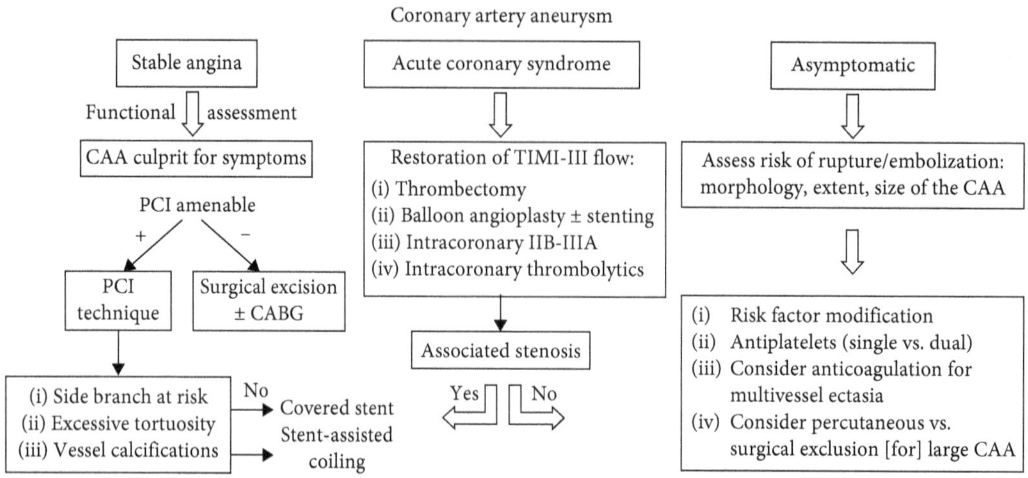

FIGURE 6: Suggested algorithm for management of coronary artery aneurysms [2].

The most common cause of CAA is atherosclerosis in North America and Europe, and Kawasaki disease in Japan and China. Other causes include inflammatory disorders, trauma, bacterial endocarditis, and complications following percutaneous intervention. Most of all patients with the atherosclerosis type will present with greater than 75% narrowing of the artery [6]. Some presentations will have multiple small aneurysms. The development of atherosclerotic CAA will usually mirror clinical features and risk factors related to coronary artery disease. Symptoms of angina will correlate with areas related to coronary artery stenosis, and consequently, aneurysm.

Coronary computed tomography angiography is currently the best modality for imaging of atherosclerotic CAA due to being able to perform a complete evaluation of coronary artery plaques, vessel patency, and overall visualization of the actual aneurysm and any resulting thrombus formation [7]. During cardiac catheterization, aneurysms will likely be underestimated because there is only an endoluminal view [7]. Although definitive diagnosis requires a histopathological sample, it is difficult to obtain unless the patient is postmortem or open-heart surgery is performed.

Presently, data is lacking for the prevalence of giant CAAs in the United States. There has been a slight increase in research; however, expanding data is primarily in Asiatic countries likely due to having a higher incidence of Kawasaki disease, which is endemic in this population [8]. Furthermore, prevalence data for giant CAAs is practically nonexistent to be able to predict the possible incidence in the United States population, independent of knowledge of known risk factors. Between 2005 to 2011, there were only a few angiography studies in the United States which reported a 0.2% CAA prevalence, whereas in Taiwan, it was found that there were approximately 200 cases per year within that time frame, with no increase in the incidence of CAA [8]. Another report speculated that the occurrence of CAA may be due to a complication of angioplasty and drug-eluting stent implantation [6]. As one would gather, treatment of this condition, particularly if it is giant, is currently done on a case-by-case basis.

Rupture of an aneurysmal coronary artery can lead to thrombus formation, embolization, ischemia, acute pericarditis, or pericardial effusion, which may progress to cardiac tamponade, as was seen in this case [9]. Incidence and prognosis of these phenomena are currently unknown. What has been noted is that the 5-year survival rate was 71% for aneurysms greater than 8 mm in diameter, and that the prognosis of CAAs greater than 20 mm is currently unknown and are at an increased risk of rupture [10]. Other complications noted were mycotic aneurysms that followed a myocardial ischemia and increased incidence in the septic or the immunecompromised [10].

Assessment and treatment for CAA is not currently standardized; however, asymptomatic patients with aneurysms should receive treatment, especially if they are greater than 30 mm in diameter [1]. Appropriate therapy is uncertain. Current options are surgical resection, coil embolization, and percutaneous approaches with covered stents, and pharmacotherapy (Figure 6) [2]. There is a question as to whether conservative management or surgery is the best approach. Two common interventions are coronary artery bypass grafting that may or may not include aneurysm ligation or resection and polytetrafluoroethylene-covered stents [11]. One study reported that polytetrafluoroethylene-covered stents are effective for aneurysms of 6-10 mm in diameter. Surgical intervention is the first line when the left main is involved or if the aneurysm is "giant" [2]. In this case, a JOSTENT GraftMaster coronary stent graft system was used, as surgical repair was not found to be a viable option. It consists of a single polytetrafluoroethylene layer that is sandwiched between two coaxial, 316 L stainless steel, slotted-tube, balloon-expandable stents [12]. It is available for diameters of 2.75-5 mm, lengths of 12, 16, 19, and 26 mm, and has an overall 96% procedure success rate when it is purposed for its intended manufactured use [12]. Strategic management of CAA is not definitive and should be coordinated based on each individual patient and their clinical findings until further research data is available to provide a cohesive approach to therapy.

4. Conclusion

The diagnosis and management of giant CAAs are challenging. Detailed physical examination and careful interpretation of chest X-ray and/or computed tomography angiography findings are extremely important in asymptomatic patients or in those who have complaints of chest pain. Treatment with a percutaneous intervention-covered stent is the most common treatment method at this time, particularly since the outcomes after percutaneous intervention have been historically favorable when not associated with myocardial infarction. We described a unique case in how to intervene on a giant CAA that was unexpectedly longer than the longest covered stent in the setting of a pericardial effusion. Further research in the United States is essential to increase the knowledge on how CAAs are managed, with a standardized assessment that would lead to an early diagnosis of this rare disease process.

Authors' Contributions

Osayi Lawani's contributions consisted of conceptualization, visualization, data curation, and original draft production, review, and editing. Rick Ganim's contributions consisted of supervision, conceptualization, procedural methodology, validation, investigation, resource utilization, and revision and editing of the original draft.

Acknowledgments

Special thanks to Anjelica Alvarado, Misty Jennings, and Richard Shannon for their support and assistance.

References

[1] N. K. Jha, H. Z. Ouda, J. A. Khan, G. P. Eising, and N. Augustin, "Giant right coronary artery aneurysm- case report and literature review," *Journal of Cardiothoracic Surgery*, vol. 4, no. 1, p. 18, 2009.

[2] A. Kawsara, I. J. Núñez Gil, F. Alqahtani, J. Moreland, C. S. Rihal, and M. Alkhouli, "Management of coronary artery aneurysms," *JACC: Cardiovascular Interventions*, vol. 11, no. 13, pp. 1211–1223, 2018.

[3] A. H. Yonace, "Morgagni's letters," *Journal of the Royal Society of Medicine*, vol. 73, no. 2, pp. 145–149, 2018.

[4] P. Eshtehardi, S:. Cook, I. Moarof, H. J:. Triller, and S. Windecker, "Giant coronary artery Aneurysm: Imaging findings before and after treatment with a polytetrafluoroethylene-covered stent," *Circulation: Cardiovascular Interventions*, vol. 1, no. 1, pp. 85-86, 2008.

[5] S. Jarcho, "Bougon on coronary aneurysm (1812)," *The American Journal of Cardiology*, vol. 24, no. 4, pp. 551–553, 1969.

[6] I. J. Núñez-Gil, P. M. Alberca, N. Gonzalo, L. Nombela-Franco, P. Salinas, and A. Fernández-Ortiz, "Giant coronary aneurysm culprit of an acute coronary syndrome," *Revista Portuguesa de Cardiologia*, vol. 37, no. 2, pp. 203.e1–203.e5, 2018.

[7] J. Jeudy, C. S. White, S. J. Kligerman et al., "Spectrum of coronary artery Aneurysms:From the radiologic pathology archives," *Radiographics*, vol. 38, no. 1, pp. 11–36, 2018.

[8] C. T. Fang, Y. P. Fang, Y. B. Huang, C. C. Kuo, and C. Y. Chen, "Epidemiology and risk factors of coronary artery aneurysm in Taiwan: a population based case control study," *BMJ Open*, vol. 7, no. 6, article e014424, 2017.

[9] H. Mori, K. Wakabayashi, and H. Suzuki, "Rapidly growing coronary artery aneurysm associated with pericarditis," *Coronary Artery Disease*, vol. 29, no. 2, pp. 168–170, 2018.

[10] S. Hiramori, K. Hoshino, H. Hioki et al., "Spontaneous rupture of a giant coronary artery aneurysm causing cardiac tamponade: a case report," *Journal of Cardiology Cases*, vol. 3, no. 3, pp. e119–e122, 2011.

[11] F. Gundoğdu, S. Arslan, E. Buyukkaya, and H. Senocak, "Treatment of a coronary artery aneurysm by use of a covered stent graft - a case report," *International Journal of Angiology*, vol. 16, no. 1, pp. 31-32, 2007.

[12] Abbott, "Graftmaster RX Coronary Stent System," 2019, https://www.cardiovascular.abbott/us/en/hcp/products/percutaneous-coronary-intervention/graftmaster-rx-stent-graft-system.html.

16

Cardiac Excrescences of Unusual Origin

Jason R. Stuck[1] **and Amgad N. Makaryus**[2,3]

[1]*PinnacleHealth CardioVascular Institute, 1000 North Front Street, Wormleysburg, PA 17043, USA*
[2]*Donald and Barbara Zucker School of Medicine at Hofstra/Northwell, Department of Cardiology, North Shore University Hospital, 300 Community Drive, Manhasset, NY 11030, USA*
[3]*Department of Cardiology, NuHealth, Nassau University Medical Center, 2201 Hempstead Turnpike, East Meadow, NY 11554, USA*

Correspondence should be addressed to Amgad N. Makaryus; amakaryu@numc.edu

Academic Editor: Ertugrul Ercan

Mesothelial/monocytic incidental cardiac excrescences (cardiac MICE) are a rare finding that are most often discovered incidentally either upon echocardiography or invasive cardiovascular procedures. In total, less than 50 known cases have been reported since first being discovered over 30 years ago. They are typically benign lesions; however, there has been a reported case of cardiac MICE being responsible for severe cardiopulmonary compromise and another case of the lesion embolizing leading to cerebral infarctions and ultimately death. Cardiac papillary fibroelastomas are also uncommon lesions found in the heart though they are not as rare as cardiac MICE. They are also benign and are typically attached to valvular surfaces; however, they also can be found as mobile masses. Just as cardiac MICE, they are capable of causing turbulent flow and thrombus formation and have been reported as the cause of ischemic events due to their ability to embolize. We present a case of cardiac MICE and cardiac papillary fibroelastoma in an individual who initially presented with neurologic symptoms concerning for a cerebrovascular accident. The patient was found to have a left ventricular mass composed of both cardiac MICE and cardiac papillary fibroelastomas.

1. Introduction

Cardiac masses are frequently noted on echocardiogram studies; however, primary neoplastic cardiac tumors are rare. The most frequent etiology of cardiac masses is either a normal variant or a result of an infectious etiology, such as infective endocarditis. The most common cause of a primary cardiac tumor is a myxoma; the second most common is a cardiac lipoma. In spite of being rare, primary cardiac tumors are often thought of, but rarely proven to be, the cause of an embolic event in patients.

Cardiac MICE is a rare primary cardiac mass and is typically a benign incidental finding noticed either through imaging of the heart, invasive cardiac procedures, or at the time of an autopsy. They are solid lesions and are a hypercellular admixture of mesothelial cell clusters, with some degree of mesothelial hyperplasia, histiocytes, fibrin, and macrophages. This mixture is embedded within abundant fibrin, and there are large aggregates of histiocytes and strips of bland mesothelial cells [1, 2].

Their exact origin is not yet confirmed; however, two theories exist to explain their existence. The first hypothesis attests that they are originated by damage to the endocardium, due to trauma or an invasive process such as cardiac catheterization [1–4]. A second hypothesis holds that they are iatrogenically deposited during a cardiac intervention. The masses have most frequently been found in the left cardiac chambers and have been predominantly reported in the left ventricle or on the valves themselves. However, there have been cases describing cardiac MICE in multiple other areas in the heart such as free floating in the left atrium, within an ascending aortic aneurysm, pericardial sac, celiac artery, atrioventricular groove, and right atrium [1, 5].

Cardiac papillary fibroelastomas are rare and are the third most common primary cardiac tumors. They also are found primarily through imaging of the heart, most commonly echocardiography, as well as incidentally during surgery or autopsy. In the majority of the cases of cardiac papillary fibroelastoma, the lesion is found on a valvular surface, most often in the left side of the heart. It has most commonly been reported on the aortic valve (close to half of the time), followed by the mitral valve, then the tricuspid valve, and finally the pulmonary valve. Their origin and pathogenesis are currently not completely understood, but they are hypothesized to be the result of organization of fibrin deposits in the endocardium. As with cardiac MICE, they are free moving masses and therefore have the capability to embolize causing potentially catastrophic events [3, 6].

Here, we discuss the case of an individual who, after presenting with symptoms concerning for a cerebrovascular accident, was found to have a mass in her left ventricle. Pathologic analysis revealed tissue consistent with cardiac MICE and cardiac papillary fibroelastoma.

2. Case Summary

The patient is a 77-year-old woman with a past medical history of diabetes, cerebrovascular disease, and coronary artery disease. Her past surgical history is significant for the placement of three coronary stents, which were placed on three separate occasions, the most recent having been placed 6 years prior. The patient initially presented to her primary care physician with "occasional shakes," which were concerning for a transient ischemic attack. After detecting a carotid bruit on exam, the patient was sent for a bilateral carotid Doppler exam which revealed right carotid artery stenosis. Shortly after this, an echocardiogram was preformed which revealed a 2.0 cm x 0.5 cm mass in the left ventricular outflow tract. The patient was then sent to our institution for further evaluation. After the initial evaluation, the patient was scheduled for carotid endarterectomy.

The surgery was uneventful; however, after the procedure, the patient sustained a cerebrovascular accident. Imaging of the brain suggested an embolic etiology for the cerebrovascular accident, and the patient underwent an echocardiogram to rule out the possibility of a cardiac origin for the embolus. The echocardiogram showed a large mobile mass attached to the undersurface of the posterior mitral apparatus with extension into the left ventricular outflow tract. Additional findings included severe mitral annular calcification, mild to moderate central mitral valve regurgitation with calcified mitral leaflets, calcified trileaflet aortic valve with normal opening, concentric left ventricular remodeling, and an ejection fraction of 70%.

The mass was felt to be at a high risk for remobilization and was considered the cause of her recent cerebrovascular accident. Prior to removing the mass, the patient then underwent coronary angiography which showed severe stenosis of the left anterior descending artery as well as the ostial circumflex artery. Due to her past history of diabetes, as well as multiple vessel disease, the patient and physicians elected to proceed with double vessel coronary artery bypass grafting and concurrent excision of the mass. During the coronary artery bypass, the patient's left anterior descending artery was bypassed using the left internal mammary artery and reversed saphenous vein graft was used to bypass the circumflex marginal branch. An intraoperative transesophageal echocardiogram was completed to better visualize the mass. The findings were an approximately 2.0 cm × 0.5 cm calcified independently mobile echodensity attached to the ventricular side of the mitral annulus extending into the left ventricular outflow tract during ventricular systole. Additional findings included mitral annular calcification and mild-moderate mitral regurgitation, which were nearly identical to the preoperative echocardiogram. The mass was identified by the surgeon at its attachment with the subvalvular chordal apparatus of the posterior mitral leaflet. It was approximately 2.5 cm in diameter and consisted of soft yellowish material with several strands attached to it. Initially, it was thought to be, due to its appearance, either old endocarditis or degenerated calcium.

The mass was resected without complications and sent for pathology. To rule out an infectious etiology of the mass, it was cultured and tested for the presence of acid fast bacilli, all of which were negative. Blood cultures were also sent at this time. The patient was placed on antibiotics due to the possibility of endocarditis, but they were discontinued shortly afterwards as the patient demonstrated no other signs of infection and was afebrile, and all blood cultures were negative. Unexpectedly, the pathology report returned with a diagnosis of cardiac MICE and papillary fibroelastoma. Both of these components comprised the mass that was resected. The patient was discharged and, to date, is alive and doing well.

3. Discussion

Our case highlights the unexpected pathologic diagnosis of cardiac MICE. On echocardiography, it is not possible to diagnose cardiac MICE separately from fibroelastoma especially as in this case where the portions/components of the mass were contiguous. In our case, the diagnosis of cardiac MICE was unexpected and was made based on the pathologic analysis of the resected specimen. It is the pathologic findings that allow for the differentiation on the histological level of cardiac MICE from fibroelastoma.

Mesothelial/monocytic incidental cardiac excrescences were first reported in 1979. Due to their apparent origin, the endothelium and its morphologic similarity to histoid hemangiomas found at other locations were initially described as histiocytoid hemangiomas [5, 7–9]. Prior to their discovery, in 1975, Rosai and Dehner reported extravascular lesions, found in 13 different hernia sacs, whose composition was similar to that of MICE and were described as nodular mesothelial hyperplasia. Since that time, additional cases detailing similar lesions have been reported in the pleural and abdominal cavities [10]. In 1997, Chan et al. reported pathologic findings in the pleural cavity and considered the lesions to be nodular mesothelial hyperplasia, induced by inflammatory response as opposed to artifacts, and speculated that a similar hyperplastic change of the mesothelial cells might also occur in the pericardial cavity [7].

The actual term cardiac MICE was not first proposed until a 1994 case report describing four cases resembling a

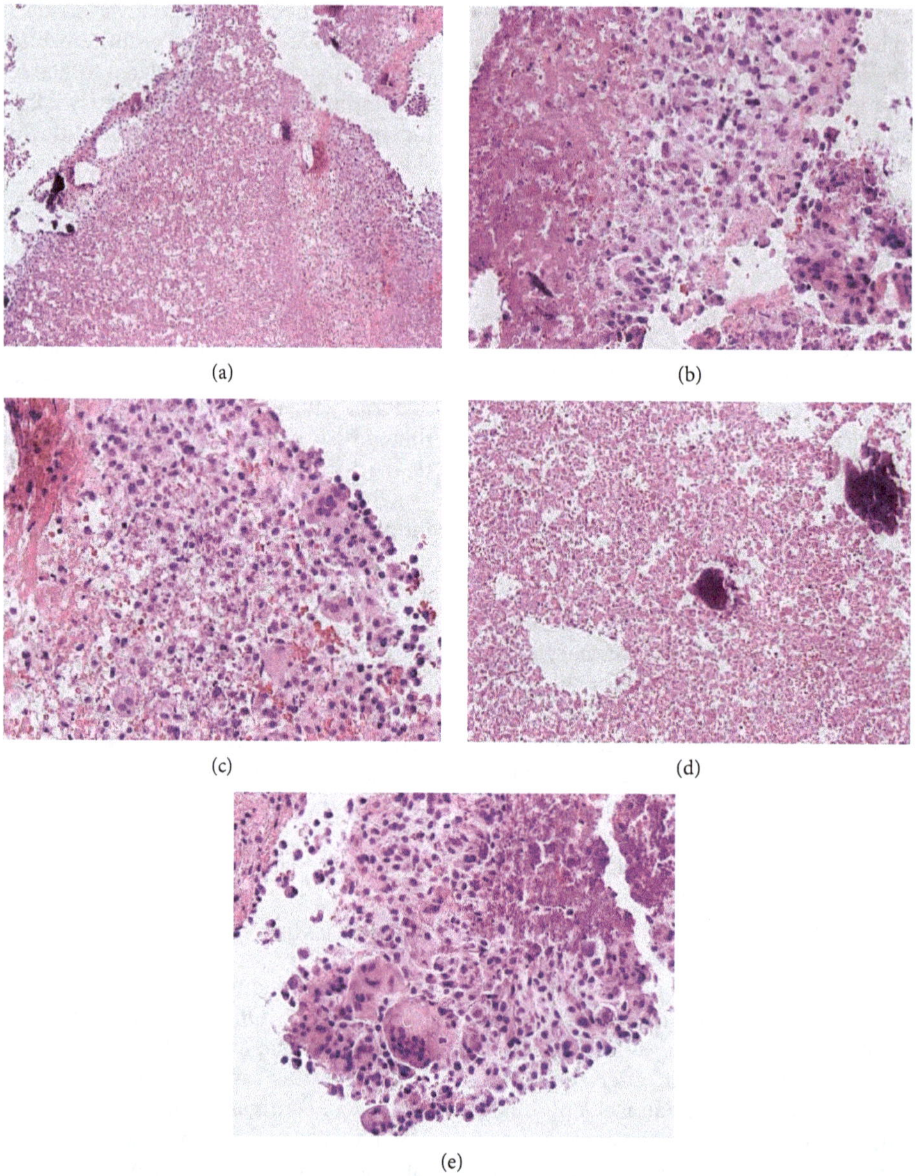

FIGURE 1: Cardiac MICE.

histiocytoid hemangioma was discovered while retrospectively examining surgical pathology files from 1970 to 1992 [1]. Immunohistochemistry concluded that their composition was that of cuboidal cells (exhibiting cytokeratin positivity) and histiocytes (exhibiting CD68 positivity), and examination of the cells for malignancy, by a use of carcinoembryonic antigen and Leu-M1, was negative, leading to the conclusion that the lesions were of benign origin. Additionally, as three out of the four cases had undergone cardiac catheterization, it was first postulated that the lesions were of an iatrogenic nature and in some way related to these previous interventions [1, 11–13].

Since that time, a 2008 article on cardiac MICE reported that the known number of cases were 35, though the true number of cases is uncertain and likely underreported [3]. As more cases of cardiac MICE surfaced, their epidemiology became more complex, but patterns started to emerge. The lesions have typically been found in the left cardiac chambers, with the masses predominantly being detected in the left ventricle or on the valves themselves; however, they have also been reported as free floating in the left atrium, within an ascending aortic aneurysm, pericardial sac, celiac artery, atrioventricular groove, and right atrium [1, 5, 14, 15].

Pathologically, cardiac MICE (Figure 1) are solid lesions and are a hypercellular admixture of mesothelial cell clusters, with some degree of mesothelial hyperplasia and histiocytes. This mixture is embedded within abundant fibrin, and there are large aggregates of histiocytes and strips of bland mesothelial cells [1, 2].

The origin of cardiac MICE remains up for debate, but two leading theories have arisen to explain their existence, although it is necessary to mention that neither theory by itself is sufficient to fully account for and accurately describe all reported cases of cardiac MICE.

The first theory to be described referred to as the "reactive" theory suggests that these lesions arise secondary to trauma, most often of an iatrogenic etiology. It has been proposed that, after the initial injury to the endocardium occurs, the mesothelial cells are exposed to the bloodstream and aggregate with histiocytes and fibrin beginning the formation of the mass. At least one other case has also been presented that supports the involvement of the adhesion cell process [4, 7, 16]. Of the reported cases of cardiac MICE, a number of them describe cases in which prior instrumentation preceded their discovery and support the reactive theory. It is hypothesized that it was this trauma or microperforation during the instrumentation that lead to mesothelial cell hyperplasia and cell ingrowth from pericardium to endocardium and the development of the lesion [2].

Though prior cardiac intervention is the most common cause of endothelial trauma thus setting into place the chain of events that lead to cardiac MICE formation, at least one case has been reported with a unique underlying catalyst. In 1997, a case of a 38-year-old woman with cardiac MICE was described; although she had no prior cardiac interventions, she was discovered to have a lung adenocarcinoma which involved the hilum but not the pericardium. During surgery, a small fragment of free-floating tissue was found in the pericardial cavity. Upon pathological examination of the specimen, microscopic examination demonstrated a composite of cells indicative of cardiac MICE (clusters of histiocytes, mesothelial cells, and fibrin). In addition to these findings, the sample contained rare pleomorphic adenocarcinoma cells. These cells tested positive for stains confirming their underlying malignant composition. It was then proposed that the surrounding mesothelial cells, histiocytes, and fibrin were formed in response to the invasion of the pericardial space by the adenocarcinoma [2]. In addition, it has been postulated that cardiac MICE may have been induced at least partially by the procoagulant activity of invasive adenocarcinoma. This case again alludes to the concept that adhesion molecules or an adhesive process may play a role in the process [4, 16].

An alternative to the reactive theory is often described as the "artifactual" theory and postulates that cardiac MICE is merely an amalgamation of debris iatrogenically deposited during an invasive cardiac procedure [3, 17]. In 1994, Courtice et al. reported cases of cardiac MICE in which perforation of major cardiac structures at catheterization had not been found in their subject patients [17]. For their study, they examined a material found in extracorporeal bypass pumps and a material adherent to mediastinal and pericardial drains. They found samples consistent with cardiac MICE in 18 of 22 cases of extracorporeal bypass pump filters investigated, and 2 of 15 of mediastinal and pericardial drains following cardiac surgery. They and others suggested that lesions produced during cardiac surgery by the cardiotomy suction and compaction of friable mesothelial strips and other tissue debris and fibrin into tumor-like fragments, may be transported around the operative site on the suction tip. The fragments that are not removed from the cardiac chambers after an intervention are transferred by the suction catheter tips to the intravascular space during heart surgery, and the cellular components may aggregate and form a free-floating mass in the heart [14, 15, 17].

Although most often thought of as an incidental finding, there has been at least one reported case of cardiac MICE causing severe acute cardiopulmonary failure [4]. The patient presented with what initially seemed like a chronic obstructive pulmonary disease exacerbation but decompensated due to severe acute pulmonary edema which was believed to be secondary to severe aortic regurgitation. Prior to the patient's acute decompensation, a transthoracic echocardiogram was completed which showed a 2.0 cm mobile mass on the aortic valve prolapsing into the left ventricular outflow tract. The patient underwent aortic valve repair, and in addition to the mass being visualized on the aortic valve, a soft tissue mass was seen free-floating in the left ventricular outflow tract. Perforation of the left coronary leaflet and adjacent erosion of the endocardium were also noted. Contrary to all previous cases, cardiac MICE in this instance was not incidental, rather it was responsible for the severe acute aortic valve regurgitation, obstruction of the left ventricular outflow tract, and ultimately the patient's severe pulmonary edema and decompensation [4].

Cardiac papillary fibroelastomas are a rare cause of primary cardiac tumors, and studies have estimated that there are approximately 200 cardiac tumors in every 1 million autopsies preformed. Cardiac papillary fibroelastomas are responsible for approximately 7% of all primary cardiac tumors [6, 18–20]. A 2003 report reviewing a total of 725 cases of cardiac papillary fibroelastomas showed that 55% of the patients were male, and although the lesion was most commonly found in the 8th decade of life, there were 10 cases that were reported in children under the age of ten. Of note, the oldest patient was 92 years of age and the youngest case was reported in a newborn child. After analysis of the cases, no clear risk factor was identified for development of cardiac papillary fibroelastomas [6].

Similar to cardiac MICE, cardiac papillary fibroelastomas (Figure 2) are solid lesions most often found on the valves of the heart, and there are multiple theories that exist to suggest their origin. They have been hypothesized to be caused by turbulent blood flow across the endocardium, inflammation, and true neoplasms [21]. Histologically, cardiac papillary fibroelastomas are covered with endothelium that surrounds a layer of acid mucopolysaccharide, and they possess an inner vascular core composed of connective tissue. The connective tissue matrix that comprises the fibroelastoma is a collection of collagen, smooth muscle cells, and elastic fibers [20].

In the vast majority of the cases, nearly 80%, the lesion was found on the valvular surface, most often on the aortic valve (close to half of the time), followed by the mitral valve, then the tricuspid valve, and finally the pulmonary valve. The majority of the cases found that the mass was located in the left heart (>95% of the cases), and therefore, systemic embolization is frequent. Most often incidental findings, the manifestations of cardiac papillary fibroelastomas vary greatly, but the most common presenting manifestation was embolization to systemic, coronary, or cerebral circulation. Other initial presenting symptoms varied and included angina, syncope, and myocardial infarction and sudden death [6].

Cardiac papillary fibroelastomas are most often identified incidentally by echocardiography but other modalities, such

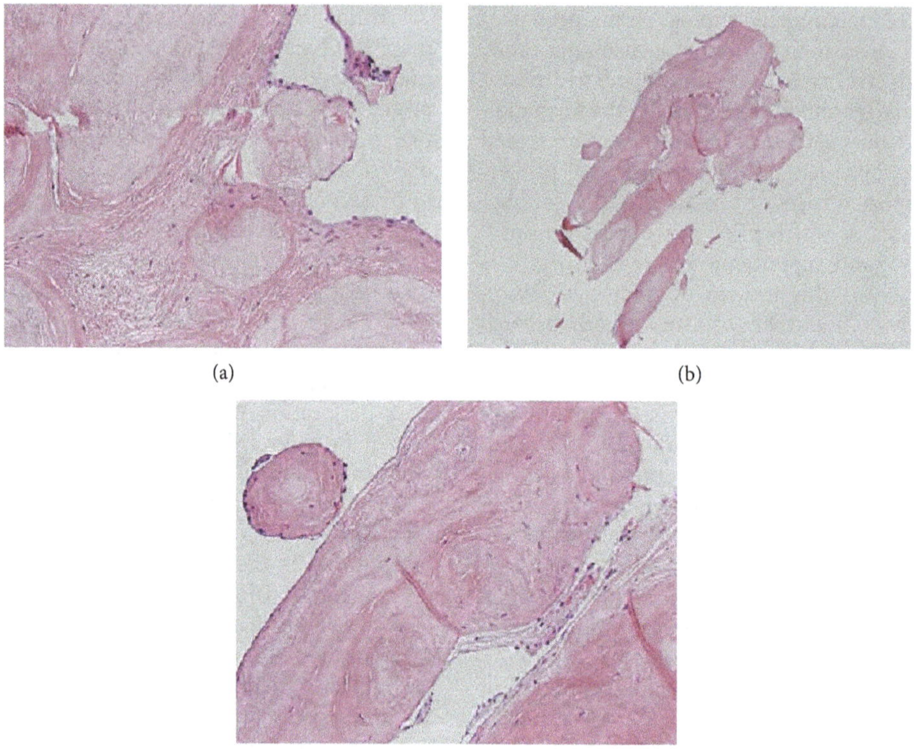

(a) (b) (c)

FIGURE 2: Cardiac papillary fibroelastoma.

as cardiac MRI and cardiac CT, have also been utilized [6]. They have also been incidentally discovered during cardiac catheterization, cardiac surgery, and autopsy [22]. Due to the potential catastrophic events that both cardiac MICE and cardiac papillary fibroelastomas have been associated with, such as sudden death, pulmonary embolism, and myocardial infarction, excision is the recommended treatment. In symptomatic patients, all previous studies have suggested that excision is the preferred treatment and should be offered to all patients who are candidates. Surgery is curative and has been shown to improve both the long and short term prognosis, and recurrence has yet to be reported in regard to both lesions [6]. If the patient is not a candidate for surgery, oral anticoagulation is the recommended treatment for cardiac papillary fibroelastomas, but there have been no randomized controlled trials to date on the efficacy of this treatment [6, 23, 24]. No previous studies have been conducted, and no interventions currently exist for cardiac MICE in patients that are not surgical candidates. Additionally, as mentioned, the challenge remains the difficulty in the echocardiographic diagnosis of cardiac MICE which leads to the necessity of cardiac MICE diagnosis based on the histopathologic specimen analysis of the resected mass.

This case illustrates a rare case of a lesion comprised of both cardiac MICE and cardiac papillary fibroelastoma. To our knowledge, although they have been presented separately, there has never been a case reported of a mass consisting of both cardiac MICE and cardiac papillary fibroelastoma. Additionally, there have been very few cases of cardiac MICE embolizing causing systemic symptoms. In the case of our patient, the likely origin of her neurologic symptoms was an embolic event caused by her left ventricular mass. The patient did have a history of prior cardiac instrumentation as she underwent cardiac catheterization on three separate occasions which would support the reactive theory of cardiac MICE and potentially an inflammatory/reactive etiology of cardiac papillary fibroelastomas.

References

[1] J. P. Veniot, H. D. Tazelaar, W. D. Edwarda, and T. V. Colby, "Mesothelial/monocytic incidental cardiac excrescences: cardiac MICE," *Modern Pathology*, vol. 7, pp. 9–16, 1994.

[2] P. Argani, S. S. Sternberg, M. Burt, N. V. Adsay, and D. S. Klimstra, "Metastatic adenocarcinoma involving a mesothelial/monocytic incidental cardiac excrescence (cardiac MICE)," *The American Journal of Surgical Pathology*, vol. 21, no. 8, pp. 970–974, 1997.

[3] S. Censi, A. Dell'Amore, R. Conti, and P. Lorenzini, "Cardiac mesothelial/monocytic-incidental-excrescence: more than an artifactual lesion?," *Interactive CardioVascular and Thoracic Surgery*, vol. 7, no. 6, pp. 1201–1203, 2008.

[4] T. T. Pham, K. Antons, R. Shishido, J. Mullvain, F. Salem, and P. Haghighi, "A case of mesothelial/monocytic cardiac excrescence causing severe acute cardiopulmonary failure," *The American Journal of Surgical Pathology*, vol. 29, no. 4, pp. 564–567, 2005.

[5] J. Rosai, J. Gold, and R. Landy, "The histiocytoid hemangiomas: a unifying concept embracing several previously described entities of skin, soft tissue, large vessels, bone and heart," *Human Pathology*, vol. 10, no. 6, pp. 707–730, 1979.

[6] R. M. Gowda, I. A. Khan, C. K. Nair, N. J. Mehta, B. C. Vasavada, and T. J. Sacchi, "Cardiac papillary fibroelastoma: a comprehensive analysis of 725 cases," *American Heart Journal*, vol. 146, no. 3, pp. 404–410, 2003.

[7] J. K. C. Chan, K. T. Loo, B. K. C. Yau, and S. Y. Lam, "Nodular histiocytic/mesothelial hyperplasia: a lesion potentially mistaken for a neoplasm in transbronchial biopsy," *The American Journal of Surgical Pathology*, vol. 21, no. 6, pp. 658–663, 1997.

[8] C. Dannaker, D. Piacquadio, C. B. Willoughby, and R. W. Goltz, "Histiocytoid hemangioma: a disease spectrum. Report of a case with simultaneous cutaneous and bone involvement limited to one extremity," *Journal of the American Academy of Dermatology*, vol. 21, no. 2 Part 2, pp. 404–409, 1989.

[9] D. J. Luthringer, R. Virmani, S. W. Weiss, and J. Rosai, "A distinctive cardiovascular lesion resembling histiocytoid (epithelioid) hemangioma evidence suggesting mesothelial participation," *The American Journal of Surgical Pathology*, vol. 14, no. 11, pp. 993–1000, 1990.

[10] J. Rosai and L. P. Dehner, "Nodular mesothelial hyperplasia in hernia sacs: a benign reactive condition simulating a neoplastic process," *Cancer*, vol. 35, no. 1, pp. 165–175, 1975.

[11] M. Wu, A. Anderson, and L. B. Kahn, "A report of mesothelial/monocytic incidental cardiac excrescences and a literature review," *Annals of diagnostic pathology*, vol. 4, no. 1, pp. 39–43, 2000.

[12] M. A. Rubin, J. A. Snell, H. D. Tazelaar, E. E. Lack, J. L. Austenfeld, and N. Azumi, "Cardiac papillary fibroelastoma: an immunohistochemical investigation and unusual clinical manifestations," *Modern Pathology*, vol. 8, no. 4, pp. 402–407, 1995.

[13] S. W. Ryu, M. S. Beom, S. R. Kim, and G. S. Kim, "Cardiac papillary fibroelastoma," *Revista Portuguesa de Cardiologia*, vol. 34, no. 7-8, pp. 507-508, 2015.

[14] Y. Ikeda, C. Yutani, M. Imakita et al., "Two cases of mesothelial/monocytic incidental cardiac excrescences of the heart," *Pathology International*, vol. 48, no. 8, pp. 641–644, 1998.

[15] C. Y. Lin, F. C. Tsai, and B. R. Fang, "Mesothelial/monocytic cardiac incidental excrescences of the heart: case report and literature review," *International Journal of Clinical Practice*, vol. 59, pp. 23–25, 2005.

[16] D. Suarez-Vilela and F. M. Izquierdo-Garcia, "Mesothelial/-Monocytic Incidental Cardiac Excrescence: A Process Mediated by Adhesion Molecules?," *The American Journal of Surgical Pathology*, vol. 29, no. 11, p. 1545, 2005.

[17] R. W. Courtice et al., "Tissue fragments recovered at cardiac surgery masquerading as tumoral proliferations: evidence suggesting iatrogenic or artefactual origin and common occurrence," *The American Journal of Surgical Pathology*, vol. 18, no. 2, pp. 167–174, 1994.

[18] K. Reynen, "Frequency of primary tumors of the heart," *The American Journal of Cardiology*, vol. 77, no. 1, p. 107, 1996.

[19] H. P. Goldberg, F. Glenn, C. T. Dotter, and I. Steinberg, "Myxoma of the left atrium: diagnosis made during life with operative and postmortem findings," *Circulation*, vol. 6, no. 5, pp. 762–767, 1952.

[20] J. P. Sun, C. R. Asher, X. S. Yang et al., "Clinical and echocardiographic characteristics of papillary fibroelastomas: a retrospective and prosepective study in 162 patients," *Circulation*, vol. 103, no. 22, pp. 2687–2693, 2001.

[21] M. J. Costa, A. N. Makaryus, and D. R. Rosman, "A rare case of a cardiac papillary fibroelastoma of the pulmonary valve diagnosed by echocardiography," *The International Journal of Cardiovascular Imaging*, vol. 22, no. 2, pp. 199–203, 2006.

[22] F. H. Edwards, D. Hale, A. Cohen, L. Thompson, A. T. Pezzella, and R. Virmani, "Primary cardiac valve tumors," *The Annals of Thoracic Surgery*, vol. 52, no. 5, pp. 1127–1131, 1991.

[23] G. Pinelli, J. P. Carteaux, P. M. Mertes, T. Civit, A. Trinh, and J. P. Villemot, "Mitral valve tumor revealed by stroke," *The Journal of Heart Valve Disease*, vol. 4, no. 2, pp. 199–201, 1995.

[24] J. Sastre-Garriga, C. Molina, J. Montaner et al., "Mitral papillary fibroelastoma as a cause of cardiogenic embolic stroke: report of two cases and review of the literature," *European Journal of Neurology*, vol. 7, no. 4, pp. 449–453, 2000.

17

Presentation and Management of a Giant Coronary Artery Aneurysm with a Fistula to the Right Ventricle

Nicholas Peterman,[1] Bradley Kaptur,[1] and Naveed Adoni[1,2]

[1]*Carle Illinois College of Medicine, University of Illinois Urbana-Champaign, Champaign, IL, USA*
[2]*Carle Foundation Hospital, Urbana, IL, USA*

Correspondence should be addressed to Bradley Kaptur; bkaptur2@illinois.edu

Academic Editor: Dirk Bandorski

A 27-year-old female presented to our emergency department in ventricular tachycardia. During her workup, she was found to have an extremely rare giant aneurysmal left anterior descending artery (LAD) ending in a coronary fistula to the right ventricle (RV). After stabilization, a variety of treatment options were considered, as there is no standard first-line treatment.

1. Introduction

A coronary artery fistula (CAF) is a rare finding that is characterized by an abnormal termination of a coronary artery into a cardiac chamber, coronary sinus, pulmonary artery, or pulmonary vein [1]. CAF is predominantly congenital and accounts for 0.4% of cardiac anomalies [1]. It is believed to be present in 0.002% of the total population and has no correlation with either race or sex [1]. CAF causes blood flow to bypass myocardial capillary networks and can subsequently lead to ischemia of the tissue distal to the malformation.

Subsequent compensation leads to progressive dilation of the proximal coronary artery [2]. Clinically significant complications of this interplay of ischemia and compensation are present in 11% of those younger than 20 and in 35% of those older than 20 [2]. Potential sequelae include atherosclerotic deposition, mural thrombosis, and rupture [2]. However, the most common complication is coronary artery aneurysm (CAA) formation, which is defined as the dilation of an arterial segment over 1.5 times that of normal [1]. In rarer cases, the CAA can be classified as a giant coronary artery aneurysm (GCAA) when its diameter is over 20 mm [3]. The overall prevalence of a GCAA in the population is 0.02–0.2%, with other potential causes including Takayasu arteritis, Kawasaki disease, and atherosclerosis [4]. Although GCAA is normally asymptomatic, the concomitant CAF that leads to its creation is not [5]. Reported complications include exertional dyspnea (60%), endocarditis (20%), and angina (3-7%) [1]. Eventual congestive heart failure is seen in nearly a fifth of older patients [1].

2. Case Presentation

A 27-year-old female presented to our emergency department with a chief complaint of ongoing chest pain that had persisted for the past 5 days. She also mentioned the onset of extreme lightheadedness, and she believed that she came close to passing out several times. Her chest pain was located at her left chest, between her shoulder blades, and with radiation to her left arm. She denied nausea, vomiting, or diaphoresis, but she noted mild shortness of breath. Her initial blood pressure was 114/78, with a temperature 98.4 degrees Fahrenheit.

Upon interview and outside chart review, it was found that the patient had a significant history of perimembranous ventricular septal defect (spontaneously closed), double-chamber right ventricle, left anterior descending to right ventricle coronary cameral fistula, right ventricular clot

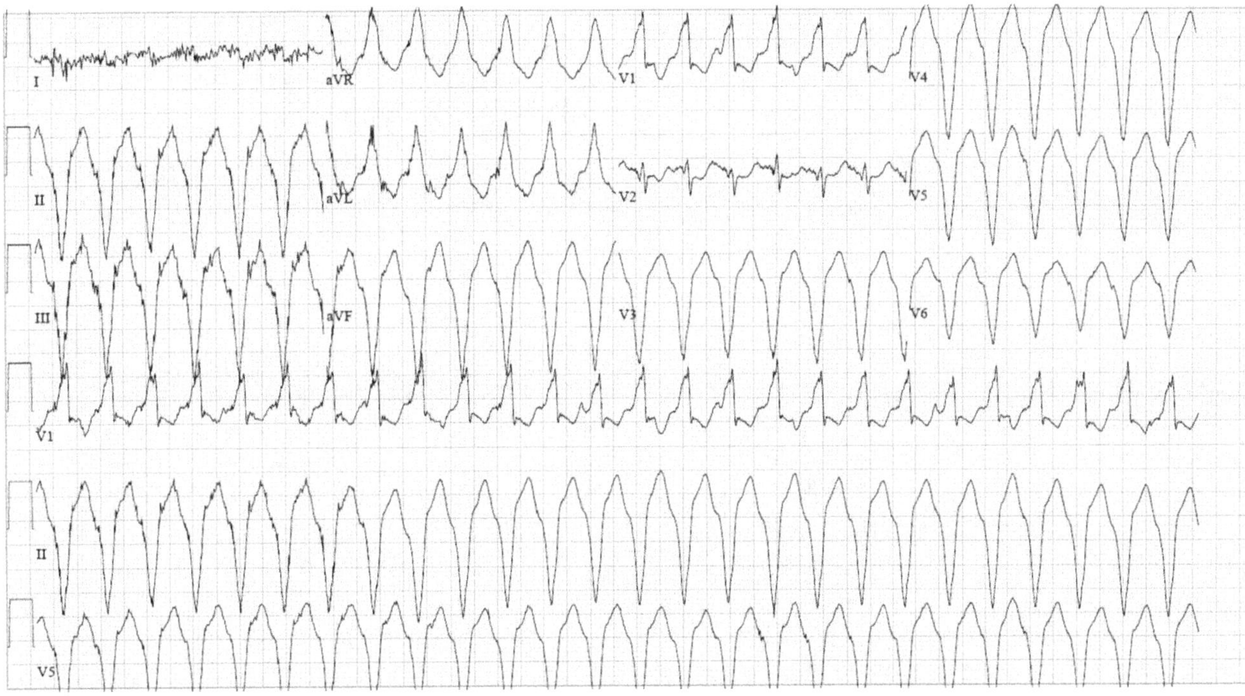

Figure 1: Initial EKG, before cardioversion, showing SMVT. 159 BPM, PR interval 38 ms, QRS duration 188 ms, QT/QTc 322/523 ms.

(managed with rivaroxaban), and ventricular tachycardia (managed with amiodarone, mexiletine, and metoprolol).

Sustained monomorphic ventricular tachycardia (SMVT) was noted on her initial EKG (Figure 1), and soon after, the patient appeared diaphoretic and ill with increasing complaints of lightheadedness and palpitations. After initial presentation and identification of VT with precipitous systolic blood pressure drop to the 80s, an IV line was started and etomidate 10 mg IV was given.

After a lack of improvement, the decision was made to cardiovert. She was cardioverted with 200 joules. Normal sinus rhythm was achieved after cardioversion, and the patient's blood pressure returned to the levels seen on presentation. An EKG postcardioversion was conducted that demonstrated likely inferior STEMI (Figure 2). Her ST elevations status postcardioversion pointed to inferior STEMI as a result of embolus from turbulent flow or reduced cardiac output from SMVT on top of CAD.

At this point, her troponins had climbed from 0.30 to 0.84 within 2 hours of admission, and the patient was brought to the catheterization lab.

Left heart catheterization (Figure 3) showed the left main, and LAD arteries were diffusely dilated and tortuous, ending in a coronary aneurysm with a fistulous connection to the right ventricular apex. The connection point was separated from the remainder of the chamber by a fibrous, C-shaped band of tissue with minor communication in the apical and upper portions of the right ventricle.

No blockage was identified, and PCI was not conducted. It was believed her VT and elevated troponins were secondary to her structural heart disease, and she was transferred to an outside hospital for surgery.

Ablation options were considered, including traditional catheter ablation, noninvasive ablation, and surgical ablation. The traditional catheter ablation was initially favored by the managing team, but the patient was against the procedure due to high-risk stratification and preference to be managed pharmacologically. A single lead ICD was ultimately implanted subcutaneously given the anatomic constraints of her apical RV and the preference of the patient. The patient was discharged without complications on sotalol, mexiletine, rivaroxaban, aspirin, and atorvastatin.

One month later, the patient had a subsequent episode of VT with ED admission. She was cardioverted to sinus rhythm and monitored for several hours. Her sotalol was changed to amiodarone, and the VT zone settings of her ICD were reprogrammed to lower the threshold for firing. Additionally, the plan to perform outpatient ablation within the next few weeks was discussed with the patient.

After discharge from the emergency department, the patient declined to schedule her ablation procedure, though she did continue with her medication regimen. She was transitioned to sotalol and mexiletine for longer-term VT suppression. Over the subsequent 18 months, she had 1 further episode of sustained tachycardic palpitations with a heart rate in the 150 s. According to the patient, this episode coincided with significant stress in her personal life. At that time, EKG demonstrated MMVT that was below the ICD therapeutic settings. Device interrogation revealed multiple episodes of antitachycardia pacing initiation preceding this episode. She was cardioverted in the ED, and her device settings were once again reprogrammed. Throughout this time, the patient has continued to decline the ablation procedure and has elected to continue with medical management.

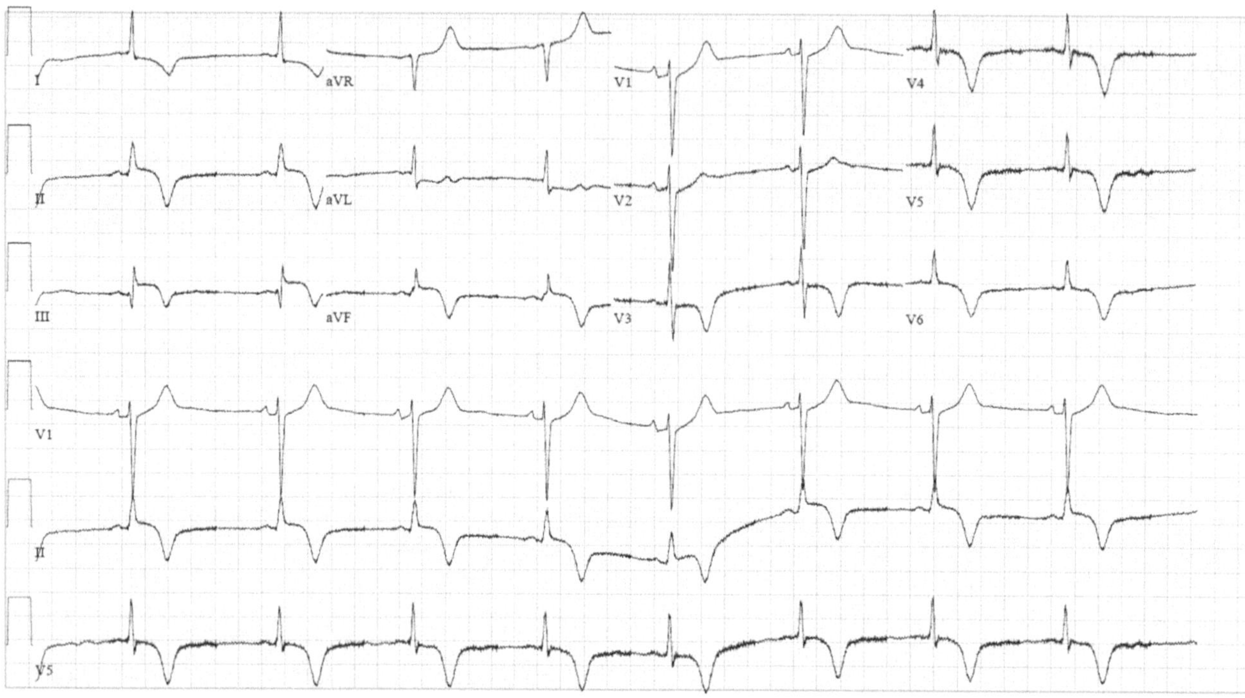

Figure 2: EKG status post cardioversion demonstrating ST elevations in II, III, and AVF. T-wave inversions noted in V3, V4, V5, and V6. 52 BPM, PR interval 106 ms, QRS duration 80 ms, QT/QTc 458/425 ms.

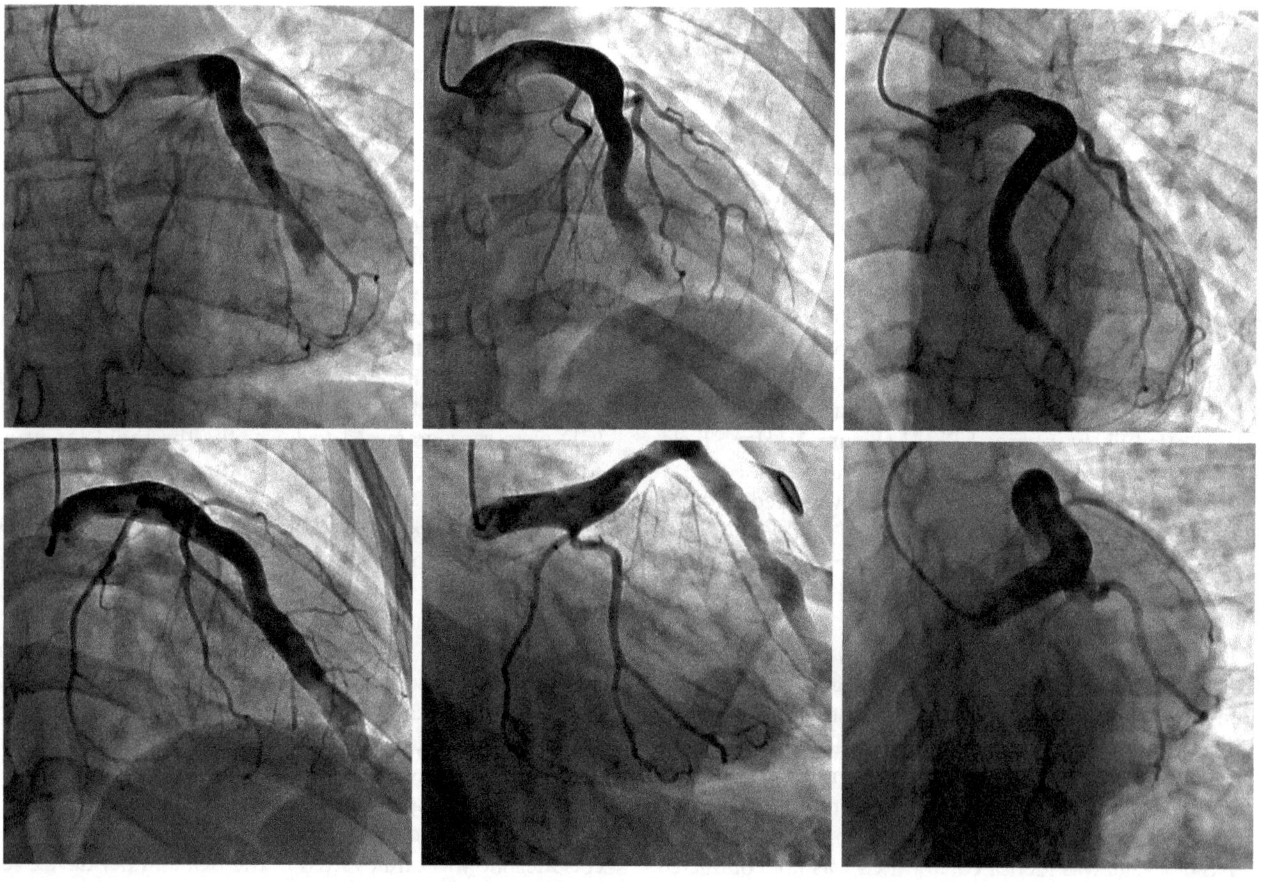

Figure 3: The left main and LAD arteries are diffusely dilated and tortuous, ending in a coronary aneurysm with a fistulous connection to the right ventricular apex. The left anterior descending artery measures 13 mm proximally with a giant aneurysm measuring 21 mm as it fistulizes to the RV apex.

3. Discussion

Clinical presentation of CAF depends on the magnitude of left-to-right shunting and the possibility of developing coronary steal syndrome [1]. Coronary steal describes the shunting of high-pressure coronary vasculature into the low-resistance circulation through the fistula. The change in pressure between the linked cavities is large enough to precipitate a high volume of flow that "steals" blood flow from the surrounding myocardium and amplifies ischemia. This is especially prominent during exercise [1].

Although rare, concomitant CAF and CAA have been treated surgically before [6]. The repair is done by closing the fistula and then forming a bypass route using a vein graft in order to supply the distal vasculature [6, 7]. However, due to both the giant nature of the aneurysm and the diffuse ectasia of the entire LAD in this patient, the best treatment plan becomes more difficult to determine [6].

Beyond the normal hemodynamics of the fistula, this patient presented with recurrent SMVT originating from the malformation that predisposed her to sudden cardiac death [8]. Along with ablation, an ICD and antiarrhythmic pharmacotherapy would be the standard of care due to VT with structural heart abnormality [1, 8]. Options for implantation are complicated due to her double right ventricle. The fibrous band bisecting her right atrium would obstruct optimal lead placement during transvenous insertion, thus leaving subcutaneous lead placement as the preferred route [9]. The natural history of aneurysms is progressive enlargement. The likely long-term management of this disease process involves intervention [10–13]. However, our patient specifically and adamantly declined catheter ablation of her VT. Thus, in the context of strong patient preference, the ICD was chosen for secondary prevention.

Regarding the choices of medication in our patient, the brief choice of amiodarone was made on the basis of the patient's history, recent AHA and NASPE guidelines, and her QRS and QT intervals. At that time, the potential adverse effects in terms of toxicity involving multiple organ systems were balanced by its superior prevention of sustained ventricular tachyarrhythmias. However, once the patient again declined long-term management in the form of ablation, medication choice in the form of sotalol and mexiletine was resumed.

The mechanism of ST elevation in this patient is another area of interest. In our patient, the EKG postcardioversion demonstrated ST elevations and she had climbing troponins. Per STEMI protocol, she was taken for left heart catheterization. At that time, concerns were high for possible embolus from turbulent follow or reduced cardiac output from SMVT on top of CAD. During the catheterization, no blockage was identified, and thus, PCI was not conducted. At the time, it was believed that her VT and elevated troponins were secondary to her structural heart disease. Coronary steal is a plausible mechanism of ST elevation in this clinical context. In retrospect, the use of fractional flow reserve (FFR) as a diagnostic tool during the initial angiography may have provided additional insight into the responsible mechanism. In the literature, coronary artery aneurysms have been previously associated with unstable angina and STEMI [14–17].

4. Conclusions

Ventricular tachycardia can present in the setting of rare structural abnormalities like CAF with GCAA. Subsequent workup requires an understanding of both the unique pathophysiology of the abnormality and an adaptation of related best practice treatments to fit the unique needs of the patient.

Consent

A written consent form was obtained from the patient for publication of this study.

References

[1] D. Challoumas, A. Pericleous, I. A. Dimitrakaki, C. Danelatos, and G. Dimitrakakis, "Coronary arteriovenous fistulae: a review," *International Journal of Angiology*, vol. 23, no. 1, pp. 1–10, 2014.

[2] M. M. Elahi, K. J. Zehr, D. Ho, and D. Stewart, "Giant aneurysmal left main coronary artery to right atrium fistula a case for surgical approach," *MOJ Surgery*, vol. 2, no. 1, 2015.

[3] R. N. Khouzam, J. D. Gardner, R. Bomb, and A. A. Holden, "Multi-vessel giant coronary artery aneurysm in an elderly female," *Annals of Translational Medicine*, vol. 5, no. 10, p. 210., 2017.

[4] P. D. Crawley, W. J. Mahlow, D. R. Huntsinger, S. Afiniwala, and D. C. Wortham, "Giant coronary artery aneurysms: review and update," *Texas Heart Institute Journal*, vol. 41, no. 6, pp. 603–608, 2014.

[5] D. Li, Q. Wu, L. Sun et al., "Surgical treatment of giant coronary artery aneurysm," *The Journal of Thoracic and Cardiovascular Surgery*, vol. 130, no. 3, pp. 817–821, 2005.

[6] N. Salehi, N. Samiei, H. Pouraliakbar, A. H. Sabet, and A. Vakili-Zarch, "Giant aneurysmal fistula of the left main coronary artery to the right atrium," *The Heart Surgery Forum*, vol. 15, no. 5, pp. E292–E293, 2012.

[7] H. Wang, X. Luo, W. Wang, X. Wang, C. Yang, and C. Zeng, "Successful transcatheter patent ductus arteriosus occluder embolization of a congenital left coronary artery aneurysm and fistulas draining into the right atrium," *Annals of Thoracic and Cardiovascular Surgery*, vol. 18, no. 6, pp. 540–543, 2012.

[8] S. R. Dukkipati, J. S. Koruth, S. Choudry, M. A. Miller, W. Whang, and V. Y. Reddy, "Catheter ablation of ventricular tachycardia in structural heart disease: indications, strategies, and outcomes–part II," *Journal of the American College of Cardiology*, vol. 70, no. 23, pp. 2924–2941, 2017.

[9] R. E. Knops, L. R. A. Olde Nordkamp, P.-P. H. M. Delnoy et al., "Subcutaneous or transvenous defibrillator therapy," *The New England Journal of Medicine*, vol. 383, no. 6, pp. 526–536, 2020.

[10] T. Uzuka, M. Nakamura, T. Nakajima, N. Watanabe, and Y. Fukazawa, "Surgery of giant right coronary artery aneurysm complicated with coronary artery fistula to left ventricle," *Journal of Cardiac Surgery*, vol. 33, no. 2, pp. 95-96, 2018.

[11] E. Beckmann, S. Rustum, S. Marquardt et al., "Surgical treatment of coronary artery aneurysms," *Journal of Cardiac Surgery*, vol. 32, no. 11, pp. 674–679, 2017.

[12] Y. Wang, Y. Yang, L. Xia, W. Ding, Q. Ji, and C. Wang, "Surgical correction of coronary artery ectasia combining congenital coronary artery fistula," *Congenital Heart Disease*, vol. 16, no. 1, pp. 95–106, 2020.

[13] H. R. Khan, M. A. Shajar, and S. K. Naik, "Giant right coronary artery aneurysm," *Journal of Cardiac Surgery*, vol. 31, no. 8, pp. 527-528, 2016.

[14] F. Er, H. Çakır, B. Erdolu, and D. Ay, "Left main coronary artery aneurysm presenting with unstable angina," *Journal of Cardiac Surgery*, vol. 33, no. 8, pp. 440-441, 2018.

[15] A. Bath, F. Shaikh, and J. K. Kalavakunta, "Coronary artery aneurysm presenting as STEMI," *BMJ Case Reports CP*, vol. 12, no. 6, article e231013, 2019.

[16] B. Seguy, E. A. Osborn, M. Pernot, and E. Gerbaud, "A giant coronary artery aneurysm and recurrent ST-segment elevation myocardial infarction: a management dilemna," *Cardiology Journal*, vol. 26, no. 2, pp. 212–214, 2019.

[17] J. P. Monteiro, E. Flores-Umanzor, and S. Brugaletta, "STEMI with a massive coronary aneurysm: a rare finding with a management dilemma," *JACC Case Reports*, vol. 2, no. 3, pp. 477–479, 2020.

18

Caseous Intracardiac Calcification: A Diagnostic Enigma

Simon G. Findlay,[1] **Nicholas M. Child,**[1] **and Douglas F. Muir**[2]

[1]*North Tees and Hartlepool NHS Trust, Stockton-on-Tees, UK*
[2]*The James Cook University Hospital, Middlesbrough, UK*

Correspondence should be addressed to Simon G. Findlay; simon.findlay@newcastle.ac.uk

Academic Editor: Assad Movahed

Intramyocardial calcification is a rare phenomenon often only discovered on postmortem. We describe the case of a healthy 69-year-old lady diagnosed with idiopathic caseous intracardiac calcification extending from the mitral valve annulus. We present high-quality images and propose an investigatory template for future cases.

1. Introduction

A 69-year-old lady was admitted to the acute medical unit with a several-month history of progressive, exertional breathlessness and atypical chest pain. Cardiac risk factors were hypertension, hyperlipidaemia, and a positive family history of ischaemic heart disease. Drug therapy on admission was simvastatin and amlodipine.

Clinical examination revealed a grade 3 pansystolic murmur radiating to the apex, with no signs of cardiac failure, organomegaly, or lymphadenopathy. The pulse was regular at 81 bpm, BP was 119/90 mmHg, and oxygen saturations were 100% on room air. EKG demonstrated sinus rhythm with fixed, lateral T-wave inversion and ST depression. Serial troponin-Is were 44, 44, and 31 ng/L (normal range: 0-14). Haematology and blood biochemistry were normal including d-dimer, liver function tests, and serum amylase. Chest X-ray demonstrated normal lung fields; however, subtle intracardiac calcification within the cardiac silhouette was visible and comparable to a radiograph in 2015.

A transthoracic echocardiogram (echo) demonstrated mobile valve leaflets with an echo-bright structure in the region of the posterior mitral annulus suggestive of calcification. However, views were limited due to poor echogenicity with incomplete visualisation of the myocardium. A transoesophageal echocardiogram (TOE) revealed a heavily calcified mitral annulus but no mitral stenosis. A bidirectional jet of moderate mitral regurgitation (MR) was noted secondary to extensive mitral annular calcification (MAC) with tethering of the leaflet tips, particularly the anterior mitral valve leaflet. No other valvular heart disease was present, and the left ventricle (LV) retained good contractility throughout with overall normal function.

A CT coronary angiogram (CTCA) (Siemens' SOMATOM Definition Flash CT) showed extensive MAC which infiltrated the left ventricular myocardium resulting in widespread intramyocardial calcification, predominantly in the septum and anterior wall and also in the apex and apical lateral wall (Figure 1). Maximal septal LV wall thickness measured 28 mm and similarly around the infiltrative lesions. The calcified lesions were heterogenous in appearance and extended from the mitral annulus. The external layer of the lesions was calcific, whilst the internal portion was of a heterogenous lower density signal, suggesting caseation. The myocardium contracted normally around the lesions with the estimated ejection fraction of 57%. Calcification of the coronary arteries was apparent with moderate mid-left anterior descending artery (LAD) disease and moderate stenosis of the proximal first diagonal vessel. Thoracic CT screening for extracardiac calcification and carcinoma was unremarkable.

Due to the extent of the intramyocardial calcification, we sought to determine the aetiology and screen for metabolic disease. Serum calcium, phosphate, and eGFR were normal. PTH levels were slightly raised at 8.6 pmol/L (normal range: 1.3-7.3); the vitamin D level was low at 21 nmol/L (normal

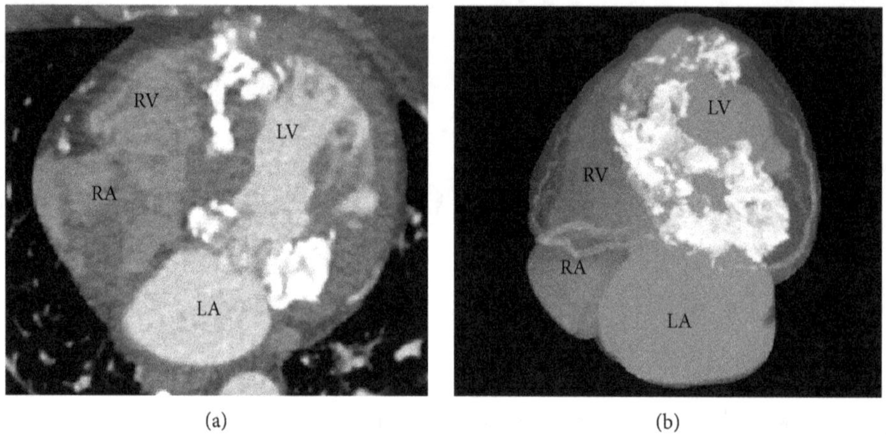

Figure 1: Computed tomography ((a) multiplanar reformatted (MPR) and (b) maximal intensity projection (MIP)) demonstrated extensive infiltrative calcification, circumferentially around the mitral annulus, extending posteriorly and septally into the myocardial apex. RA: right atrium; RV: right ventricle; LA: left atrium; LV: left ventricle.

range: 100-200) indicating vitamin D deficiency. Hb was 119 g/L (normal: 120-160) with negative haemolytic and haematinic screenings. Lipid profile revealed a triglyceride level of 5.0 mmol/L (normal: 0.12-2.10) and HDL of 0.99 mmol/L (normal: 1.2-1.8) with the total cholesterol measuring 5.7 mmol/L. There was an isolated raised bilirubin of 38 microm/L (range: 0-17), but the direct Coombs test and haptoglobin levels did not suggest haemolytic anaemia. Autoantibody screens (immunoglobulins, ANA, ANCA, dsDNA) were negative. Serum iron levels were slightly low; however, the total iron binding capacity was normal. Serum ACE levels were 24 U/L (normal: 8-52). Abdominal ultrasound confirmed fatty liver infiltration. Tuberculosis exposure was excluded through careful history taking and supported with a negative acid-fast bacilli sputum sample.

Although still experiencing exertional breathlessness, the patient's symptoms improved with low-dose furosemide, and given the presence of coronary artery disease on CTCA, she was discharged with dual antiplatelet therapy added to her current medication regimen.

Cardiac MRI was performed (Figure 2), and similar to the CT, this showed extensive calcification extending into the myocardium from the mitral valve annulus, evidenced by the absent signal on T1- and T2-weighted imaging. The lesions enhanced on late gadolinium imaging suggesting the presence of an extracellular matrix within the calcium, but they were not encased entirely by calcium and were in communication with the surrounding myocardium. The findings were consistent with an aggressive caseating, calcific process extending into the left ventricular myocardium from the mitral valve annulus. The infiltrated myocardium was thickened with reduced contractility, whilst the noninfiltrated myocardium contracted well and compensated to maintain an overall normal left ventricular ejection fraction.

Coronary angiography showed moderate mid and distal LAD disease, in addition to severe distal posterior descending artery (PDA) disease (Figure 3); this was not felt sufficient to explain the aetiology of her breathlessness.

PET CT was requested to further examine the calcified lesions within the myocardium and evaluate for metastatic calcific phenomenon. This scan demonstrated no abnormal uptake nor metabolic activity outside of the heart, therefore providing reassurance for our patient with exclusion of metastatic infiltrative disease. Interestingly, there was some evidence of metabolic activity around the calcified lesions within the heart; however, it is uncertain whether this represents an active disease process or the chronic inflammatory process described in the caseating tissue.

Given her symptomatic improvement and normal left ventricular function, ongoing surveillance was arranged with interval scanning.

2. Discussion

Myocardial calcification may be described in three principle forms: dystrophic, pericarditic, or metastatic. This classification may be useful in identifying the precipitating cause and reaching a unifying diagnosis.

2.1. Dystrophic. Dystrophic calcification derives from degenerative myocardial disease, culminating in deposition of calcium salts along the myocardial tissue [1]. Aortic and mitral valves are recognised susceptible areas through their exposure to high degrees of mechanical force and endothelial disruption. This damaged myocardial tissue creates a calcium-philic surface for the calcium salt deposition usually associated with rheumatic heart disease or ageing [2, 3].

Dystrophic calcification can even be divided into endothelial or intramyocardial causes of cardiac endothelial disruption, with ensuing pathological myocardial calcification [3, 4]. Pathologies of myocardial tissue degeneration initiating this endothelial calcification include myocardial infarction, ventricular aneurysms, or preexisting valvular heart disease [3].

Whilst intramyocardial and endothelial calcifications can share identical pathological processes, principally through extensive myocardial ischaemia or mixed valvular heart disease, mechanisms unique to intramyocardial calcification have also been described in the literature. Simonson et al. present a case of myocardial calcification secondary to

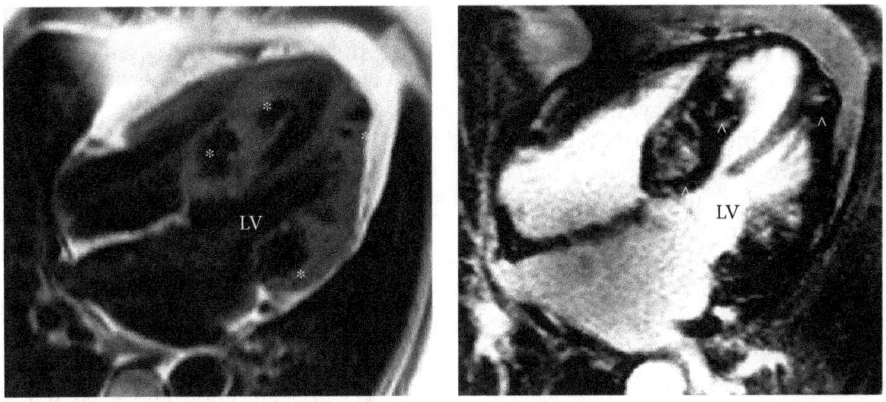

(a) (b)

Figure 2: (a) Magnetic resonance T1-weighted spin echo demonstrating multiple low signal lesions throughout the left ventricular myocardium (*), consistent with extensive infiltrative calcification of the myocardium. (b) Magnetic resonance phase-sensitive inversion recovery late gadolinium enhancement demonstrating a heterogenous composition to the intramyocardial lesions within the nulled myocardium (^), suggestive of caseating calcification within the myocardium (four-chamber view Siemens Avanto 1.5 Tesla).

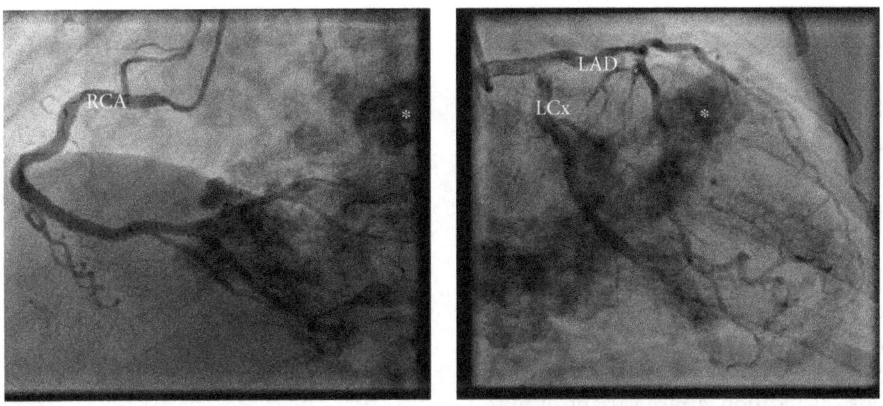

(a) (b)

Figure 3: Coronary angiography illustrating the absence of significant obstructive coronary artery disease and highlighting extensive myocardial calcification (*), particularly prominent around the mitral valve annulus: (a) left anterior oblique view and (b) right anterior oblique view. RCA: right coronary artery; LCx: left circumflex artery; LAD: left anterior descending artery.

profound septicaemia, with the acute hypotension triggering diffuse myocardial damage. They hypothesise that causes of catecholamine excess and myofibrillar degeneration can initiate an inflammatory cascade which culminates in intramyocardial calcification [4]. CT can further differentiate these intramyocardial aetiologies with its ability to delineate calcification patterns; infarction produces focal curvilinear calcification within the scarred myocardium, in contrast to systemic sepsis which reveals a typically diffuse picture [4]. CT has even identified rare cases of intramyocardial calcification secondary to hypertrophic cardiomyopathy (HCM), cardiac tumours, and systemic sarcoidosis [1].

2.2. Pericarditic. Intramyocardial and pericarditic causes of MAC can be unified through the diagnosis of tuberculosis. Whilst focal myocardial inflammation associated with previous active tuberculosis can become a precursor for calcific change [5], rarer causes of pericarditis-related calcification progressing to the myocardium are attributed to irradiation, ventricular aneurysms, systemic lupus erythematosus (SLE), and viral aetiologies. These patients typically present with pericardial constriction or from incidental imaging findings [6, 7].

2.3. Metastatic. Whereas dystrophic and pericarditic calcifications exhibit a normal calcium-phosphate metabolism, metastatic calcification ensues from a derangement of this balance and originates in the previously healthy myocardium [6]. Vascular calcification is a recognised complication of end-stage renal failure, with hyperparathyroidism, hyperuricaemia, and secondary hyperparathyroidism as important contributors. MAC has been demonstrated in patients with renal failure, especially dialysis-dependent patients, and develops due to increased levels of serum calcium caused by hyperphosphataemia. Whilst abnormal calcium-phosphate metabolism due to renal failure accounts for a high incidence of structural cardiac calcification, primary hyperparathyroid hormone excess must first be excluded [8].

Through careful consideration of this classification, we sought to identify the underlying aetiology of our patient's myocardial calcification. Our CT series ruled out pericardial extension and its attributed pathology, however demonstrated caseation of the calcified lesions. Cardiac MRI also suggested an aggressive caseating calcific process extending from the mitral valve annulus. Our images revealed a thickened, infiltrated myocardium with normal surrounding myocardium and overall preserved left ventricular ejection fraction, rather than a restrictive defect seen in endomyocardial fibrosis or pericardial disease [8]. Given these appearances of caseous calcification, a complete medical history and comprehensive serology were obtained therefore excluding inflammatory and metabolic aetiologies of myocardial calcification. Furthermore, imaging with thoracic CT and PET CT helps to rule out infiltrative disease and carcinomatous pathologies.

Cardiac sarcoid is a recognised differential of myocardial calcification; however, the absence of systemic sarcoidosis together with negative serum ACE and normal calcium levels, in addition to our imaging, sufficiently excluded this diagnosis. Increased sensitivity for diagnosing cardiac sarcoid can be achieve through endomyocardial biopsy which reveals a noncaseating granulomatous pattern, whilst cardiac MRI typically demonstrates subepicardial late gadolinium enhancement with extracardiac uptake evidenced on PET CT [9].

The literature identifies dystrophic calcification as the most prevalent aetiology of mitral annular calcification. The presence of calcific deposits extending from our patient's mitral valve annulus is certainly in keeping with dystrophic calcification secondary to degenerative valve disease. However, caseous calcification, a rare variant of mitral annular calcification, has also been recognised with an estimated prevalence of less than 1% of MAC cases [10, 11]. In contrast to the dense calcific deposition of dystrophic calcification, caseous calcification exhibits central areas of lucency within the calcific envelope and is therefore acknowledged as a separate entity. On a cellular level, microscopy has helped further differentiate the two pathologies, with caseous calcification representing an amorphous, acellular mass with a mild chronic inflammatory reaction stimulated by macrophages and lymphocytes. This perhaps explains our CT PET appearances which demonstrated metabolic activity around the calcified lesions. Though echocardiography may suggest the diagnosis of CMAC through identification of echolucency within the calcification, the limited visualisation we experienced ultimately enhanced the value of the advanced imaging modalities utilised and negated the need for biopsy [11, 12].

Cases of intramyocardial calcification are usually discovered on postmortem; therefore, it is rare for us to identify such a case in a minimally symptomatic patient. Strong emphasis should be placed upon establishing the underlying cause of intramyocardial calcification and differentiating the unifying diagnosis from cardiac tumours, myocardial abscesses, or hydatid cysts, given their prognostic implications. In the case of caseous MAC (CMAC), complications of arrhythmia, coronary events, and sudden cardiac death though rare intensify its significance as a diagnostic and prognostic entity [10, 12].

Despite establishing the diagnosis of "idiopathic intramyocardial calcification with caseous mitral annular calcification," the pertinent question remains: *How can we best treat our patients?* No consensus has been reached on the management of CMAC; one school of thought favours conservative management given the dynamic physiological yet benign process and reported spontaneous resolution of intramyocardial calcification, whilst the other favours surgical decalcification and even mitral valve replacement especially in the context of symptomatic valvular pathology [10, 11, 13]. Dietl et al. even makes the case for elective surgical resection of CCMA in asymptomatic patients [14]. Their review evaluated the prevalence of cerebral embolisation associated with CMAC, with CMAC patients at an increased risk of cardioembolic stroke (19.2%) especially when compared to MAC patients (11.8%, $p = 0.018$). This may originate from spontaneous fistulisation and embolisation of caseous necrotic material from the CMAC lesion, rendering anticoagulation ineffective for prevention of cardioembolic stroke [14]. With the ever increasing availability and value of cardiac CT, we expect many physicians to face the challenge of managing this complex condition; therefore, we aim to stimulate further research into the optimal management. For our patient, given the presence of coronary artery disease, we commenced antiplatelet therapy, continued primary cardiovascular prevention with the aim of attenuating the calcific process, and continued with diuretic therapy. She remained stable on clinical follow-up and is awaiting interval scanning.

Our case illustrates well the diagnostic enigma of idiopathic intramyocardial calcification. The atypical presentation coupled with the inconclusive first-line investigations posed a diagnostic dilemma. Furthermore, despite establishing a diagnosis of CMAC-associated mitral regurgitation, identifying the aetiology and improving patient symptoms provided additional clinical challenge. This manuscript describes our experience of idiopathic intramyocardial caseous calcification which should guide physicians encountering this condition, as well as stimulate further research into this rare, though fascinating, diagnosis.

Consent

Informed consent was obtained from all individual participants included in the study.

Authors' Contributions

All authors were involved with the clinical case, manuscript write-up, and revision. NC and DM provided the clinical imaging modalities and interpretation.

References

[1] D. Patterson, D. Gibson, R. Gomes et al., "Idiopathic calcified myocardial mass," *Thorax*, vol. 29, no. 5, pp. 589–594, 1974.

[2] P. K. Fulkerson, B. M. Beaver, J. C. Auseon, and H. L. Graber, "Calcification of the mitral annulus: etiology, clinical associations, complications and therapy," *The American Journal of Medicine*, vol. 66, no. 6, pp. 967–977, 1979.

[3] D. C. Barnard, L. Pape, J. Missri, and J. E. Dalen, "Massive myocardial calcification and normal coronary arteries," *Texas Heart Institute Journal*, vol. 12, no. 4, pp. 363–365, 1985.

[4] S. Simonson, W. T. Miller, A. Perl, and D. A. Torigian, "Diffuse left ventricular myocardial calcification in the setting of sepsis on CT imaging," *Journal of Thoracic Imaging*, vol. 22, no. 4, pp. 343–345, 2007.

[5] T. Butz, M. van Bracht, A. Meissner et al., "Mitral valve disease as well as uncommon extensive epipericardial and intramyocardial calcification secondary to massive mitral annular calcification," *European Journal of Echocardiography*, vol. 11, pp. 85–88, 2010.

[6] D. Aras, S. Topaloglu, B. Demirkan, B. Deveci, O. Ozeke, and S. Korkmaz, "Porcelain heart: a case of massive myocardial calcification," *The International Journal of Cardiovascular Imaging*, vol. 22, no. 1, pp. 123–126, 2006.

[7] Y. Molad, N. Levin-Iaina, M. Vaturi, J. Sulkes, and A. Sagie, "Heart valve calcification in young patients with systemic lupus erythematosus: a window to premature atherosclerotic vascular morbidity and a risk factor for all-cause mortality," *Atherosclerosis*, vol. 185, no. 2, pp. 406–412, 2006.

[8] A. E. Kempf, M. G. Momeni, and F. Saremi, "Myocardial calcinosis in chronic renal failure," *Journal of Radiolgy Case Report*, vol. 3, no. 2, pp. 16–19, 2009.

[9] K. Kusano and K. Satomi, "Diagnosis and treatment of cardiac sarcoidosis," *Heart*, vol. 102, no. 3, pp. 184–190, 2015.

[10] H. Arora, P. Madan, L. Simpson, and R. F. Stainback, "Caseous calcification of the mitral annulus," *Texas Heart Institute Journal*, vol. 35, no. 2, pp. 211–213, 2008.

[11] D. Harpaz, I. Auerbach, V. Zvi, M. Motro, A. Tobar, and S. Rosenblatt, "Caseous calcification of the mitral annulus: a neglected, unrecognised diagnosis," *Journal of the American Society of Echocardiography*, vol. 14, no. 8, pp. 825–831, 2001.

[12] I. Y. Elgendy and C. R. Conti, "Caseous calcification of the mitral annulus: a review," *Clinical Cardiology*, vol. 36, no. 10, pp. E27–E31, 2013.

[13] W. J. Barson, J. Craenen, D. M. Hosier, R. L. Brawley, and M. D. Hilty, "Survival following myocarditis and myocardial calcification associated with infection by Coxsackie virus B-4," *Pediatrics*, vol. 68, no. 1, pp. 79–81, 1981.

[14] C. Dietl, C. Hawthorn, and V. Raizada, "Risk of cerebral embolization with caseous calcification of the mitral annulus: review article," *The Open Cardiovascular Medicine Journal*, vol. 10, no. 1, pp. 221–232, 2016.

19

Statin-Induced Triad of Autoimmune Myocarditis, Myositis and Transaminitis

Muhammad Ajmal,[1] Amitoj Singh,[1] Saad Kubba,[1] Michelle Hershman,[2,3] and Tushar Acharya[1,2,3]

[1]*Division of Cardiology, Department of Internal Medicine, USA*
[2]*Department of Medical Imaging, University of Arizona College of Medicine, Tucson, USA*
[3]*Banner University Medical Center, Tucson, USA*

Correspondence should be addressed to Tushar Acharya; tacharya@shc.arizona.edu

Academic Editor: Takatoshi Kasai

Despite well-established cardiovascular benefits, statins have been associated with myopathic side effects ranging from myalgias to rhabdomyolysis and autoimmune necrotizing myositis. Statins have not been previously shown to cause myocarditis. Our case highlights this rare entity.

1. History of Presentation

A 70-year-old male presented to the emergency department (ED) with shortness of breath and generalized body aches associated with muscle weakness in all extremities. These symptoms dated back a few months; however, there was an acute decompensation in the past 1 week which led to the hospital visit. Shortness of breath was associated with orthopnea and chest discomfort. At the time of presentation to the ED, there was severe limitation of daily activities including inability to get out of bed, stand from a sitting position, and perform personal grooming. Presenting vitals were stable (pulse 84 beats per minute, blood pressure 134/60 mmHg). Physical examination demonstrated diffuse tenderness and objective weakness in all four extremities (3/5 strength). Reflexes were intact, and there were no focal neurological deficits. Cardiorespiratory examination demonstrated bibasilar crackles, an elevated JVP, and bilateral lower extremities pitting edema. An electrocardiogram demonstrated a normal dual-chamber function with ventricular pacing and atrial sensing.

2. Past Medical History

The patient had known diffuse nonobstructive coronary artery disease (CAD) (by coronary angiography). Other comorbidities included chronic kidney disease stage III and complete heart block status postdual-chamber pacemaker (implanted 1 year ago). His medications included atorvastatin 80 mg daily (6 months), metoprolol tartrate 25 mg twice daily, aspirin 81 mg, and glipizide 5 mg daily.

3. Differential Diagnosis

Clinically, the patient had signs and symptoms of a combined skeletal (proximal muscle weakness) and myocardial insult (acute heart failure with evidence of elevated filling pressures). While statins were suspected to at least be partially responsible for the clinical presentation, a unifying pathophysiology was sought and would require further testing. Subsequently, focused laboratory testing, imaging, and eventual pathological testing were performed as described below.

4. Investigations

Laboratory examination revealed rhabdomyolysis with acute kidney injury, transaminitis, and myocardial injury (elevated hs-troponin and NT-pro BNP). Rheumatologic workup yielded an abnormally elevated anti-HMGCR-Ab, which was suggestive of autoimmune necrotizing myositis with moderate significance (Table 1). Skeletal muscle biopsy (gastrocnemius) confirmed necrotizing myopathy and neurogenic atrophy.

Magnetic resonance imaging (MRI) of the upper and lower extremities demonstrated diffuse muscular edema in keeping with acute myositis (Figure 1). Due to myocardial injury (elevated serum hs-cTnT and NT-pro BNP), cardiac involvement was suspected. An echocardiogram and subsequently a cardiac MRI were obtained. Echocardiography demonstrated normal biventricular size and function without regional wall motion abnormalities and no significant valvular abnormalities. Cardiac MRI confirmed normal biventricular size and overall LV function as seen on the echocardiogram. On tissue characterization, myocardial T1 was significantly elevated (Figure 1(a)) in the midanterolateral and inferolateral left ventricular walls suggesting expanded extracellular compartment due to edema/inflammation or fibrosis. T2 mapping images also demonstrated mildly increased values corresponding to these same areas in keeping with myocardial edema (Figure 1). On dynamic perfusion imaging, there was a resting perfusion defect in these areas, presumably due to perivascular edema or direct vascular injury. Late gadolinium enhancement imaging was diagnostic for myocarditis and showed enhancement in a midwall distribution involving the midantero- and inferolateral walls and in an epicardial distribution in the apical anterior wall (Figures 1(d), 2, 3). Our proposed algorithm for evaluating statin-induced myocarditis is shown in Figure 4.

TABLE 1: Laboratory findings.

Laboratory	Patient's results	Normal value
White blood cells	7.3 K/mm^3	4-11 K/mm^3
Hemoglobin	10.7 g/dL	13.5-17 g/dL
Platelets	230 K/mm^3	130-450 K/mm^3
Sodium	141 mmol/L	134-147 mmol/L
Potassium	5.3 mmol/L	5.3 mmol/L
Chloride	110 mmol/L	95-108 mmol/L
Bicarbonate	17 mmol/L	>19 mmol/L
BUN	67 mg/dL	8-25 mg/dL
Creatinine	1.8 mg/dL	<1.5 mg/dL
Anion gap	14	
AST	716 U/L	<50 U/L
ALT	907 U/L	<60 U/L
ALP	389 U/L	<140 U/L
hs-troponin	1577 ng/L – >1619 ng/L–>1538 ng/L	<11 ng/L
NT-pro BNP	2427 pg/mL	<124 pg/mL
CK	29,200 U/L	<355 U/L
CK-MB	525 ng/ml	<6.7 ng/mL
Serum aldolase	130 IU/L	<7.6 IU/L
ESR	85	<30
HMGCR-Ab	59	<20
ANA	Negative	Negative
ASMA	Negative	Negative
Anti-Jo1 antibodies	Negative	Negative

AST: aspartate aminotransferase; ALT: alanine transaminase; ALP: alkaline phosphatase; NT-pro BNP: N-terminal probrain natriuretic peptide; CK: total creatine kinase; CK-MB: creatine kinase-myocardial band; ESR: erythrocyte sedimentation rate; HMGCR-Ab: β-hydroxy β-methylglutaryl-CoA reductase antibody; ANA: antinuclear antibodies; ASMA: antismooth muscle antibodies.

5. Management

The initial suspicion for statin-induced myositis and rhabdomyolysis was confirmed with an elevated HMGCR antibody, abnormal MRI of extremities, and inflammatory myocyte necrosis on skeletal muscle biopsy. Atorvastatin was discontinued, and patient was resuscitated with intravenous normal saline. Close cardiac monitoring and electrolyte replacement were undertaken given acute myocarditis. Through the initial week of his hospitalization, the patient's renal function improved but neuromuscular weakness and pain continued. Once fulminant necrosis was confirmed on biopsy, given persistent skeletal weakness, immunosuppressive therapies were instituted. These included intravenous Solu-Medrol (125 mg daily × 3 days) and intravenous immunoglobulin (IVIG) (2 mg/kg IVIG × 1 dose). Despite this regimen, the patient remained clinically and chemically symptomatic (total CK and liver enzymes remained elevated). This prompted a trial of intravenous rituximab (1 g). Due to ongoing need for IV immunosuppression and slow improvement in muscle strength, the patient had a protracted hospital course lasting 4 weeks. Once clinically stable, he was discharged to a short-term rehabilitation facility. His laboratory work at discharge showed an improvement in CK (2815 U/L), AST (182 U/L), ALT (411 U/L), and ALP (172 U/L). He did not develop arrhythmias during the hospital stay.

6. Discussion

Despite its multiple, well-documented beneficial effects in atherosclerotic cardiovascular disease, statin use has been associated with side effects like muscle and liver injury [1, 2]. Myalgias have been commonly reported with statins but only 1 out of 10,000 patients develops objective muscle injury with CK elevation [3]. Most of these resolve spontaneously with statin cessation. In contrast, statin-induced autoimmune necrotizing myositis (ANM) is very rare but

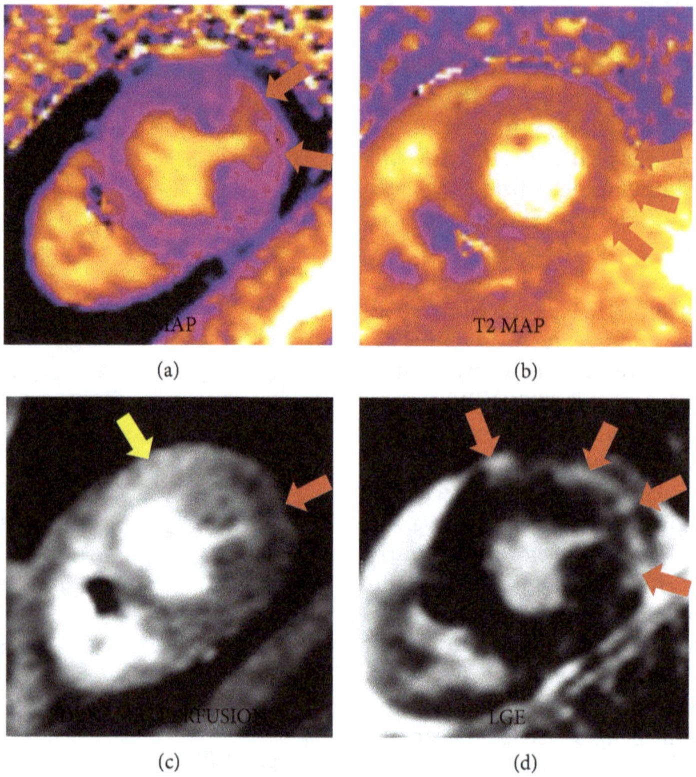

Figure 1: (a) Bright signal intensity on T1 map showing increased extracellular compartment due to inflammation/fibrosis. (b) Bright signal intensity on T2 map corresponding to inflammation/edema. (c) Normal (yellow arrow) and abnormal (red arrow) perfusion due to vascular injury/myocardial edema in the areas corresponding to (d) late gadolinium enhancement (LGE).

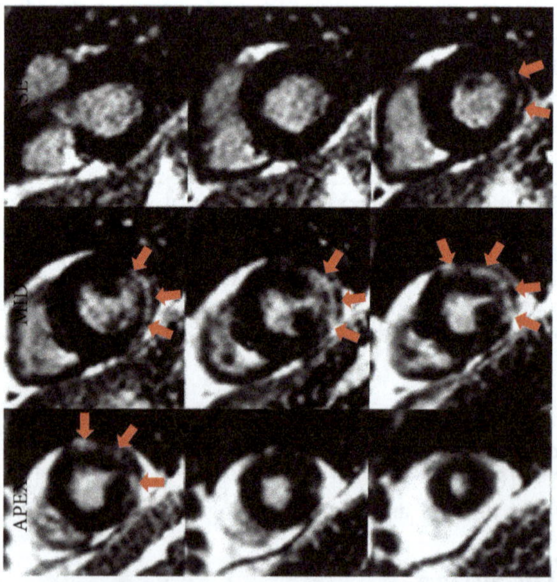

Figure 2: Late gadolinium enhancement (red arrows) in a midwall and epicardial distribution involving the inferolateral, anterolateral, and anterior walls consistent with myocarditis (short axis stack).

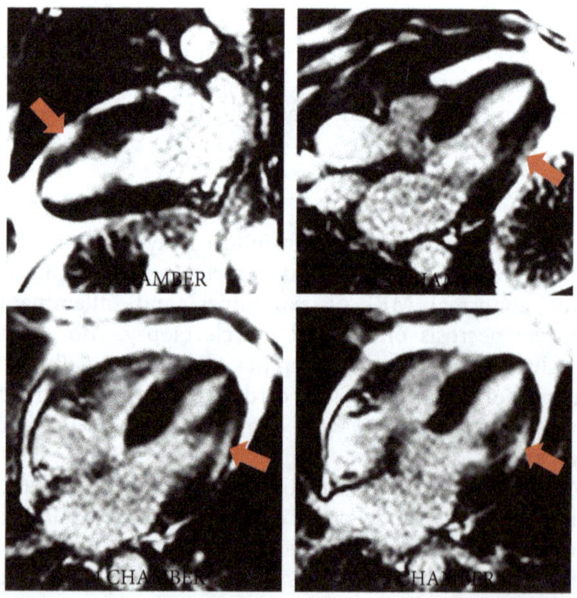

Figure 3: Late gadolinium enhancement (red arrows) in a midwall and epicardial distribution involving the inferolateral, anterolateral, and anterior walls consistent with myocarditis (long axes).

potentially life-threatening. It is diagnosed with antibodies to HMGCR and muscle necrosis on biopsy. ANM requires aggressive immunosuppression in addition to statin cessation [4–6].

Statin-induced myocarditis with or without associated autoimmune necrotizing myositis has not been reported in literature before. In fact, some reports suggest that statins may be helpful in treating myocarditis and postmyocarditis

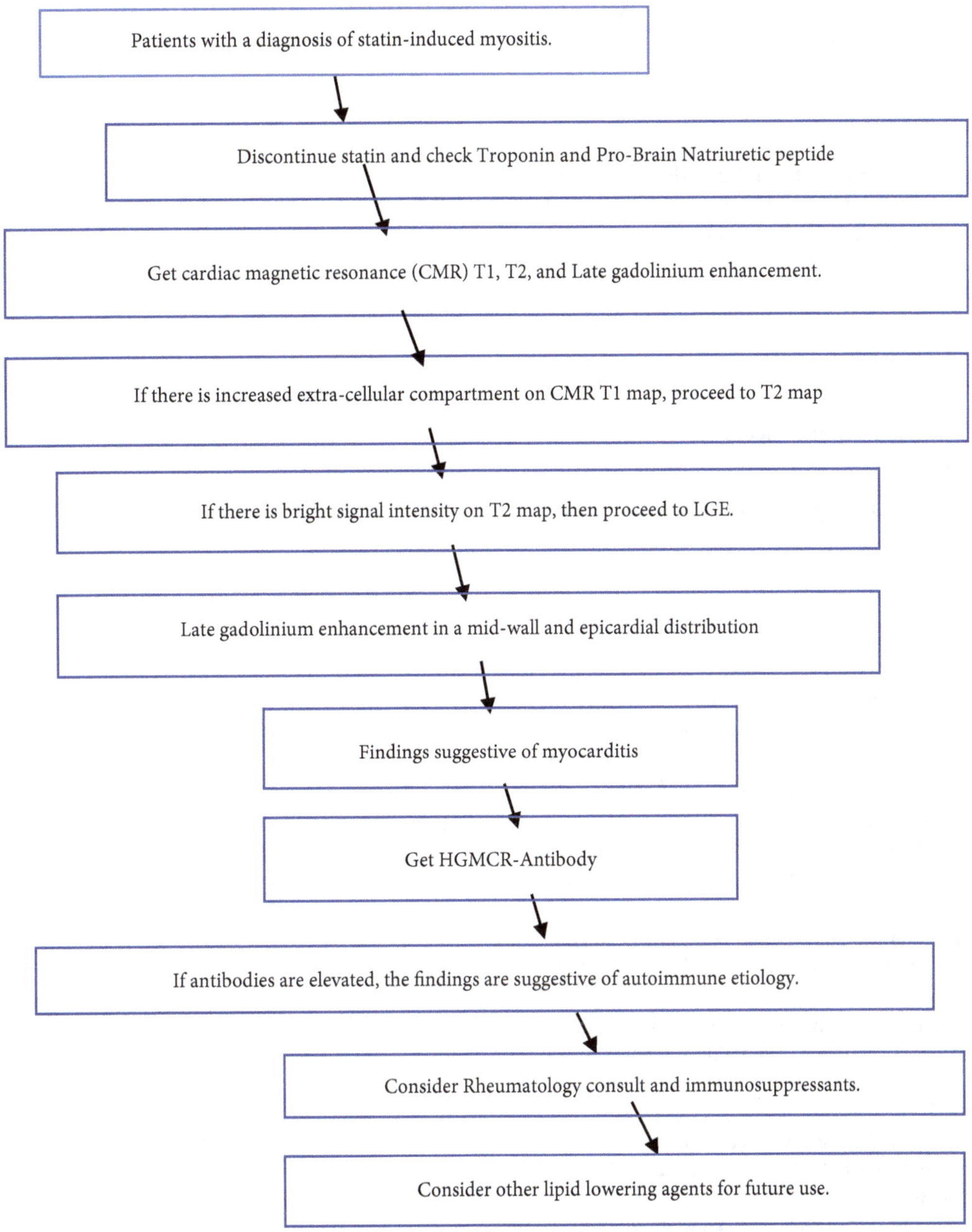

FIGURE 4: Algorithm for evaluating statin-induced myocarditis (LGE (late gadolinium enhancement)).

dilated cardiomyopathy [7]. This beneficial effect in myocarditis and particularly autoimmune myocarditis is thought to be due to anti-inflammatory/pleotropic effects of statins and possibly mediated by inhibition of antigen-presenting cells and lymphocytes leading to quiescence of an inflammatory surge and reduction in inflammatory biomarkers [8].

Contrary to these reports, our case represents a rare instance where statins can act as an offender and result in autoimmune myocarditis. Myocarditis is likely mediated by direct tissue injury not too different in its pathogenesis from the necrotizing myositis of the skeletal muscle. It is hypothesized that statin-induced overexpression of HMGCAR in genetically susceptible individuals may lead to autoimmunity against HMGCAR causing muscle injury. Since injured muscles produce more HMGCAR, this may perpetuate a cycle that may not be abated by discontinuation of statin and require immunosuppression [5].

Readers should familiarize themselves with this extremely rare adverse effect, especially in setting of elevated cardiac enzymes, which can be misinterpreted as acute coronary syndrome instead of myocarditis.

7. Follow-Up

The patient was an outpatient in the cardiology and rheumatology clinic 4-week posthospital discharge and continued to show clinical improvement (he could now walk without support). His steroid regimen is gradually being tapered over 6 months with close rheumatologic follow-up.

8. Conclusion

This is the first reported case of statin-induced myocarditis. Myocarditis in this patient is likely a part of the larger spectrum of statin-induced autoimmune necrotizing myositis, a very rare condition managed with aggressive immunosuppressants.

9. Learning Objectives

(1) Recognize autoimmune necrotizing myositis and myocarditis as a rare complication of statin use

(2) Diagnosis and management of this life-threatening myopathy

References

[1] S. Grundy, M. Stone, A. L. Bailey et al., "2018 AHA/ACC/AACVPR/AAPA/ABC/ACPM/ADA/AGS/APhA/ASPC/NLA/PCNA guideline on the management of blood cholesterol: a report of the American College of Cardiology/American Heart Association task force on clinical practice guidelines," *Circulation*, vol. 139, no. 25, pp. e1082–e1143, 2019.

[2] W.-S. Lee and J. Kim, "Statin-induced liver and muscle toxicities," *Molecular & Cellular Toxicology*, vol. 15, no. 1, pp. 9–17, 2019.

[3] M. Law and A. R. Rudnicka, "Statin safety: a systematic review," *The American Journal of Cardiology*, vol. 97, no. 8A, pp. 52C–60C, 2006.

[4] S. Nazir, S. Lohani, N. Tachamo, D. Poudel, and A. Donato, "Statin-associated autoimmune myopathy: a systematic review of 100 cases," *Journal of Clinical Rheumatology*, vol. 23, no. 3, pp. 149–154, 2017.

[5] A. L. Mammen, "Statin-associated autoimmune myopathy," *The New England Journal of Medicine*, vol. 374, no. 7, pp. 664–669, 2016.

[6] P. Sharma, B. Timilsina, J. Adhikari, P. Parajuli, R. Dhital, and N. Tachamo, "Statin-induced necrotizing autoimmune myopathy: an extremely rare adverse effect from statin use," *J Community Hosp Intern Med Perspect*, vol. 9, no. 6, pp. 503–506, 2019.

[7] P. E. Lazzerini, P. L. Capecchi, and F. Laghi-Pasini, "Statins as a new therapeutic perspective in myocarditis and postmyocarditis dilated cardiomyopathy," *Cardiovascular Drugs and Therapy*, vol. 27, no. 5, pp. 365–369, 2013.

[8] J. L. Wu, S. Matsui, Z. P. Zong et al., "Amelioration of myocarditis by statin through inhibiting cross-talk between antigen presenting cells and lymphocytes in rats," *Journal of Molecular and Cellular Cardiology*, vol. 44, no. 6, pp. 1023–1031, 2008.

20

Heart Team Intervention for Calcified Left Main Coronary Disease and Jeopardized Left Internal Mammary Artery Graft

Nobunari Tomura,[1] Masashi Fujino,[1] Yu Kataoka,[1] Shuichi Yoneda,[1] Hiroaki Sasaki,[2] and Teruo Noguchi[1]

[1]*Department of Cardiovascular Medicine, National Cerebral and Cardiovascular Center, 6-1 Kishibe-Shimmachi, Suita, Osaka, Japan*
[2]*Department of Cardiovascular Surgery, National Cerebral and Cardiovascular Center, 6-1 Kishibe-Shimmachi, Suita, Osaka, Japan*

Correspondence should be addressed to Masashi Fujino; fujinom@ncvc.go.jp

Academic Editor: Aiden Abidov

It is sometimes difficult to identify the culprit lesion and treatment strategy in patients with acute coronary syndrome who have complex coronary lesions and jeopardized left internal mammary artery graft. This report describes a heart team approach for a non-ST-segment elevation myocardial infarction case with complex coronary vasculature. A 73-year-old man presented to the emergency department with crescendo angina. He had a history of total aortic arch replacement with concomitant coronary artery bypass graft using left internal mammary artery. Emergent coronary angiography demonstrated severe stenosis at left main trunk bifurcation caused by calcified nodule. While the bypass graft to left anterior descending coronary artery was patent, the proximal segment of left subclavian artery was occluded. Following the prompt discussion with our heart team, we performed percutaneous coronary intervention in the first step for treating the left main stenosis using rotational atherectomy into the unprotected left circumflex artery. After clinical recovery, stress myocardial scintigraphy identified the presence of anteroseptal ischemia, which indicated coronary subclavian steal syndrome due to left subclavian artery occlusion. Contrast-enhanced CT visualized that the occlusion originated from the anastomosis, suggesting the potential procedural risk of endovascular treatment by dilatation. Our heart team discussed again and decided to undergo axillo-axillary artery bypass surgery. He was discharged 8 days after the surgery without any sequelae. This is the rare case report of non-ST-segment elevation myocardial infarction who had similar condition to coronary subclavian steal syndrome after total aortic arch replacement. This case highlights the importance of a collaborative approach of the heart team to identify the best therapeutic strategy in a patient with complex coronary vasculature.

1. Introduction

It is sometimes difficult to identify the culprit lesion and appropriate treatment strategy in patients with acute coronary syndrome who undergo coronary artery bypass grafting (CABG). A previous study of percutaneous coronary intervention (PCI) in patients with prior CABG demonstrated that the target vessel was a native coronary artery in 73.4% of cases and a bypass graft in the remaining 26.6% (saphenous vein graft, 25.0%; arterial graft, 1.5%) [1]. The coronary subclavian steal syndrome (CSSS) was first described in 1974 and is caused by retrograde or insufficient blood flow through the internal mammary artery graft, with subsequent myocardial ischemia. Proximal atherosclerotic stenosis of the ipsilateral subclavian artery is the most frequent cause of CSSS, and its consequences include angina or acute coronary syndrome [2, 3]. Although one case report discussed the endovascular treatment of CSSS complicated with coronary artery disease [4], the current case report describes the rare occurrence of non-ST-segment elevation myocardial infarction (NSTEMI) after total aortic arch replacement (TAR) in which a jeopardized left internal mammary artery (LIMA) graft resulted in a condition similar to CSSS.

2. Case Presentation

A 73-year-old man presented to the emergency department with crescendo angina. The patient had a past medical history of hypertension and diabetes mellitus. Four years earlier, he had undergone TAR with concomitant CABG using the LIMA to treat a thoracic aortic aneurysm and severe stenosis of the left anterior descending artery (LAD). The branch of the trifurcated graft for aortic arch replacement was sutured end-to-end to the left subclavian artery (LSA), and the LIMA was anastomosed to the LAD.

On admission, he had a blood pressure of 117/75 mmHg, pulse rate of 66 beats/min, and arterial oxygen saturation of 97%. Physical examination was unremarkable, with no cardiac murmurs, respiratory sounds, or facial or leg edema. Chest X-ray revealed no pulmonary edema or cardiomegaly. Electrocardiography demonstrated ST-segment depression in leads II, aVF, and V4-V6 and ST-segment elevation in lead aVR (Figure 1). Echocardiography showed hypokinetic posterior wall motion (left ventricular ejection fraction 55%). The troponin T level was 2.45 ng/ml (reference < 0.014 ng/ml). We diagnosed the patient with NSTEMI. Despite the fact that he had a moderate GRACE risk score of 135 points, we performed emergent coronary angiography due to his medical history and electrocardiography results.

Coronary angiography revealed severe stenosis with a calcified nodule at the left main bifurcation (Figure 2(a)). The proximal segment of the LSA was occluded (Figure 2(b)), although the LIMA bypass to the LAD was patent (Figure 2(c)). Angiography indicated myocardial ischemia in the region of the unprotected left circumflex artery (LCX), as well as suspected insufficient supply in the region of the LAD with concomitant LSA occlusion, a condition that resembled CSSS.

Our heart team of cardiovascular interventionists and surgeons promptly discussed potential treatments. PCI with a two-stent strategy for the calcified left main bifurcation lesion was thought to have potentially worse clinical outcomes than a one-stent strategy in terms of target lesion revascularization and stent thrombosis. The risk of re-CABG was estimated to be high, since the Society of Thoracic Surgeons risk score for mortality was 10.1%. Our heart team decided to perform PCI from the left main lesion to the LCX using a one-stent strategy and to then discuss elective revascularization of the occluded LSA.

We performed the ad hoc PCI for the lesions from the left main stenosis to the LCX. While the guidewire crossed successfully, an intravascular ultrasound (IVUS) catheter did not due to severe calcification. After balloon angioplasty with a 1.0 mm balloon, debulking was performed using a 1.5 mm rotational atherectomy burr, allowing subsequent IVUS catheter passage. IVUS images revealed a calcified nodule (Figure 3(a)). After additional balloon angioplasty with a 3.0 mm noncompliant balloon, a 3.5/28 mm sirolimus-eluting stent (Ultimaster, Terumo, Tokyo, Japan) was successfully implanted (Figure 3(b)).

Stress myocardial scintigraphy performed 7 days after PCI identified anteroseptal ischemia (Figure 4(a)), which indicated CSSS due to LSA occlusion. Contrast-enhanced CT visualized LSA occlusion at the anastomosed site (Figure 4(b)), suggesting procedural risk associated with endovascular treatment. Our heart team decided to perform axillo-axillary artery bypass surgery.

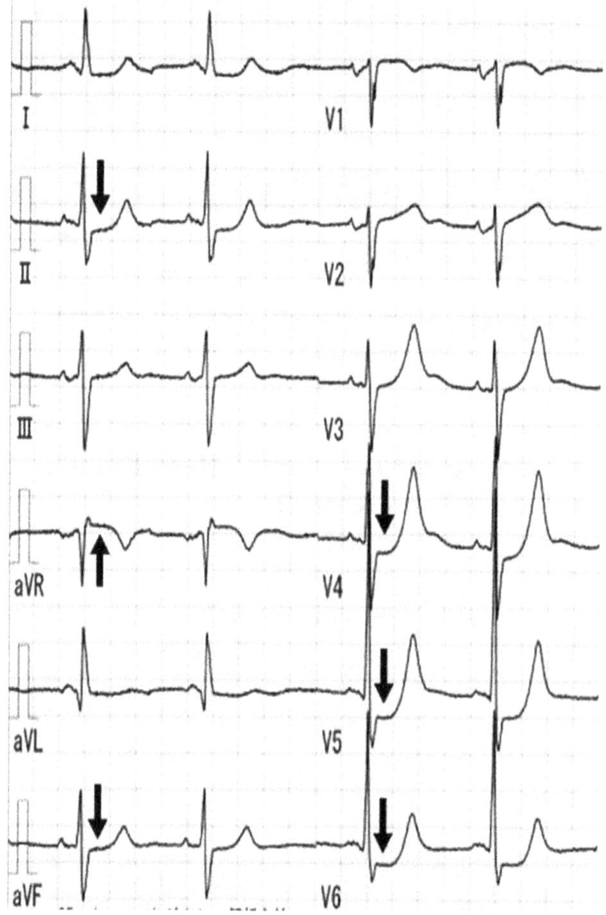

Figure 1: Electrocardiogram. Electrocardiogram showed ST-segment depression in leads II, aVF, and V4-V6 and ST-segment elevation in lead aVR.

Stress myocardial scintigraphy performed 3 days postoperatively showed an improvement in anteroseptal ischemia (Figure 4(c)). The patient was discharged without chest pain 8 days postoperatively. Contrast-enhanced CT performed 21 days postoperatively showed patency of the bypass graft (Figure 4(d)).

3. Discussion

We experienced a case of NSTEMI with complex left main coronary lesions and a jeopardized LIMA graft after TAR. There were three main challenges: identifying the culprit lesion; determining the optimal PCI treatment of the left main coronary bifurcation lesion with the calcified nodule; and deciding how to treat the jeopardized LIMA graft after TAR, which resulted in a condition that resembled CSSS. Our heart team performed emergent PCI for the lesions from the left main stenosis to the LCX and conducted elective surgery for the LSA occlusion to treat the jeopardized LIMA graft.

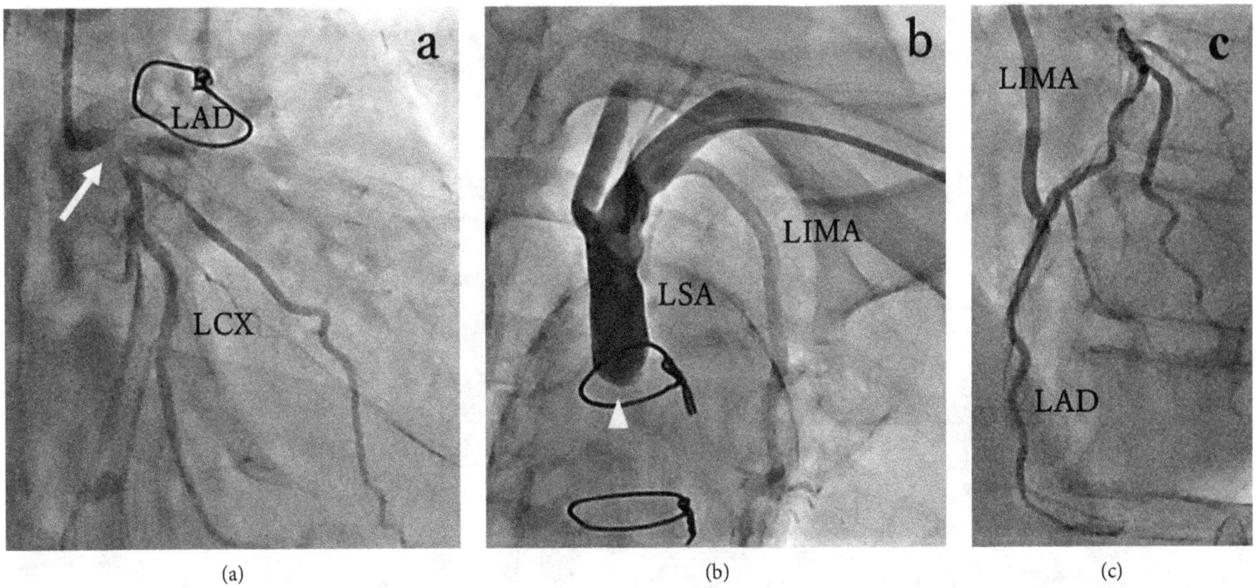

FIGURE 2: Angiography. Coronary angiography showed severe stenosis with a calcified nodule (arrow) at the left main coronary bifurcation (a). Subclavian angiography revealed occlusion of the proximal subclavian artery (arrowhead) (b). A left internal mammary artery bypass to the left anterior descending coronary artery was patent (c). LAD: left anterior descending artery; LCX: left circumflex artery; LIMA: left internal mammary artery; LSA: left subclavian artery.

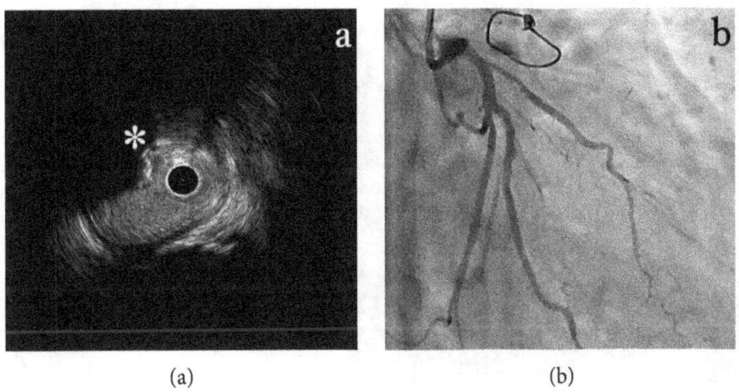

FIGURE 3: Intravascular imaging and final coronary angiography. Intravascular ultrasonography after rotational atherectomy revealed the presence of a calcified nodule (asterisk) (a). Final coronary angiography revealed TIMI3 flow to the left circumflex coronary artery after deployment of a drug-eluting stent.

Although it was difficult to identify the culprit lesion, we chose the optimal treatment from among three options: re-CABG, PCI for the left main bifurcation lesion with a two-stent strategy, or hybrid PCI therapy for the lesions from the left main stenosis to the LCX and revascularization for the occluded LSA. Re-CABG was estimated to carry high surgical risk. PCI for a calcified nodule is challenging despite advances in coronary intervention procedures. Previously, we reported that acute coronary syndrome attributable to a calcified nodule was associated with an increased risk of target lesion revascularization [5]. Furthermore, the bifurcation two-stent strategy was associated with higher rates of target lesion revascularization and stent thrombosis than the one-stent strategy [6]. Since angiography suggested that the LSA was chronically occluded, a single-stent strategy for the left main bifurcation lesion with the calcified nodule was deemed preferable.

The American College of Cardiology (ACC) guidelines state that revascularization using the ipsilateral internal mammary artery is reasonable in asymptomatic patients with subclavian artery stenosis (Class IIa) when performed either by extra-anatomic bypass surgery or subclavian angioplasty and stenting [7]. The technical success rate of the percutaneous approach can be >90%, with 5-year patency rates of 85% [8]. Surgical revascularization has a patency rate in excess of 70% at 5 years [9]. Since there were concerns about procedural risks of endovascular treatment for LCA occlusion at the anastomosed site, our heart team prioritized surgical treatment.

It is important that complex coronary artery disease be treated following meticulous evaluation of target lesions by a heart team. In this case, our heart team successfully performed emergent PCI for left main stenosis with a one-stent strategy, as well as selective surgery for the jeopardized

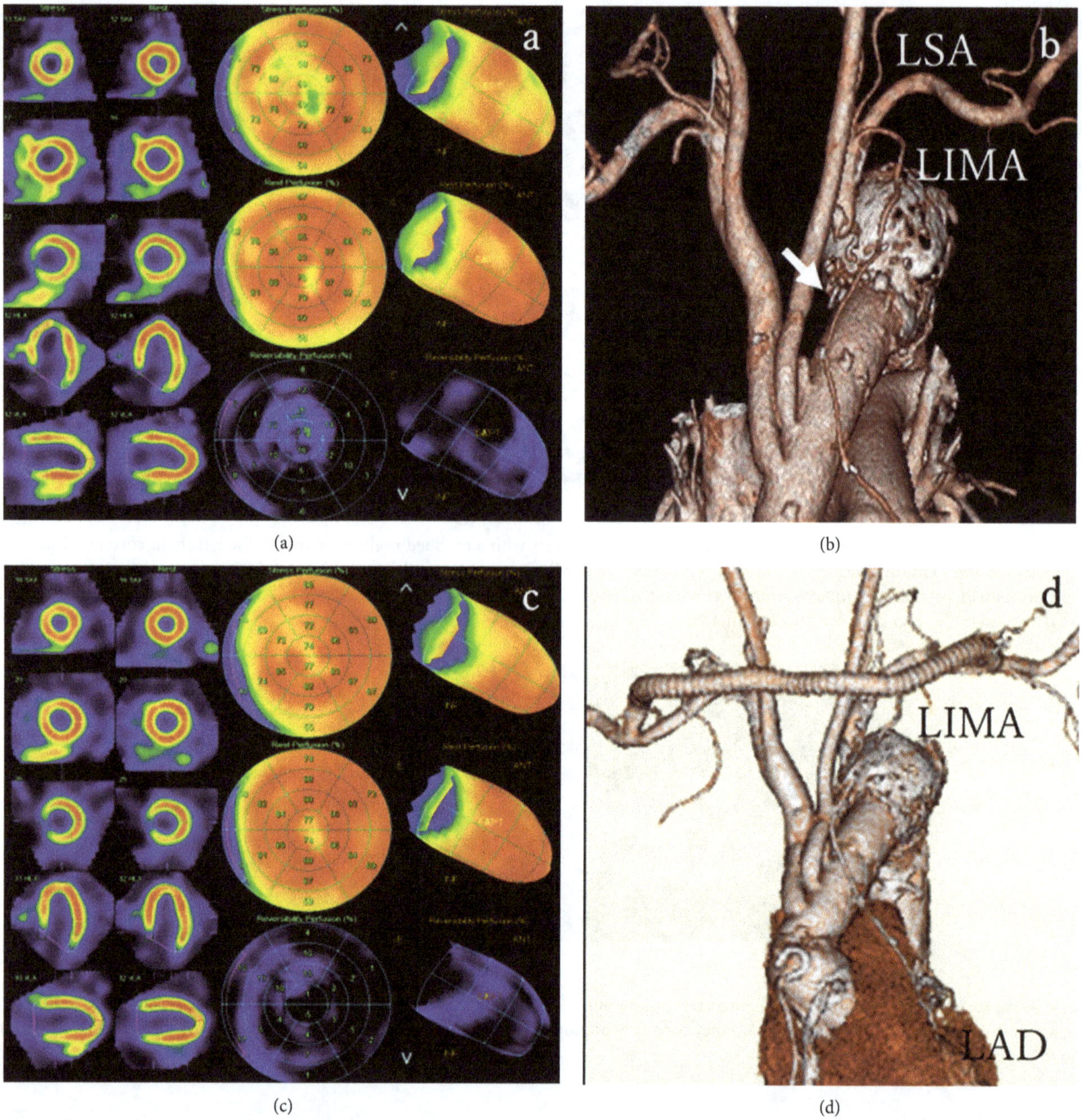

FIGURE 4: Myocardial scintigraphy and contrast-enhanced CT. Stress myocardial scintigraphy 7 days after the PCI procedure showed anteroseptal ischemia (a). Contrast-enhanced CT confirmed left subclavian artery occlusion at the anastomosed site (arrow) (b). Stress myocardial scintigraphy 3 days after axillo-axillary artery bypass surgery revealed improvement of myocardial ischemia (c). Contrast-enhanced CT 21 days postoperatively showed patency of the bypass graft (d). LAD: left anterior descending artery; LIMA: left internal mammary artery; LSA: left subclavian artery.

LIMA graft. The ACC expert consensus document on PCI without on-site surgery also states that patients with high-risk lesions should not undergo nonemergent PCI at facilities without the capacity for on-site surgical procedures [10]. We should immediately collaborate with surgeons even when we treat such patients at these facilities.

Abbreviations

ACC:	American College of Cardiology
CABG:	Coronary artery bypass grafting
CSSS:	Coronary subclavian steal syndrome
IVUS:	Intravascular ultrasound
LAD:	Left anterior descending artery
LCX:	Left circumflex artery
LIMA:	Left internal mammary artery
LSA:	Left subclavian artery
NSTEMI:	Non-ST-segment elevation myocardial infarction
PCI:	Percutaneous coronary intervention
TAR:	Total aortic arch replacement.

Consent

The patient gave written consent to participate in this report.

Acknowledgments

Dr. Fujino is supported by a Grant-in-Aid for Young Scientists from the Japan Society for the Promotion of Science (20K17138).

References

[1] E. S. Brilakis, C. I. O'Donnell, W. Penny et al., "Percutaneous coronary intervention in native coronary arteries versus bypass grafts in patients with prior coronary artery bypass graft surgery: insights from the veterans affairs clinical assessment, reporting, and tracking program," *JACC. Cardiovascular Interventions*, vol. 9, no. 9, pp. 884–893, 2016.

[2] P. T. Harjola and M. Valle, "The importance of aortic arch or subclavian angiography before coronary reconstruction," *Chest*, vol. 66, no. 4, pp. 436–438, 1974.

[3] B. Cua, N. Mamdani, D. Halpin, S. Jhamnani, S. Jayasuriya, and C. Mena-Hurtado, "Review of coronary subclavian steal syndrome," *Journal of Cardiology*, vol. 70, no. 5, pp. 432–437, 2017.

[4] C. Machado, L. Raposo, S. Leal et al., "Coronary-subclavian steal syndrome: percutaneous approach," *Case Reports in Cardiology*, vol. 2013, Article ID 757423, 4 pages, 2013.

[5] H. Sugane, Y. Kataoka, F. Otsuka, et al., "Cardiac outcomes in patients with acute coronary syndrome attributable to calcified nodule," *Atherosclerosis*, vol. 318, pp. 70–75, 2021.

[6] M. Ohya, K. Kadota, M. Toyofuku et al., "Long-term outcomes after stent implantation for left main coronary artery (from the multicenter assessing optimal percutaneous coronary intervention for left main coronary artery stenting registry)," *The American Journal of Cardiology*, vol. 119, no. 3, pp. 355–364, 2017.

[7] T. G. Brott, J. L. Halperin, S. Abbara et al., "2011 ASA/ACCF/AHA/AANN/AANS/ACR/ASNR/CNS/SAIP/SCAI/SIR/SNIS/SVM/SVS guideline on the management of patients with extracranial carotid and vertebral artery disease. a report of the American College of Cardiology Foundation/American Heart Association Task Force on Practice Guidelines, and the American Stroke Association, American Association of Neuroscience Nurses, American Association of Neurological Surgeons, American College of Radiology, American Society of Neuroradiology, Congress of Neurological Surgeons, Society of Atherosclerosis Imaging and Prevention, Society for Cardiovascular Angiography and Interventions, Society of Interventional Radiology, Society of NeuroInterventional Surgery, Society for Vascular Medicine, and Society for Vascular Surgery," *Circulation*, vol. 124, no. 4, pp. e54–130, 2011.

[8] K. Q. Wang, Z. G. Wang, B. Z. Yang et al., "Long-term results of endovascular therapy for proximal subclavian arterial obstructive lesions," *Chinese Medical Journal*, vol. 123, no. 1, pp. 45–50, 2010.

[9] B. J. Potter and D. S. Pinto, "Subclavian steal syndrome," *Circulation*, vol. 129, no. 22, pp. 2320–2323, 2014.

[10] G. J. Dehmer, J. C. Blankenship, M. Cilingiroglu et al., "SCAI/ACC/AHA expert consensus document: 2014 update on percutaneous coronary intervention without on-site surgical backup," *Circulation*, vol. 129, no. 24, pp. 2610–2626, 2014.

21

Pulmonary Artery and Pulmonic Valve Vegetations in a Young Pregnant Filipino with Patent Ductus Arteriosus

Valerie R. Ramiro, Jezreel L. Taquiso, Stephanie Martha O. Obillos, Charlene F. Agustin, Jose Donato A. Magno, and Eric Oliver D. Sison

Section of Cardiology, Department of Medicine, University of the Philippines-Philippine General Hospital, Philippines

Correspondence should be addressed to Valerie R. Ramiro; vrramiro@yahoo.com

Academic Editor: Aiden Abidov

Background. Infective endocarditis (IE) involving the pulmonic valve and/or the pulmonary artery is rare. An unrepaired patent ductus arteriosus (PDA) is a risk factor for IE. A previous IE is also a risk factor that predisposes to IE recurrence. Discriminating between IE recurrence and a persistence of a vegetation from a previously treated IE can be difficult. We present the case of a 19-year-old primigravid with an unrepaired PDA and a history of IE treated 7 years prior, with positive blood cultures and vegetations on the pulmonic valve and pulmonary artery seen on transthoracic echocardiogram (TTE). *Methods and Results.* On TTE, a small-sized PDA with a Qp : Qs of 1.18 and vegetations on the pulmonic valve and pulmonary artery were documented. Despite the paucity of symptoms, she was empirically treated as culture-negative IE and given 2 weeks of ceftriaxone. Repeat TTE done after 2 weeks only showed a slight decrease in the vegetation size. Due to the paucity of symptoms of infection, lack of growth of the vegetation, and absence of embolic events, the vegetations were deemed to be persistent remnants from the previous IE rather than a recurrent IE. She was advised surgical PDA closure and harvest of vegetations after delivery, but the patient did not consent. The rest of her perinatal course was uneventful. *Conclusion.* Persistence of vegetations despite successful medical treatment occurs in some cases and has not been reported to be associated with increased morbidity. Therefore, a follow-up of IE after treatment should be guided by the clinical course and response to therapy as well as the echocardiographic morphology of vegetations over time.

1. Introduction

The involvement of the pulmonic valve and the pulmonary artery in infective endocarditis (IE) is rare. Unrepaired congenital heart disease (CHD), including patent ductus arteriosus (PDA), is a risk factor for IE. A previous IE is likewise a significant risk factor that predisposes to IE recurrence. Discriminating between IE recurrence and a persistence of a vegetation from a previously treated IE can be difficult. This paper is aimed at describing a case of pulmonic valve and pulmonary artery vegetations in a pregnant patient with an unrepaired PDA and a distant history of IE treatment. This is the first documented case of pulmonic valve and pulmonary artery vegetation in a patient with a PDA in our institution.

2. Case

This is the case of 19-year-old primigravid with an unrepaired PDA who was incidentally found to have vegetations on the pulmonary artery and pulmonic valve on routine prenatal transthoracic echocardiogram (TTE).

She had an unremarkable childhood until 10 years old when she was diagnosed with moderate patent ductus arteriosus, presenting as exertional dyspnea. She was lost to follow-up until 2 years later, at 12 years old, when she was admitted at the emergency room for edema, exertional dyspnea, and orthopnea. On physical examination, she was in respiratory distress, tachypneic with alar flaring, and had bilateral crackles. She was initially treated for community-acquired pneumonia and pulmonary tuberculosis, with initial

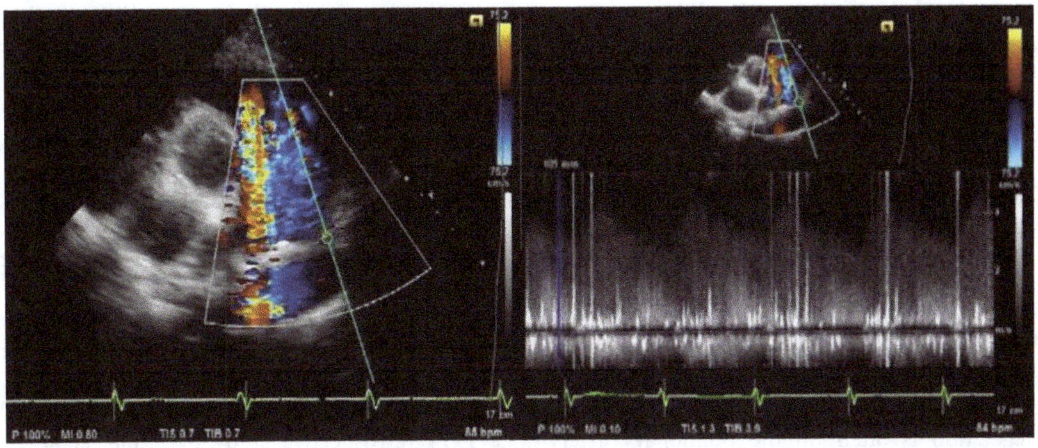

FIGURE 1: In the short axis view at the level of the aortic valve, there is a retrograde mosaic jet entering the distal pulmonary artery from the posterolateral direction, indicative of patent ductus arteriosus, with the following measurements: PSAX 9 mm, 10 mm (with color); suprasternal 8.1 mm, 1 mm (with color). Continuous flow across the defect is demonstrated on spectral Doppler. Computed Qp : Qs is 1.18.

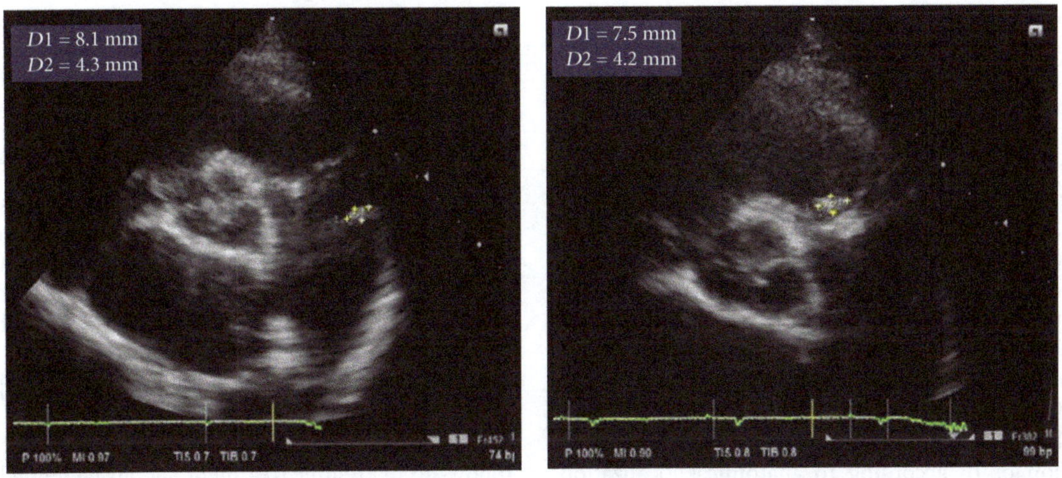

(a) (b)

FIGURE 2: In the short axis view at the level of the aortic valve, there are mobile echogenic vegetations attached to the pulmonary artery (a) measuring 8.1 × 4.3 mm and on the pulmonic valve (b) measuring 7.5 × 4.2 mm.

blood cultures yielding *Streptococcus viridans*. This was treated with Penicillin G. However, despite improvement of pneumonia, she was persistently febrile. Repeat blood cultures were positive for *Pseudomonas putida*. A TTE revealed multiple vegetations at the pulmonary artery and pulmonic valve. The IE was then treated with a 6-week course of intravenous meropenem. Furosemide, digoxin, and enalapril were also initiated for the heart failure. Surgery to close the PDA and remove the vegetations was offered but was not done due to the lack of consent and funds. Serial TTE done during the following year did not show a significant decrease in the size of the pulmonary artery masses. She was again lost to follow-up but continued taking furosemide, digoxin, and enalapril.

She returned to our institution for prenatal care. She discontinued taking furosemide, enalapril, and digoxin at the start of pregnancy. Given her history of a congenital heart disease, a TTE was ordered as part of the prenatal work-up. The TTE was done on her 29th week AOG, and it revealed a PDA with a computed Qp : Qs of 1.18 (see Figure 1), as well as vegetations on the pulmonic valve and pulmonary artery (see Figure 2).

Despite the absence of fever and signs of worsening heart failure, she was preemptively admitted and treated empirically for IE with intravenous ceftriaxone. During this period, she did not have fever nor signs of decompensation. Serial blood cultures were negative. On repeat TTE after 2 weeks, there was only a slight decrease in the size of the vegetation and it was treated as a persistent vegetation from her previous bout of IE at 12 years old. She was advised surgery, for closure of the PDA and harvest of vegetations, after delivery, but the patient did not consent. The rest of her perinatal course was uneventful.

3. Discussion

According to the European Society of Cardiology (ESC), at present, 0.2 to 4% of all pregnancies in western industrialized countries are complicated by cardiovascular diseases. Maternal heart disease, in general, is now said to be the major cause of maternal death during pregnancy. Because of improved treatment of CHD during childhood, more of these patients reach child-bearing age. In western countries, CHD is the most frequent cardiovascular disease present during pregnancy (75–82%) [1]. In our institution, rheumatic heart disease is still the predominant cardiac complication among pregnant patients followed by CHD [2]. Another study done in our institution showed that among pregnant patients with CHD, PDA (20%) was one of the most common lesions encountered [3]. Patients with small-sized PDA, without Eisenmenger syndrome, may tolerate pregnancy well [1].

An unrepaired PDA is a risk factor for IE, and when it occurs, the vegetation is often on the pulmonary artery side of the PDA [4]. The proposed pathogenesis of IE associated with CHD involves complex interactions among the damaged valvular or mural endocardium exposing the matrix proteins to thromboplastin and tissue factor, formation of a nonbacterial thrombotic endarteritis, and eventual microbial adherence, colonization, and replication [4]. The turbulent blood flow through the aorta and pulmonary artery which causes endothelial injury and subsequent seeding of pathogens onto the injured endothelium is central to the proposed pathogenetic mechanisms for the development of vegetations particularly in patients with PDA [5].

IE involving the pulmonic valve is rare. The estimated incidence of IE associated with PDA was reported to be 1% per year with the decline in recent years attributed to early treatment with routine closure of PDA, improved dental care, and prevalent use of antibiotics both for prophylaxis and for IE treatment [4]. A review done by Knirsch and Nadal in 2011 on IE in CHD presented pooled percentages of distribution of IE according to anatomical localization based on data of retrospective clinical studies. Affectation of the pulmonic valve was 8.8%, the pulmonary artery was 2.3%, and the PDA was 2.7% [6]. A retrospective study done in our institution by Javier et al. reviewed 135 cases of patients with TTE findings consistent with IE from 2004 to 2009. Of these, 91 cases fulfilled Duke's criteria for definite IE. On their review, they found that CHD was the second most common underlying cardiac abnormality (17.5%), 21.1% of which was PDA [7].

There have been several case reports on IE involving either the pulmonary artery or the pulmonic valve, but their outcomes have either been unknown as the patient was lost to follow-up [8] or documented to be resolved by surgical resection or antibiotics [5, 9–11]. In our patient's case, the vegetation persisted despite completion of culture-guided antibiotic therapy during her initial episode of IE at 12 years old. A surgical harvest of the vegetation with concomitant closure of the PDA was not performed at the time as the patient was lost to follow-up.

A previous IE is a significant risk factor that predisposes to IE recurrence. A prospective cohort study by Alagna in 2013 reported a 4.8% rate of repeat IE. A previous IE was one of the associated risk factors, with odds ratio of 2.8 (95% CI 1.6-5.4) [12]. However, in patients with poor documentation or recall of their past medical history, discriminating between IE recurrence and a persistent or residual vegetation from a previously treated IE may be difficult.

There is no strong recommendation for the closure of a PDA to prevent an initial attack especially for small or silent PDA [13]. However, in our patient who had a history of previous IE, a surgical closure of the PDA with concomitant harvest of vegetations was warranted. Unfortunately, the patient did not consent to the procedure despite being advised of the risk of embolization of the vegetation and the risk of Eisenmenger syndrome.

Resolution of the vegetation after antibiotic treatment is one of the indications of successful treatment of IE. However, a 1994 retrospective study by Vuille et al. describing the natural course of vegetations after medical therapy found that out of 41 vegetations, 29 vegetations persisted at the end of treatment (59% of which had no significant change in size, and 52% appeared denser). This led to the conclusion that despite successful medical treatment, persistence of vegetations is still commonly demonstrated echocardiographically and that treatment of IE should be guided by the clinical evolution or response to therapy, rather than the echocardiographic changes of a vegetation [14]. In recent years, this concept is still maintained. The 2010 ESC recommendations for the practice of echocardiography in IE also acknowledge the difficulty of interpreting an unchanged or reduced vegetation size with antibiotic treatment. However, the progressive growth of a vegetation and increasing valvular regurgitation foreshadow poor prognosis as they are risk factors for embolic events and morbidity [15]. The mere persistence of a vegetation despite paucity of supportive evidence for IE, such as symptoms or positive blood cultures, is not associated with increased morbidity [16]. Therefore, a follow-up of IE after treatment should be guided mainly by the clinical course and response to therapy and not only by the change over time of the echocardiographic morphology of vegetations.

Disclosure

This case report has been presented in the following conferences: (i) poster presentation, Echo ASE ASEAN Symposium, Manila, Philippines, March 2018; (ii) poster presentation, Asian Pacific Society of Cardiology Congress, Taipei, Taiwan, May 2018; and (iii) third place, oral presentation, Philippine General Hospital Annual Research Forum, October 2018.

References

[1] European Society of Gynecology (ESG), Association for European Paediatric Cardiology (AEPC), Association for European Paediatric Cardiology (AEPC) et al., "ESC Guidelines on the management of cardiovascular diseases during pregnancy: The task force on the management of cardiovascular diseases during pregnancy of the European Society of Cardiology (ESC)," *European Heart Journal*, vol. 32, no. 24, pp. 3147–3197, 2011.

[2] J. E. D. L. Duya, A. D. C. Javier, M. A. Vicente et al., "Pregnancy in adults with congenital heart disease," in *Philippine General Hospital Adult Congenital Heart Disease*, p. 162, Section of Cardiology, Department of Medicine, University of the Philippines Manila - Philippine General Hospital, 2nd edition, 2016.

[3] J. T. Reyes, R. B. Capito, and F. R. Punzalan, "Clinical profile and outcomes of pregnant patients with congenital heart diseases at the University of the Philippines-Philippine General Hospital (UP-PGH)," *Philippine Journal of Cardiology*, vol. 40, no. 1, pp. 31–35, 2013, 2012.

[4] D. J. Schneider and J. W. Moore, "Patent ductus arteriosus," *Circulation*, vol. 114, no. 17, pp. 1873–1882, 2006.

[5] K. N. Choi, T. H. Yang, B. S. Park et al., "A case with patent ductus arteriosus complicated by pulmonary artery endarteritis," *Journal of Cardiovascular Ultrasound*, vol. 16, no. 3, pp. 90–92, 2008.

[6] W. Knirsch and D. Nadal, "Infective endocarditis in congenital heart disease," *European Journal of Pediatrics*, vol. 170, no. 9, pp. 1111–1127, 2011.

[7] A. C. Javier, F. E. Punzalan, N. S. Abelardo, E. M. Salvana, and K. Leyritana, "P031 The changing face of infective endocarditis in the adult Filipino: a six year review (2004-2009) at the Philippine General Hospital," *International Journal of Cardiology*, vol. 147, Supplement 1, pp. S17–S18, 2011.

[8] R. Kadakia, J. Giullian, and H. Dokainish, "Patent ductus arteriosus complicated by pulmonary artery endarteritis in an adult," *Echocardiography*, vol. 21, no. 7, pp. 665–667, 2004.

[9] L. R. Cuenza, A. A. Adiong, and L. W. S. Rondilla, "Pulmonary endarteritis in a patient with patent ductus arteriosus and a bicuspid aortic valve," *Philippine Journal of Internal Medicine*, vol. 52, no. 4, pp. 1–3, 2014.

[10] Y. Sugimura, M. Katoh, and M. Toyama, "Patent ductus arteriosus with pulmonary endarteritis," *Internal Medicine*, vol. 52, no. 18, pp. 2157-2158, 2013.

[11] A. Yanýk, E. Yetkin, M. Lleri, G. Yetkin, K. Penen, and S. Göskel, "Vegetation due to *Streptococcus viridans* in the pulmonary artery in a child with patent ductus arteriosus," *International Journal of Cardiology*, vol. 72, no. 2, pp. 189–191, 2000.

[12] L. Alagna, L. P. Park, B. P. Nicholson et al., "Repeat endocarditis: analysis of risk factors based on the International Collaboration on Endocarditis – Prospective Cohort Study," *Clinical Microbiology and Infection*, vol. 20, no. 6, pp. 566–575, 2014.

[13] E. B. Fortescue, J. E. Lock, T. Galvin, and D. B. McElhinney, "To close or not to close: the very small patent ductus arteriosus," *Congenital Heart Disease*, vol. 5, no. 4, pp. 354–365, 2010.

[14] C. Vuille, M. Nidorf, A. E. Weyman, and M. H. Picard, "Natural history of vegetations during successful medical treatment of endocarditis," *American Heart Journal*, vol. 128, no. 6, pp. 1200–1209, 1994.

[15] G. Habib, L. Badano, C. Tribouilloy et al., "Recommendations for the practice of echocardiography in infective endocarditis," *European Journal of Echocardiography*, vol. 11, no. 2, pp. 202–219, 2010.

[16] S. D. Solomon, J. Wu, and L. Gillam, "Chapter 14 Echocardiography," in *Braunwald's Heart Disease*, p. 236, Elsevier/-Saunders, Philadelphia, PA, USA, 10th edition, 2015.

22

Rotational Atherectomy-Assisted Crossing of a Complex Right Coronary Artery Lesion using the Retrograde Approach

Abdul-Subulr Yakubu,[1] **Xiaoqiang Zhang**,[2] **and Bin Zhang**[3]

[1]*Tamale Teaching Hospital, Tamale, Ghana*
[2]*Chengdu 2nd People Hospital, China*
[3]*Second Division of the Cardiology Department, Guangdong Cardiovascular Institute, Guangdong General Hospital, Guangdong, China*

Correspondence should be addressed to Abdul-Subulr Yakubu; subulr87@gmail.com

Academic Editor: Yigit Canga

Chronic total occlusion lesions present a major challenge for the interventional cardiologist. In this case, we report the successful use of rotational atherectomy to facilitate retrograde percutaneous coronary intervention of a complex totally occluded right coronary artery after modification of the proximal cap of the lesion to enable placement of the RotaWire in the vessel architecture.

1. Introduction

The results of percutaneous coronary interventions (PCI) have dramatically improved in the last decades. Despite this improvement, chronic total occlusion (CTO) lesions still remain a major challenge of interventional cardiology due to the complexity of these lesions. As CTO equipment and techniques continue to improve, so has the success of wiring occlusive lesions [1]. Rotational atherectomy (RA) in CTO has found use in situations where balloon or microcatheter advancement poses a challenge following successful guide wire crossing. This approach has been found to be feasible and safe and to increase the procedural success rate in these tough CTO lesions with heavy calcification [2]. However, its role in heavily calcified wire-uncrossable lesions is less well established and RA is generally considered contraindicated in these situations.

2. Case Presentation

The patient is a 68-year-old male with chronic kidney disease on peritoneal dialysis for 3 years. He presented with recurrent exertional chest pain at a local facility where he underwent coronary angiography showing complex 3-vessel disease with severe diffuse calcification of all coronary arteries. The proximal left anterior descending (LAD) and left circumflex (LCX) arteries showed 99% stenosis, and the right coronary artery (RCA) was totally occluded (Figure 1). A broken coronary guide wire was left in situ following a failed attempt at RCA revascularization.

The patient was referred to the Guangdong Cardiovascular Institute for angioplasty. The RCA was engaged with a 7-French Amplatz left 0.75 guiding catheter and the left coronary artery (LCA) with 7-French XB 3.5 catheter. Antegrade crossing of the RCA chronic total occlusion (CTO) lesion with various guide wires including Pilot 150 and 200, UB3, and Conquest Pro failed necessitating a switchover to the retrograde strategy. The LAD lesion was prepared with rotational atherectomy, and the proximal segment was stented with a $3.0 * 24$ mm drug-eluting stent (DES). The RCA was approached retrogradely through the first septal collateral using SION blue guide wire through a 150 cm Corsair microcatheter (Asahi Intecc, Nagoya, Japan) and advanced to the distal cap of the CTO lesion. A Pilot 150, Pilot 200, UB3, and Conquest Pro guide wires failed to cross to the proximal true lumen. Through the antegrade

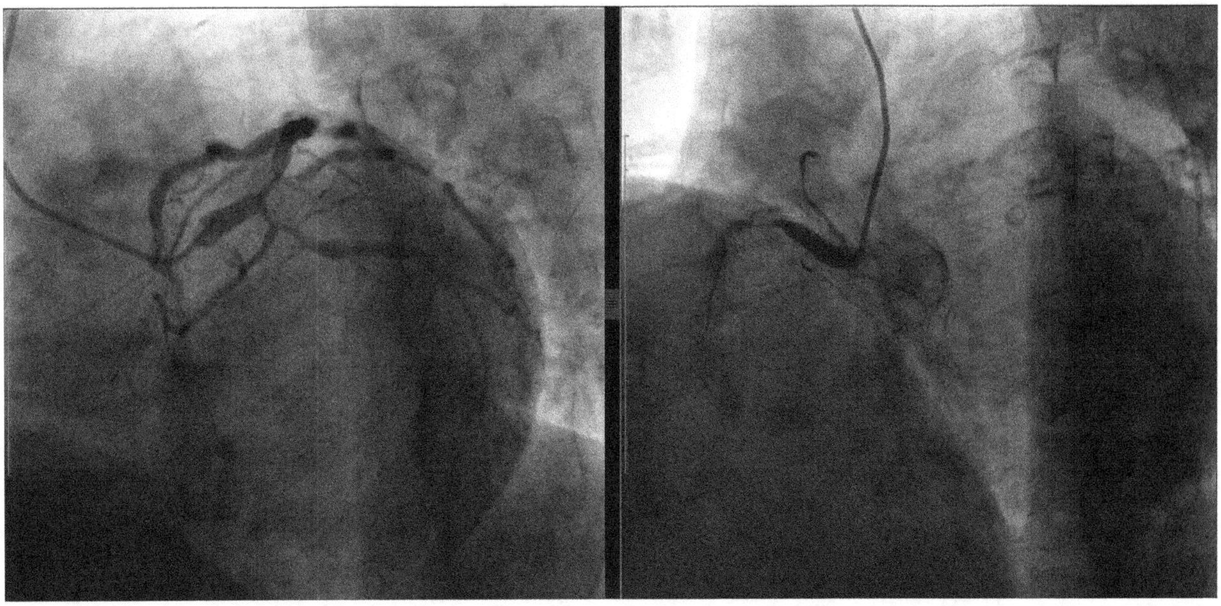

FIGURE 1: (a) Coronary angiogram of the LCA showing a severe bifurcation lesion involving the proximal LAD and LCX. (b) RCA angiogram shows a proximal CTO with a diffusely calcified vessel. There is a broken guide wire tip in the mid portion of the RCA from the previously failed PCI attempt.

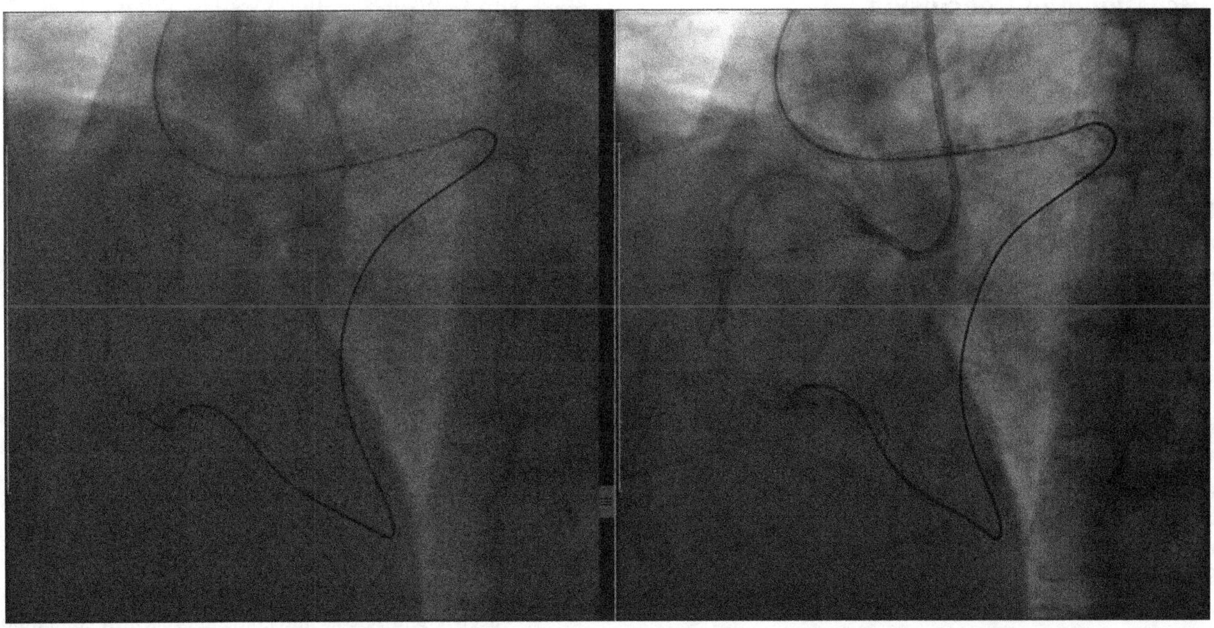

FIGURE 2: (a) Rotational atherectomy through the vessel architecture of the proximal segment of the RCA CTO lesion. (b) Guide extension catheter (Guidezilla) placed through antegrade guiding catheter helps with tracking the retrograde guide wire into the antegrade guiding catheter.

guide and with the help of stiffer guide wires (Pilot 200, Conquest Pro), the proximal cap of the CTO lesion was punctured and modified. This eventually facilitated the placement of a RotaWire (Boston Scientific, Marlborough, MA, USA) through the architecture of the occluded vessel followed by rotational atherectomy with a small-sized (1.25 mm) burr. Repeated cycles of proximal cap modification with further advancement of the RotaWire and rotational atherectomy through the vessel architecture facilitated passage of the antegrade gear (microcatheter and guide extension catheter) through the long CTO segment (Figure 2).

Reverse controlled antegrade and retrograde subintimal tracking (reverse CART) facilitated passage of the retrograde guide wire into the antegrade guide extension (Guidezilla, Boston Scientific) and guiding catheter. A successful "rendezvous" between the retrograde microcatheter and an antegrade RotaWire (Boston Scientific, Marlborough, MA) was achieved, followed by further rotational atherectomy into

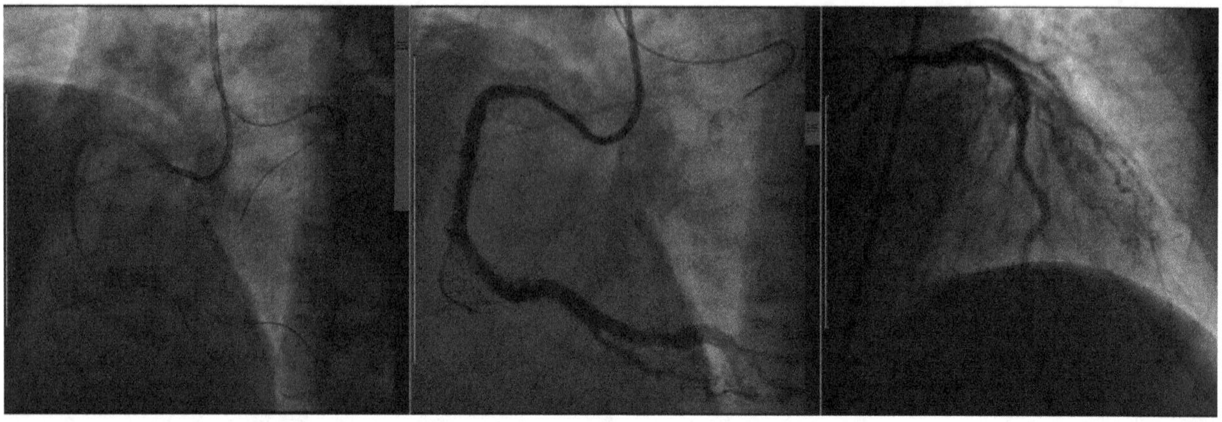

Figure 3: (a) Successful wiring of RCA into PD and PL blanches. PD = posterior descending; PL = posterolateral. (b) RCA angiogram postprocedure. (c) Left angiogram postprocedure.

the distal true lumen. The procedure was completed using standard techniques after exchanging for a workhorse guide wire. Three DES were implanted into the RCA with satisfactory final results (Figure 3). The whole procedure lasted 03:04 hours of which 02:11 hours were spent on the RCA lesion. About 260 milliliters of contrast agent was used.

3. Discussion and Conclusion

Flexibility, creativity, and patience are often required to achieve success in CTO PCI as each CTO lesion is unique. Retrograde CTO PCI has revolutionized CTO percutaneous coronary intervention and in experienced operators is as effective and safe as an antegrade approach [3–5].

Rotational atherectomy has found use in balloon or microcatheter uncrossable lesions, which are a relatively common occurrence in CTO PCI. Whilst the feasibility of RA in CTO PCI has already been suggested, current practice and recommendations dictate that an attempt at RA should follow confirmation of placement of the guide wire in the true lumen [6]. Rotational atherectomy through a dissection plane is generally contraindicated because of concerns of expansion of the dissection plane and vessel perforation. Recently, however, it has been demonstrated that RA can be used successfully provided one remains in the vessel architecture and employs a small- to medium-sized burr [7, 8]. Rotational atherectomy in CTO has been found to be safe and effective with outcomes not adversely affected by the presence of a prior dissection [9].

Not infrequently, particularly in long, tortuous, and calcified lesions, as in our case, a true-to-true lumen wiring is unsuccessful. The concept of "vessel architecture" is based on the distinction between coronary structures (plaque, intima, media, and adventitia) and the extravascular space and represents a safe work environment for guide wire and device manipulation [10]. Hence, the ability to manage the subadventitial space is invaluable in contemporary CTO PCI. In the absence of intravascular imaging, the location of the guide wire within the vessel architecture in our case was guided by the tactile feedback of the wire as well as the contralateral angiogram. Operator experience in such situations is key to producing a successful outcome as RA in the adventitia (versus subintimal or intraplague) is associated with a higher likelihood of perforation. The operator in our case is a very experienced interventionist who has performed over one thousand retrograde PCI procedures.

Our case demonstrates the successful use of RA through a calcified and totally occluded RCA segment to facilitate retrograde PCI after an initial failure of the traditional antegrade and retrograde techniques. The proximal cap of the CTO lesion was modified with high tip-load guide wires to facilitate placement of the RotaWire (Boston Scientific) within the vessel architecture of CTO segment followed by successful RA and retrograde crossing by reverse CART.

References

[1] T. DeMartini, "Advances in retrograde technique for coronary chronic total occlusions," *Current Cardiology Reviews*, vol. 10, no. 2, pp. 158–160, 2014.

[2] W.-C. Huang, H.-I. Teng, W.-L. Chan, and T.-M. Lu, "Short-term and long-term clinical outcomes of rotational atherectomy in resistant chronic total occlusion," *Journal of Interventional Cardiology*, vol. 31, no. 4, pp. 458–464, 2018.

[3] A. P. Kotsia, G. C. Christopoulos, and E. S. Brilakis, "Use of the retrograde approach for treating a "balloon-uncrossable" coronary chronic total occlusion," *Interventional Cardiology*, vol. 6, no. 3, pp. 261–264, 2014.

[4] C. K. Lee, Y. H. Chen, M. S. Lin et al., "Retrograde approach is as effective and safe as antegrade approach in contemporary percutaneous coronary intervention for chronic total occlusion: a Taiwan single-center registry study," *Acta Cardiologica Sinica*, vol. 33, no. 1, pp. 20–27, 2017.

[5] O. Kwon, P. H. Lee, S.-W. Lee et al., "Retrograde approach for the percutaneous recanalisation of coronary chronic total occlusions: contribution to clinical practice and long-term outcomes," *EuroIntervention*, vol. 15, no. 4, pp. e354–e361, 2019.

[6] S. K. Sharma, M. I. Tomey, P. S. Teirstein et al., "North American expert review of rotational atherectomy," *Circulation. Cardiovascular Interventions*, vol. 12, no. 5, article e007448, 2019.

[7] G. Touma, D. Ramsay, and J. Weaver, "Chronic total occlusions – Current techniques and future directions," *IJC Heart & Vasculature*, vol. 7, pp. 28–39, 2015.

[8] G. Capretti, M. Carlino, A. Colombo, and L. Azzalini, "Rotational atherectomy in the subadventitial space to allow safe and successful chronic total occlusion recanalization: pushing the limit further," *Catheterization and Cardiovascular Interventions*, vol. 91, no. 1, pp. 47–52, 2018.

[9] C. Brinkmann, A. Eitan, C. Schwencke, D. G. Mathey, and J. Schofer, "Rotational atherectomy in CTO lesions: too risky? Outcome of rotational atherectomy in CTO lesions compared to non-CTO lesions," *EuroIntervention*, vol. 14, no. 11, pp. E1192–E1198, 2018.

[10] L. Azzalini, M. Carlino, E. S. Brilakis et al., "Subadventitial techniques for chronic total occlusion percutaneous coronary intervention: the concept of "vessel architecture"," *Catheterization and Cardiovascular Interventions*, vol. 91, no. 4, pp. 725–734, 2018.

23

Sibutramine as a Cause of Sudden Cardiac Death

Miguel Rodriguez-Guerra,[1] Mayank Yadav,[1,2] Manoj Bhandari,[1] Archna Sinha,[3] Jonathan N. Bella,[1,2] and Eduard Sklyar[1,2]

[1]*BronxCare Health System, New York, USA*
[2]*Icahn School of Medicine at Mount Sinai, New York, USA*
[3]*St. Charles Hospital, Port Jefferson, New York, USA*

Correspondence should be addressed to Miguel Rodriguez-Guerra; m.rodriguezg.md@gmail.com

Academic Editor: Manabu Shirotani

Importance. Sibutramine was withdrawn from the US market due to association with adverse cardiovascular outcomes especially with patients having preexisting cardiac disease. However, continued presence of sibutramine in herbal medications is a concern to public safety. *Results.* We report a case of a patient with no evidence of previous coronary heart disease, who presented with non-ST elevation acute coronary syndrome (NSTE-ACS). Urgent coronary catheterization showed nonobstructive coronaries. However, patient died unexpectedly within 24 hours of admission. The patient denied toxic habits but was taking over-the-counter weight loss herbal supplements. Complete autopsy was performed which showed sibutramine in the toxicology. Patient died due to complications of acute inadvertent intoxication of sibutramine. *Conclusion and Relevance.* This is the first case report in literature showing association of sibutramine to sudden cardiac death in patients with no prior cardiac history. The continued presence of sibutramine in some over-the-counter weight loss formulations is a very concerning public health issue.

1. Introduction

Obesity is one of the modifiable cardiovascular risk factors, and its incidence has increased exponentially over the years. Sibutramine is a combined norepinephrine and serotonin reuptake inhibitor used to reduce appetite and promote weight loss in combination with diet and exercise [1]. At a daily dose of 10–20 mg, it was initially considered to have an excellent safety profile [1, 2]. However, the Sibutramine Cardiovascular Outcomes (SCOUT) trial showed that it has adverse cardiovascular outcomes, especially with patients having preexisting cardiac disease [3]. Based on this report, sibutramine was withdrawn from the US market after the Food and Drug Administration (FDA) recommendations in October 2010. We report a case of a patient who was taking inadvertently sibutramine as a component of over-the-counter weight loss herbal medications who later developed non-ST elevation acute coronary syndrome (NSTE-ACS) and sudden cardiac death.

2. Case

A 59-year-old Hispanic female presented to the emergency department (ED) with abdominal pain, nausea, and vomiting that began early in the morning on the day of the presentation. She was drowsy but arousable. She denied any chest pain, shortness of breath, fever, cough, or headache. On further questioning, she denied any history of travel or sick contacts—no history of smoking, drugs, or excessive alcohol use. The patient's medications included benazepril, calcium, alendronic acid, and a "tomato extract herbal supplement" for the weight loss. The previous night she had a vegetable soup before going to sleep and had been in apparently good health until the day of the presentation.

On examination, she was afebrile with an irregularly irregular pulse rate of 60/minute, blood pressure of 130/80 mmHg, respiratory rate of 16/minute, and oxygen saturation of 90% at room air, which improved to 95% with 28% oxygen supplementation. Her complete blood count

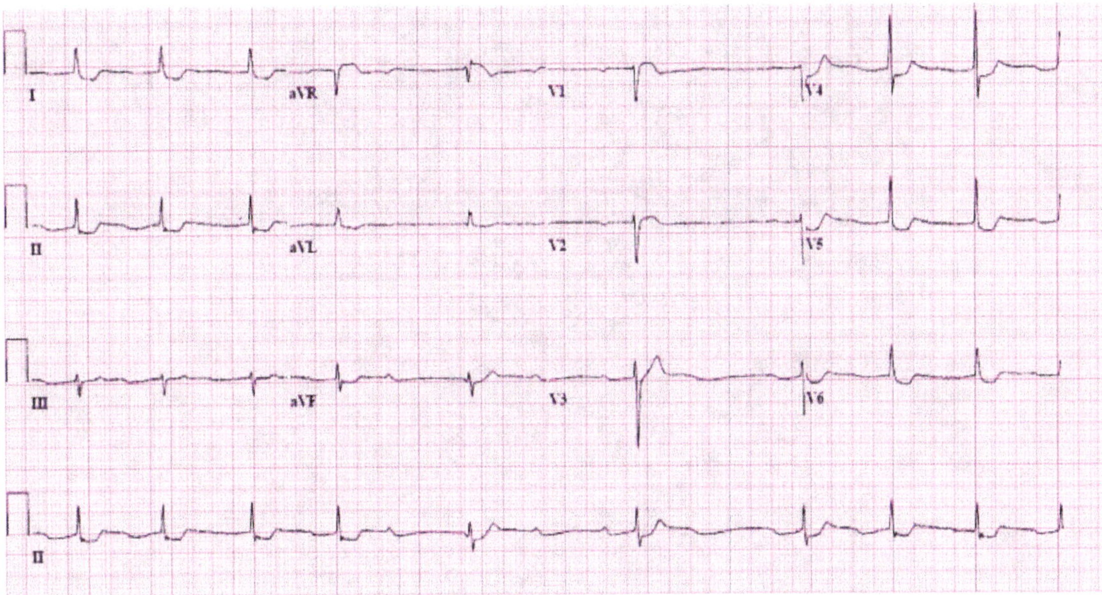

FIGURE 1: ECG at presentation showed normal sinus rhythm with ST elevation in lead aVR and ST depressions in multiple leads with high-degree atrioventricular (AV) block. ECG: electrocardiogram.

showed leukocytosis of 23.4 cells/dL. The chest X-ray was normal. Electrocardiogram (ECG) showed normal sinus rhythm with ST elevation in lead aVR and ST depressions in multiple leads with high-degree atrioventricular (AV) block (Figure 1). Echocardiogram showed normal left ventricular function and size, with no wall motion abnormalities. The cardiac enzymes, troponin T, and creatinine kinase were elevated, leading to the diagnosis of NSTE-ACS. However, cardiac catheterization showed only 50% stenosis of the proximal left anterior descending artery that could not explain the elevated cardiac enzyme and ECG changes (Figures 2(a) and 2(b)). She was subsequently transferred to the coronary care unit (CCU). In the CCU, the patient was tachypneic with rate 18-22/minute, with an oxygen saturation of 92-94% on 2 liters of oxygen, with a fluctuating mental status. Given elevated leukocyte count of 34.9 cells/dL on repeat complete blood count, broad-spectrum antibiotics (vancomycin, piperacillin-tazobactam, and metronidazole) were started. Computed tomography (CT) scan of the head was normal, and CT abdomen, which also included the lung bases, showed bilateral lower lobe airspace consolidation, possibly pneumonia, and normal finding on the abdominal scan. About 14 hours from her presentation to the hospital, she developed an episode ventricular tachycardia, which reverted spontaneously back to her usual rhythm. Later, she became bradycardic and went into asystole. The patient could not be resuscitated, and she died 15 hours after presentation to the hospital. Because of unexplained death within 24 hours of hospital admission, a complete autopsy was done. At autopsy, there was no evidence of pulmonary embolism or acute myocardial infarction. However, her forensic serum toxicology screen showed sibutramine levels of 0.27 ng/mL, and its metabolized forms of desmethylsibutramine and didesmethylsibutramine were at 0.59 ng/mL and 0.44 ng/mL, respectively. The cause of death was determined as "Complications of Acute Sibutramine Intoxication."

3. Discussion

Sibutramine is a combined norepinephrine and serotonin reuptake inhibitor used as an antiobesity agent to reduce appetite and promote weight loss in combination with diet and exercise [1]. FDA approved it in 1997 in the United States. It initially showed good safety profile [2]. It was shown to improve insulin resistance, glucose metabolism, dyslipidemia, and inflammatory markers, which led to the hypothesis that it may have antiatherogenic properties [1]. However, it also exerts a peripheral sympathomimetic effect, which induces a moderate increase in heart rate and attenuates the reduction in BP attributable to weight loss or even slightly increases BP [1, 4]. It was also shown to prolong QT interval, which could potentially increase the risk of cardiac arrhythmias [1].

Our patient presented with the NSTE-ACS, which on coronary angiography did not show any culprit lesion. The similar presentation was reported by previous case reports [5–7]. All except one case report [8], no coronary lesion was found on coronary angiogram. In all the case reports [5–8], patients were overweight but did not have any comorbidity, including known cardiac disease. However, in the randomized studies, sibutramine was attributed being a high risk of cardiac events only in patients with either known to have cardiac disease or high risk due to comorbidities [3]. The possible explanation for the above presentation can be coronary vasospasm, which is plausible, given the sympathomimetic effects of sibutramine.

We could not find any case report directly attributing sibutramine to sudden cardiac death. Our patient died within 15 hours of presentation and has one episode of ventricular

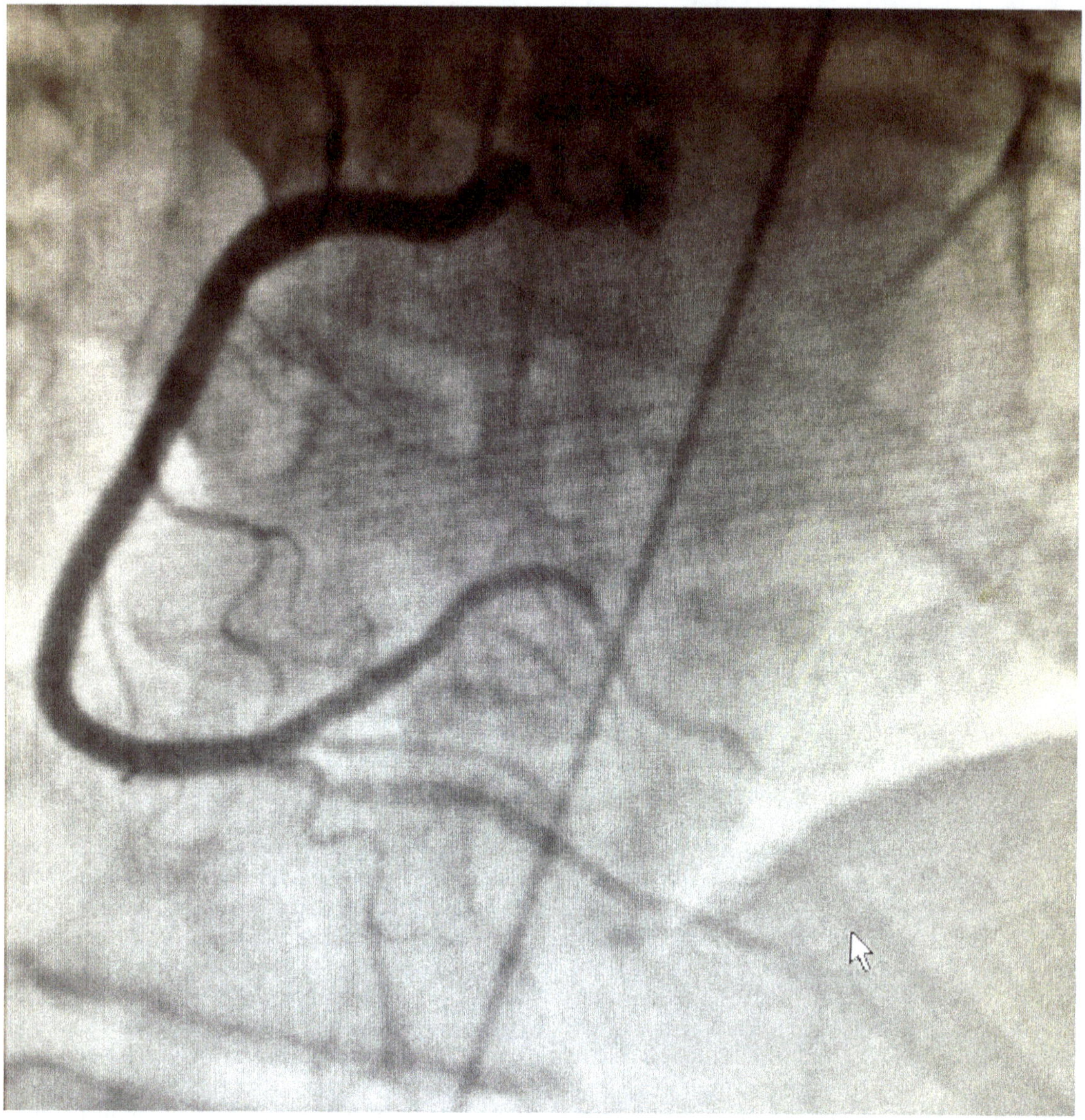

(a)

Figure 2: Continued.

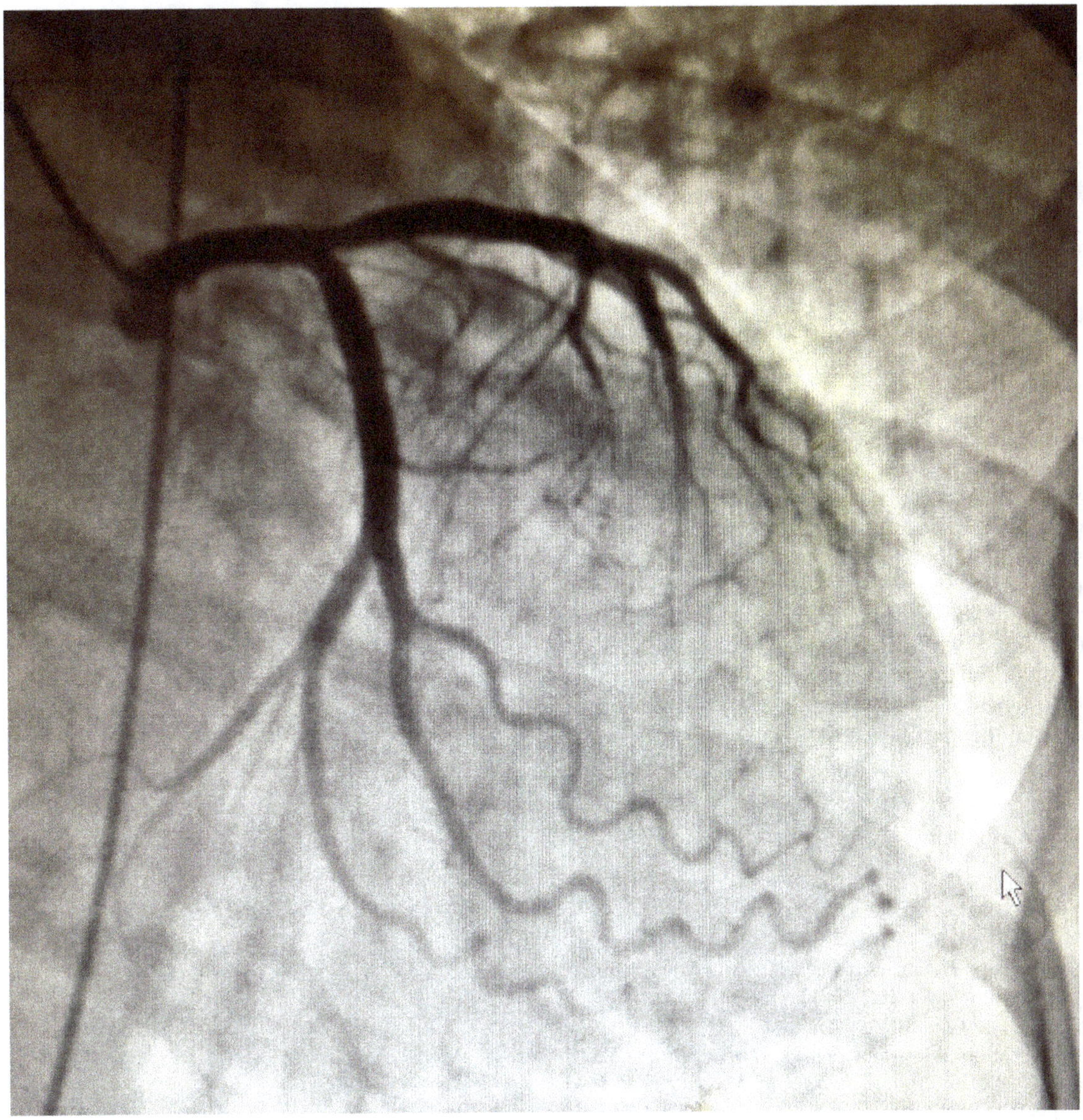

(b)

Figure 2: (a) The right coronary angiogram in the left anterior oblique cranial view showing the patent right coronary artery. (b) The left coronary angiogram in the right anterior oblique caudal view showing 50% lesion in the proximal left anterior descending artery, which is not consistent with the presentation as non-ST segment elevation acute coronary syndrome.

tachycardia, which reverted to normal sinus rhythm. Later, the patient was noted to be bradycardic and hypoxic before demise. The autopsy done did not show anything that could explain the cause of death. However, toxicology studies found significant levels of sibutramine and its metabolites desmethylsibutramine and didesmethylsibutramine. As per the autopsy report, the cause of death was determined as "Complications of Acute Sibutramine Intoxication."

Since 2002, several cardiovascular adverse events (hypertension, tachycardia, arrhythmias, and myocardial infarction) were reported in sibutramine-treated patients. This led to SCOUT trial evaluating the long-term effects of sibutramine treatment combined with diet and exercise on the rates of cardiovascular events and cardiovascular death among subjects who were at high cardiovascular risk [3]. It showed that in patients with preexisting cardiovascular conditions receiving long-term sibutramine treatment, there was an increased risk of nonfatal myocardial infarction and nonfatal stroke but not of cardiovascular death or death from any cause [3]. Because the benefit of sibutramine as a weight loss drug seems not to outweigh the cardiovascular risks, it was withdrawn from the US and European markets. However, the continued presence of sibutramine in some over-the-counter weight loss formulations is a very concerning public health issue. The FDA has now implemented stricter guidelines for the control of dietary supplements, which is a welcome step to ensure public safety [10]. Aggressive internet-based marketing plays a vital role in capturing customers for over-the-counter supplements; unfortunately, despite its withdrawal from the market since

2010, sibutramine continues to be present in many antiobesity food supplements sold on the Internet [11]. The current FDA website search for sibutramine mentions 250 results of public notice of the supplements which contain sibutramine. Still, one recent study showed that 66.7% of recalled supplements still available for purchase at least six months after FDA recalls remained adulterated with banned ingredients [12]. Further investigations are as needed to determine the effectiveness of policies on public safety, given the continued presence of some banned substances in some dietary supplements.

4. Conclusion

This case, though unfortunate eventual outcome, has few unique aspects that are worth reporting and sharing, so that knowledge thus gained can help to save other patients. First, to the best of our knowledge, this is the first case report showing an association of sibutramine with sudden cardiac death. Second, it is the sixth case report in PubMed in a patient with no medical comorbidities taking sibutramine that presented with NSTE-ACS [5–9]. Third, it is the concerning fact that the drug is still available to the patient as a component of some herbal weight reduction supplements despite being withdrawn from the market [5, 6].

References

[1] A. J. Scheen, "Cardiovascular risk-benefit profile of sibutramine," *American Journal of Cardiovascular Drugs*, vol. 10, no. 5, pp. 321–334, 2010.

[2] A. Wirth and J. Krause, "Long-term weight loss with sibutramine: a randomized controlled trial," *Journal of the American Medical Association*, vol. 286, no. 11, pp. 1331–1339, 2001.

[3] W. P. James, I. D. Caterson, W. Coutinho et al., "Effect of sibutramine on cardiovascular outcomes in overweight and obese subjects," *The New England Journal of Medicine*, vol. 363, no. 10, pp. 905–917, 2010.

[4] A. Siebenhofer, K. Jeitler, K. Horvath et al., "Long-term effects of weight-reducing drugs in people with hypertension," *Cochrane Database of Systematic Reviews*, vol. 3, article Cd007654, 2016.

[5] S. M. Azarisman, Y. A. Magdi, S. Noorfaizan, and M. Oteh, "Myocardial infarction induced by appetite suppressants in Malaysia," *The New England Journal of Medicine*, vol. 357, no. 18, pp. 1873-1874, 2007.

[6] K. M. Yim, H. W. Ng, C. K. Chan, G. Yip, and F. L. Lau, "Sibutramine-induced acute myocardial infarction in a young lady," *Clinical Toxicology*, vol. 46, no. 9, pp. 877–879, 2008.

[7] J. Poss, M. Bohm, and A. Link, "32-year-old patient with acute myocardial infarction possibly induced by the appetite suppressant sibutramine," *Deutsche Medizinische Wochenschrift*, vol. 135, no. 19, pp. 965–968, 2010.

[8] E. Eroglu, G. Gemici, F. Bayrak, A. K. Kalkan, and M. Degertekin, "Acute myocardial infarction in a 24 year-old man possibly associated with sibutramine use," *International Journal of Cardiology*, vol. 137, no. 2, pp. e43–e45, 2009.

[9] P. A. Cohen, "Assessing supplement safety–the FDA's controversial proposal," *The New England Journal of Medicine*, vol. 366, no. 5, pp. 389–391, 2012.

[10] N. Bunya, K. Sawamoto, S. Uemura et al., "Cardiac arrest caused by sibutramine obtained over the Internet: a case of a young woman without pre-existing cardiovascular disease successfully resuscitated using extracorporeal membrane oxygenation," *Acute Medicine & Surgery*, vol. 4, pp. 334–337, 2017.

[11] *Food and Drug Administration*, 2020, https://www.fda.gov/consumers/consumer-updates/weight-loss-male-enhancement-and-other-products-sold-online-or-stores-may-be-dangerous.

[12] P. A. Cohen, G. Maller, R. DeSouza, and J. Neal-Kababick, "Presence of banned drugs in dietary supplements following FDA recalls," *Journal of the American Medical Association*, vol. 312, no. 16, pp. 1691–1693, 2014.

24

Sudden Cardiac Death: The Most Feared but Potentially Preventable Presentation of Wolff-Parkinson-White Syndrome

Ana Rita Pereira, Alexandra Briosa, Rita Miranda, Sofia Sequeira Almeida, Luís Brandão, and Hélder Pereira

Cardiology Department, Hospital Garcia de Orta, Avenida Torrado da Silva, 2805-267 Almada, Portugal

Correspondence should be addressed to Ana Rita Pereira; pereira.anaritaf@gmail.com

Academic Editor: Luigi Sciarra

Background. Wolff-Parkinson-White syndrome is an uncommon cardiac disorder characterized by the presence of one or more accessory pathways that predispose patients to frequent episodes of arrhythmias. The prognosis is usually good, but there is a lifetime risk of malignant arrhythmias and sudden cardiac death. *Case Summary.* A 25-year-old male presented a witnessed out-of-hospital cardiac arrest with ventricular fibrillation rhythm. Due to rapid initiation of prehospital advanced life support, return of spontaneous circulation was observed. During the transport to the hospital, an irregular wide complex tachycardia suggestive of preexcited atrial fibrillation with haemodynamic instability was also observed and a synchronized shock was applied. Baseline 12-lead electrocardiogram was compatible with sinus rhythm and ventricular preexcitation pattern. After clinical stabilization, an electrophysiological study was performed confirming the presence of a left anterolateral accessory pathway with a short antegrade effective refractory period. Successful radiofrequency catheter ablation was achieved. *Discussion.* The reported clinical case recalls fundamental features of the Wolff-Parkinson-White syndrome and outlines the increasing evidence and importance of the invasive risk stratification and even catheter ablation in asymptomatic patients who suffer from this uncommon disease that may have a dramatic and fatal initial clinical manifestation.

1. Introduction

Wolff-Parkinson-White (WPW) syndrome is an uncommon cardiac disorder characterized by the presence of one or more accessory pathways (APs) that predispose patients to arrhythmias [1–3]. The prognosis is usually good, but there is a lifetime risk of malignant arrhythmias and sudden cardiac death (SCD), which may be the first presentation of the disease [4]. The management of symptomatic patients is well established in the international guidelines for a long time [2, 3]. Otherwise, the approach of asymptomatic preexcitation patients is less defined. Herein, we present a clinical case that intends to resemble the potential lethality of the syndrome and to emphasize the importance of risk stratification of asymptomatic patients.

2. Case Presentation

A 25-year-old male with no personal or familial history of cardiovascular disease presented a witnessed out-of-hospital cardiac arrest. Prehospital emergency service was immediately activated, and cardiopulmonary resuscitation was promptly started. When the prehospital critical care team arrived, the cardiac rhythm was ventricular fibrillation (VF) and a biphasic shock of 200 J was applied with conversion to a regular wide complex tachycardia with a heart rate of 215 bpm (Figure 1). Advanced life support was proceeded. A total of four defibrillations was applied until return of spontaneous circulation. During the transport to the hospital, the patient became unstable again presenting irregular wide complex tachycardia suggestive of preexcited atrial

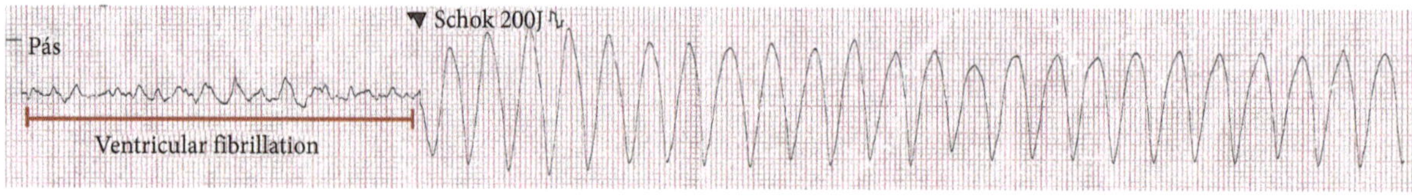

Figure 1: Twelve-lead electrocardiogram showing ventricular fibrillation. A biphasic shock of 200 J was applied with conversion to a regular wide complex tachycardia with a heart rate of 215 bpm.

fibrillation (AF) and a synchronized shock was applied (Figure 2). On arrival at the hospital, the patient was haemodynamically stable, with no significant changes on cardiopulmonary examination.

3. Investigation

No medication or drug abuse was reported. Serum potassium and magnesium levels were normal, and transthoracic echocardiogram excluded structural heart disease. However, 12-lead electrocardiogram (ECG) was compatible with sinus rhythm and ventricular preexcitation with shortened PR interval, delta waves in V3-V6 and inferior leads, and secondary ventricular repolarization abnormalities (Figure 3).

4. Diagnosis and Treatment

An electrophysiological study (EPS) was performed. Two catheters were positioned via the right femoral vein: an Inquiry decapolar 6F catheter (Abbott, St Paul, MN, USA) in the coronary sinus and a quadripolar catheter CRD 6F (St Jude Medical Inc, St Paul, MN, USA) in the right ventricle for His activity tracing and ventricular stimulation. Fluoroscopy integrated 3D-mapping using the CARTO 3 system (Biosense-Webster, Diamond Bar, CA, USA), and intracavitary recordings confirmed the presence of ventricular preexcitation via a left anterolateral AP (Figure 4) with a short antegrade effective refractory period (AERP) of 210 ms, anterograde block cycle length of 260 ms, and retrograde block cycle length of 250 ms. During the procedure, an orthodromic atrioventricular reentrant tachycardia (AVRT) was induced with a cycle length of 410 ms. Left heart cavities were approached using a fast-cath transseptal guiding introducer SL1 curve 8.5F (St Jude Medical Inc, St Paul, MN, USA) and a BRK transseptal needle (Abbott, St Paul, MN, USA). Radiofrequency ablation was performed using a ThermoCool SmartTouch DF curve catheter (Biosense-Webster, Diamond Bar, CA, USA). Conduction over the AP was successfully interrupted within 1 second of energy delivery (35 W). At the end of the procedure, there was no evidence of ventricular preexcitation. No periprocedural complications ensued.

5. Outcome and Follow-Up

The patient was discharged three days after the procedure. At discharge, 12-lead ECG showed sinus rhythm and absence of preexcitation pattern with no delta waves and PR interval at the lower limit of normal (PR 120 ms) but revealed peaked upright T waves in leads V3-V6 and inferior leads (Figure 5). At the 6-month follow-up, the patient was asymptomatic, no tachyarrhythmias were documented, and 12-lead ECG had no change relating to that at hospital discharge.

6. Discussion

WPW pattern occurs in 0.1 to 0.2% of the general population [5, 6]. The proportion of patients with WPW who are truly asymptomatic is unknown. Nonetheless, there seems to be agreement within the literature that more than 90% of children, approximately 65% of adolescents, and 40% of patients older than 30 years of age are asymptomatic [7, 8]. A rough extrapolation of the results published by Munger et al. reveals that an asymptomatic child or adolescent accumulates a 45% probability of remaining asymptomatic, with no arrhythmia, throughout their lifetime [7–9].

At the adult age, symptoms generally onset at a mean of 28 years [9]. At paediatric age, a bimodal distribution is observed with a first peak in the first month of life (including prenatally) and a secondary, more diffuse peak through the school age years [5]. Symptoms are mainly related to the occurrence of tachyarrhythmias: AVRT in 80% of the cases and AF in 20 to 30%, which is usually triggered by AVRT in the presence of high atrial vulnerability [1, 4, 7, 8]. Preexcited AF is a potentially life-threatening arrhythmia since rapid conduction to the ventricle over an AP with a short AERP may degenerate into VF and consequently cardiac arrest, as observed in the presented clinical case [1, 4]. In fact, SCD is the most feared clinical manifestation, occurring generally around the age of 20 to 30 years, as seen in our patient [7, 8, 10–12]. A 10-year risk of SCD of 0.15-0.24% [9] and an annual incidence of 0.01-0.5% in adults [9, 13] and 0.001-0.2% in children [13, 14] are estimated. Alarmingly, between 12% and 53% (average of 27%) of WPW patients presenting with cardiac arrest had no previous symptoms or knowledge of their diagnosis [7, 8, 10–12, 15]. Because of the increasing use of ECG in the general population, the number of asymptomatic patients with WPW patterns is expected to increase [5].

For the reasons above, risk assessment and management of asymptomatic preexcitation patients both in paediatric and adult age have been the focus of several recent publications [6, 11, 16–23]. Delise and Sciarra reviewed the results of these studies concluding that asymptomatic WPW is far from rare, absence of symptoms is not in itself a marker of low risk and do not predict the findings of risk stratification, electrophysiologic study has a high predictive value, and prophylactic ablation is highly effective in preventing fatal events [8]. All this new information is also reflected in the

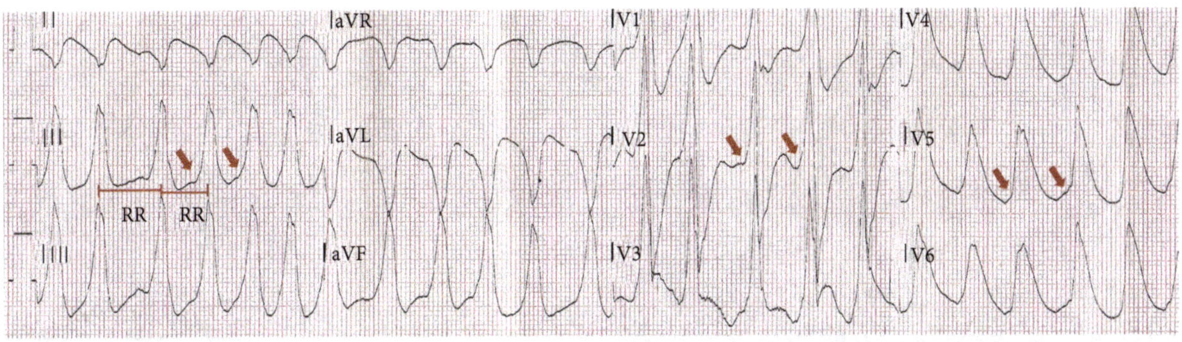

Figure 2: Twelve-lead electrocardiogram showing atrial fibrillation with a rapid preexcited ventricular response. Irregular RR intervals, wide QRS complexes with varying QRS width, and initial delta wave (arrow). The shortest preexcited RR interval is nearly 300 ms.

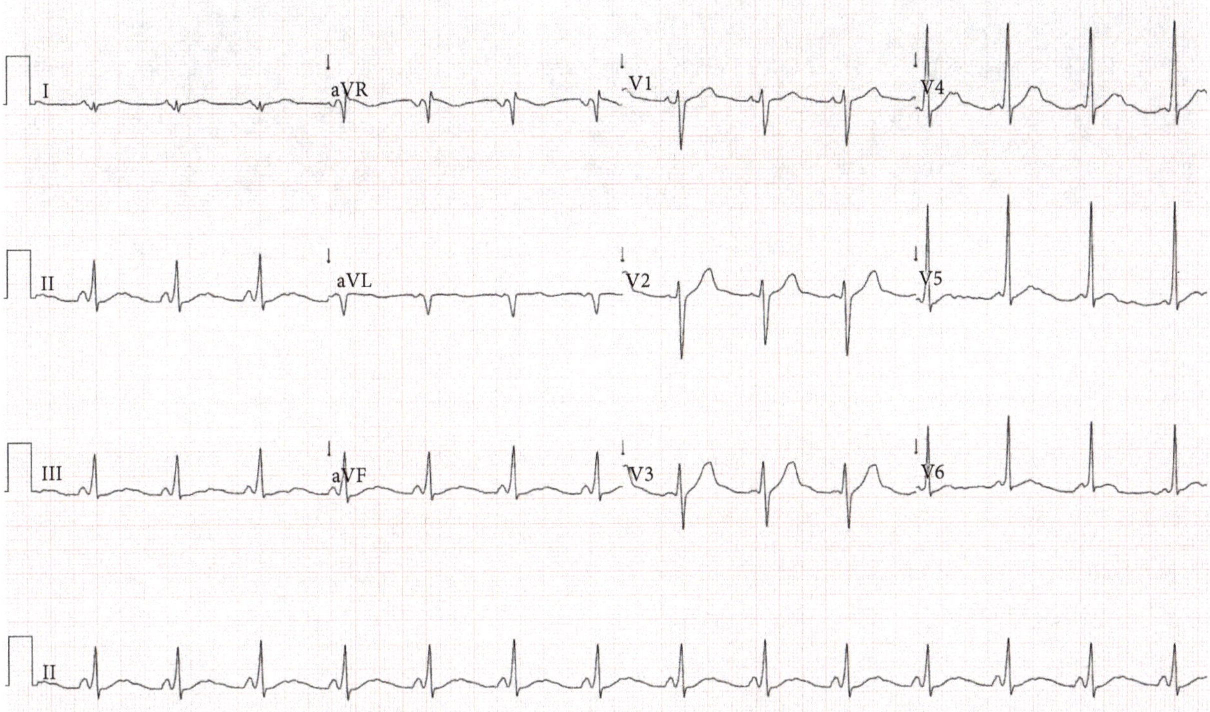

Figure 3: Twelve-lead electrocardiogram after conversion to sinus rhythm (=baseline electrocardiogram). Shortened PR interval, delta wave, and secondary repolarization abnormalities are seen. This ECG is indicative of WPW syndrome, and a left anterolateral AP is suggested by negative QRS in V1 lead, QS complex in aVL lead, and positive delta wave in V3-V6 leads and inferior leads.

2019 European Society of Cardiology (ESC) guidelines for the management of adult patients with supraventricular tachycardia [1].

Regarding risk assessment, several clinical features, invasive markers, and noninvasive markers are already recognized. Younger age and male gender are associated with an increased risk of SCD [13, 16, 20]. Invasive markers assessed by EPS of high risk comprise inducibility of AP-mediated tachycardia in the baseline state or during isoproterenol infusion [16, 20, 24], multiple APs [20], and demonstration of rapid conduction through the AP to the ventricles such as short preexcited RR interval during AF (≤250 ms) or a short AERP of the AP (≤250 ms) [16, 18, 20]. Abrupt and complete normalization of the PR interval with loss of delta wave during exercise testing or following procainamide, propafenone, or disopyramide administration has been considered a noninvasive marker of low risk [6, 9]. These risk markers are also applicable to the paediatric population since several dedicated studies have already demonstrated the validity of the noninvasive [15, 25, 26] and invasive [15, 17, 19, 27] parameters in this age.

In the 2019 ESC guidelines [1], there was no change in the symptomatic patients' approach but there was an upgrade of the asymptomatic patients' management. Invasive screening with an EPS is now recommended for patients with high-risk occupations or competitive athletes and

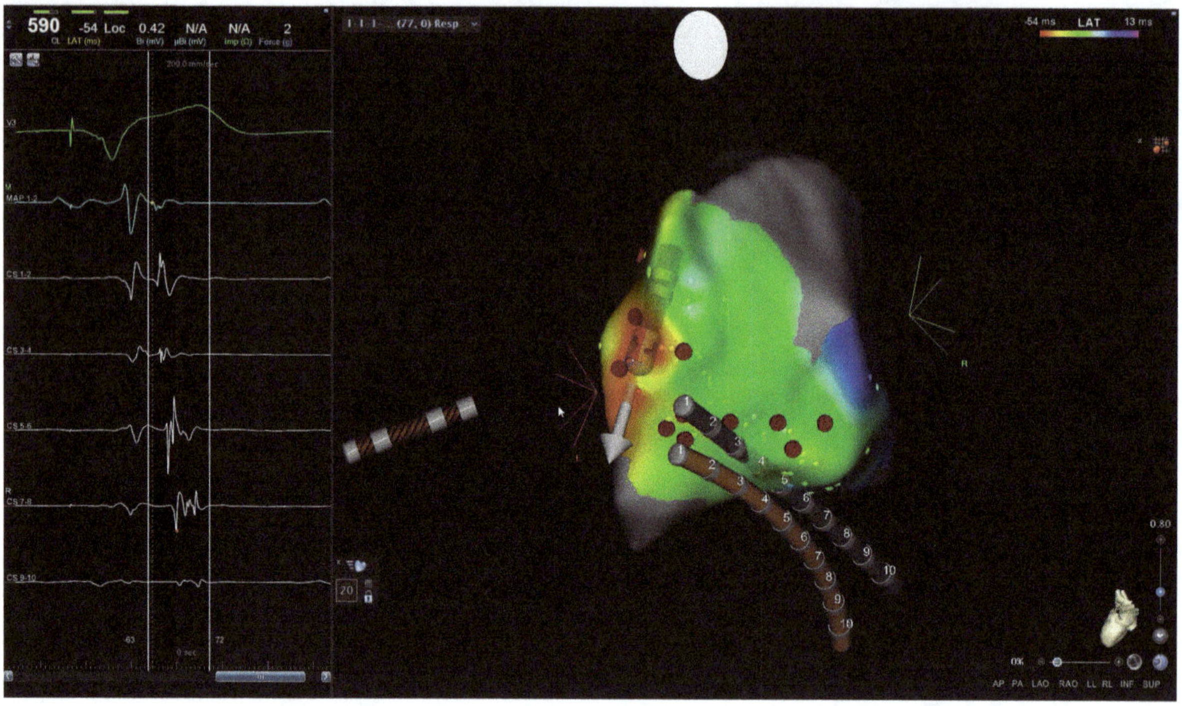

Figure 4: 3D mapping and intracavitary recordings confirming the presence of a left anterolateral AP.

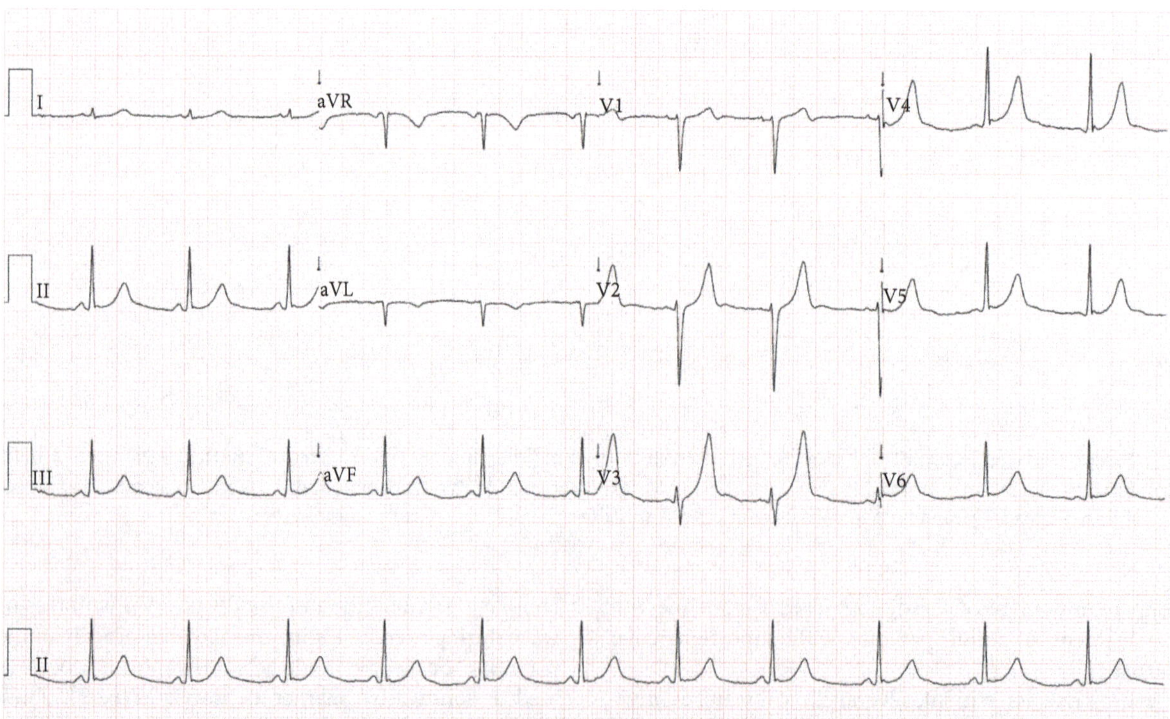

Figure 5: Twelve-lead electrocardiogram after catheter ablation. No delta waves and PR interval at the lower limit of normal but revealed peaked upright T waves in leads V3-V6 and inferior leads.

should be considered for the remaining patients. This makes the level of recommendation for EPS higher than that for noninvasive evaluation in adults' risk stratification. In contrast, an exercise stress test remains a routine part of the evaluation of asymptomatic children, and risk stratification by EPS is only recommended in those who do not have a reassuring pattern of clear loss of preexcitation during noninvasive tests [5].

Concerning management, previous guidelines [2, 3] recommended routine EPS and catheter ablation only in symptomatic patients. In the 2019 ESC guidelines [1], if a high-risk AP is diagnosed, catheter ablation is recommended and may be considered in low-risk preexcitation in appropriately experienced centres. Catheter ablation of an AP, when performed by an experienced operator, is associated with a high cure rate (>95%) and low risk (<0.5%) of major complications [16, 28]. About asymptomatic children, catheter ablation has a class IIb indication in patients 5 years and older and a class 3 indication for patients younger than 5 years since low weight and height are associated with a higher risk of complications [29]. Nevertheless, catheter ablation at paediatric age has also a high success rate (>95%) [14, 30].

Focusing on the presented clinical case, it mainly recalls WPW syndrome as a cause of SCD even in patients without previous symptoms and highlights the importance of risk stratification. The reported patient had several risk features (young age, male gender, inducibility of AVRT during EPS, and short AERP of the AP) that would have recommended AP ablation and avoid the life-threatening event if the WPW pattern had been earlier diagnosed. Nevertheless, the diagnosis of completely asymptomatic patients will remain challenging once a 12-lead ECG as a screening test for detection of cardiovascular disease in healthy and asymptomatic young people has not yet proved cost-effectiveness and therefore is not recommended [31].

An additional learning point is the revision of the different electrocardiographic features of WPW syndrome, namely, sinus rhythm with a preexcitation pattern, AVRT, and preexcited AF. A final teaching point is a discussion about the large, peaked T waves that may appear following ablation with concordant polarity in leads where the delta wave was most noticeable and/or positive. It is called a classic postablation memory T wave pattern, considered evidence of successful ablation [32].

In summary, the reported clinical case recalls fundamental features of the WPW syndrome and outlines the increasing evidence and importance of the invasive risk stratification in asymptomatic patients who suffer from this uncommon disease that may have a dramatic first clinical manifestation.

References

[1] J. Brugada, D. G. Katritsis, E. Arbelo et al., "2019 ESC guidelines for the management of patients with supraventricular tachycardiathe task force for the management of patients with supraventricular tachycardia of the European Society of Cardiology (ESC)," *European Heart Journal*, vol. 41, no. 5, pp. 655–720, 2020.

[2] C. Blomström-Lundqvist, M. M. Scheinman, E. M. Aliot et al., "ACC/AHA/ESC guidelines for the management of patients with supraventricular arrhythmias*-executive summary:," *Journal of the American College of Cardiology*, vol. 42, no. 8, pp. 1493–1531, 2003.

[3] R. L. Page, J. A. Joglar, M. A. Caldwell et al., "2015 ACC/AHA/HRS guideline for the management of adult patients with supraventricular tachycardia: a report of the American College of Cardiology/American Heart Association Task Force on Clinical Practice Guidelines and the Heart Rhythm Society," *Heart Rhythm*, vol. 13, no. 4, pp. e136–e221, 2016.

[4] B. T. Fengler, W. J. Brady, and C. U. Plautz, "Atrial fibrillation in the Wolff-Parkinson-White syndrome: ECG recognition and treatment in the ED," *The American Journal of Emergency Medicine*, vol. 25, no. 5, pp. 576–583, 2007.

[5] J. K. Triedman, "Management of asymptomatic Wolff-Parkinson-White syndrome," *Heart*, vol. 95, no. 19, pp. 1628–1634, 2009.

[6] M. W. Skov, P. V. Rasmussen, J. Ghouse et al., "Electrocardiographic preexcitation and risk of cardiovascular morbidity and Mortality," *Circulation. Arrhythmia and Electrophysiology*, vol. 10, no. 6, pp. 1–7, 2017.

[7] P. Delise and L. Sciarra, "Asymptomatic Wolff-Parkinson-White: what to do. Extensive ablation or not?," *Journal of Cardiovascular Medicine*, vol. 8, no. 9, pp. 668–674, 2007.

[8] P. Delise and L. Sciarra, "Sudden cardiac death in patients with ventricular preexcitation," *Cardiac Electrophysiology Clinics*, vol. 12, no. 4, pp. 519–525, 2020.

[9] T. M. Munger, D. L. Packer, S. C. Hammill et al., "A population study of the natural history of Wolff-Parkinson-White syndrome in Olmsted County, Minnesota, 1953-1989," *Circulation*, vol. 87, no. 3, pp. 866–873, 1993.

[10] G. Klein, T. Bashore, T. D. Sellers, E. Pritchett, W. Smith, and J. Gallagher, "Ventricular fibrillation in the Wolff-Parkinson-White syndrome," *The New England Journal of Medicine*, vol. 301, no. 20, pp. 1080–1085, 1979.

[11] P. Torner, P. Brugada, J. Smeets et al., "Ventricular fibrillation in the Wolff-Parkinson-White syndrome," *European Heart Journal*, vol. 12, no. 2, pp. 144–150, 1991.

[12] C. Timmermans, J. Smeets, L. Rodriguez, G. Vrouchos, A. van den Dool, and H. Wellens, "Aborted sudden death in the Wolff-Parkinson-White syndrome," *The American Journal of Cardiology*, vol. 76, no. 7, pp. 492–494, 1995.

[13] M. N. Obeyesekere, P. Leong-Sit, D. Massel et al., "Risk of arrhythmia and sudden death in patients with asymptomatic preexcitation: a meta-analysis," *Circulation*, vol. 125, no. 19, pp. 2308–2315, 2012.

[14] C. Pappone, F. Manguso, R. Santinelli et al., "Radiofrequency ablation in children with asymptomatic Wolff–Parkinson–White syndrome," *The New England Journal of Medicine*, vol. 351, no. 12, pp. 1197–1205, 2004.

[15] S. P. Etheridge, C. A. Escudero, A. D. Blaufox et al., "Life-threatening event risk in children with Wolff-Parkinson-White syndrome: a multicenter international study," *JACC: Clinical Electrophysiology*, vol. 4, no. 4, pp. 433–444, 2018.

[16] C. Pappone, G. Vicedomini, F. Manguso et al., "Wolff-Parkinson-White syndrome in the era of catheter ablation insights from a registry study of 2169 patients," *Circulation*, vol. 130, no. 10, pp. 811–819, 2014.

[17] V. Santinelli, A. Radinovic, F. Manguso et al., "The natural history of asymptomatic ventricular pre-excitation: a long-term prospective follow-up study of 184 asymptomatic children," *Journal of the American College of Cardiology*, vol. 53, no. 3, pp. 275–280, 2009.

[18] G. J. Klein, E. N. Prystowsky, R. Yee, A. D. Sharma, and A. Laupacis, "Asymptomatic Wolff-Parkinson-White. Should we intervene?," *Circulation*, vol. 80, no. 6, pp. 1902–1905, 1989.

[19] P. Kubuš, P. Vít, R. A. Gebauer, O. Materna, and J. Janoušek, "Electrophysiologic profile and results of invasive risk stratification in asymptomatic children and adolescents with the Wolff-Parkinson-White electrocardiographic pattern," *Circulation. Arrhythmia and Electrophysiology*, vol. 7, no. 2, pp. 218–223, 2014.

[20] V. Santinelli, A. Radinovic, F. Manguso et al., "Asymptomatic ventricular preexcitation a long-term prospective follow-up study of 293 adult patients," *Circulation. Arrhythmia and Electrophysiology*, vol. 2, no. 2, pp. 102–107, 2009.

[21] C. Pappone, G. Vicedomini, F. Manguso et al., "Risk of malignant arrhythmias in initially symptomatic patients with Wolff-Parkinson-White syndrome: results of a prospective long-term electrophysiological follow-up study," *Circulation*, vol. 125, no. 5, pp. 661–668, 2012.

[22] T. J. Bunch, H. T. May, T. L. Bair et al., "Long-term natural history of adult Wolff-Parkinson-White syndrome patients treated with and without catheter ablation," *Circulation. Arrhythmia and Electrophysiology*, vol. 8, no. 6, pp. 1465–1471, 2015.

[23] B. Brembilla-Perrot, O. Marçon, F. Chometon et al., "Supraventricular tachyarrhythmia as a cause of sudden cardiac arrest," *Journal of Interventional Cardiac Electrophysiology*, vol. 16, no. 2, pp. 97–104, 2006.

[24] J. W. Leitch, G. J. Klein, R. Yee, and C. Murdock, "Prognostic value of electrophysiology testing in asymptomatic patients with Wolff-Parkinson-White pattern," *Circulation*, vol. 83, no. 3, 1991.

[25] P. Wackel, C. Irving, S. Webber, L. Beerman, and G. Arora, "Risk stratification in Wolff-Parkinson-White syndrome: the correlation between noninvasive and invasive testing in pediatric patients," *Pacing and Clinical Electrophysiology*, vol. 35, no. 12, pp. 1451–1457, 2012.

[26] R. Bershader, C. Berul, and F. Cecchin, "Exercise testing for risk assessment in pediatric Wolff-Parkinson-White syndrome," *Heart Rhythm*, vol. 4, pp. S138–S139, 2007.

[27] G. Fazio, C. Mossuto, I. Basile et al., "Asymptomatic ventricular pre-excitation in children," *Journal of Cardiovascular Medicine*, vol. 10, no. 1, pp. 59–63, 2009.

[28] L. Bravo, F. Atienza, G. Eidelman et al., "Safety and efficacy of cryoablation vs. radiofrequency ablation of septal accessory pathways: systematic review of the literature and meta-analyses," *Europace*, vol. 20, no. 8, pp. 1334–1342, 2018.

[29] R. A. Friedman, E. P. Walsh, M. J. Silka et al., "NASPE expert consensus conference: radiofrequency catheter ablation in children with and without congenital heart disease. Report of the writing *committee*," *Pacing and Clinical Electrophysiology*, vol. 25, no. 6, pp. 1000–1017, 2002.

[30] J. D. Kugler, D. A. Danford, K. A. Houston, and G. Felix, "Pediatric radiofrequency catheter ablation registry success, fluoroscopy time, and complication rate for supraventricular tachycardia: comparison of early and recent eras," *Journal of Cardiovascular Electrophysiology*, vol. 13, no. 4, pp. 336–341, 2002.

[31] B. J. Maron, R. A. Friedman, P. Kligfield et al., "Assessment of the 12-lead ECG as a screening test for detection of cardiovascular disease in healthy general populations of young people (12-25 years of age)," *Circulation*, vol. 130, no. 15, pp. 1303–1334, 2014.

[32] M. E. Helguera, S. L. Pinski, R. Sterba, and R. G. Trohman, "Memory T waves after radiofrequency catheter ablation of accessory atrioventricular connections in Wolff-Parkinson-White syndrome," *Journal of Electrocardiology*, vol. 27, no. 3, pp. 243–249, 1994.

25

Association between Postural Orthostatic Tachycardia Syndrome and Joint Hypermobility

Alexis Javier Atuesta-Rodriguez, Yimy F. Medina-Velasquez, Orfa Motta, Maria Isabel Narvaez-Reyes, and Federico Rondon-Herrera

Rheumatology Unit, National University of Colombia, Colombia

Correspondence should be addressed to Alexis Javier Atuesta-Rodriguez; javijar2006@gmail.com

Academic Editor: Christopher S. Snyder

Joint hypermobility syndrome refers to increased joint flexibility beyond the normal range of motion. This syndrome has a benign form known as Ehlers-Danlos syndrome type 3. This is a disorder in which hypermobility is accompanied by clinical manifestations in the absence of any systemic disease. A clinical finding associated with this condition is postural orthostatic tachycardia syndrome. The following is a rare case of joint hypermobility syndrome and postural orthostatic tachycardia syndrome. The relevance of this case report lies in the impact that this disease had on the patient's quality of life and the limitation in the performance of activities of daily living.

1. Introduction

Joint hypermobility syndrome (JHS) refers to increased joint flexibility beyond the normal range of motion. Benign joint hypermobility syndrome, also known as Ehlers-Danlos syndrome (EDS) type 3, is the presence of hypermobility accompanied by clinical manifestations in the absence of a systemic disease. It is clinically diagnosed based on the maneuvers described in the Beighton score and the Brighton diagnostic criteria and after ruling out other causes [1]. The following is the report of a rare case of JHS associated with postural orthostatic tachycardia syndrome (POTS). The relevance of this case report lies in the impact that this disease had on the patient's quality of life and the limitation in the performance of activities of daily living.

2. Clinical Case

This is the case of a 16-year-old female patient with a 4-year history of snapping sound in the joints of hips, elbows, and knees, especially in extension, with noninflammatory polyarthralgia and persistent headache. Her medical history included recurrent neurocardiogenic syncopal episodes since the age of 12, along with spontaneous recovery without sequelae.

Physical examination showed joint hyperlaxity in hands, elbows, wrists, knees, and hips, with a Beighton score of 7/9 (Figures 1 and 2). Skin hyperlaxity was also observed (Figures 3 and 4). Blood pressure was 70/54 in decubitus position and 64/52 after sitting down for five minutes. Her heart rate (HR) was 80 beats per minute (bpm) when lying down and 110 bpm when sitting down. Elbow radiography showed radial head dislocation, while 24-hour Holter and blood pressure monitoring were normal. Tilt table test was compatible with mixed neurocardiogenic syncope and orthostatic intolerance syndrome.

Due to her history of neurocardiogenic syncope and joint hypermobility syndrome, after secondary causes were ruled out, she was diagnosed with JHS associated with orthostatic postural tachycardia syndrome (POTS). Nonpharmacological treatment was initiated, as well as increased fluid intake, sodium, postural therapy, among others. Clinical

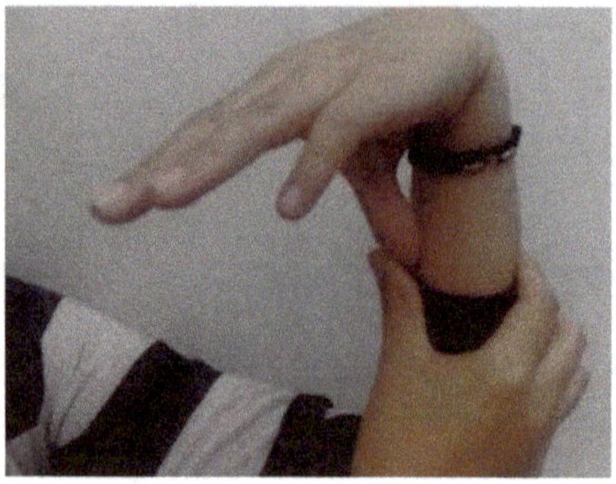

Figure 1: Hyperlaxity in the thumb.

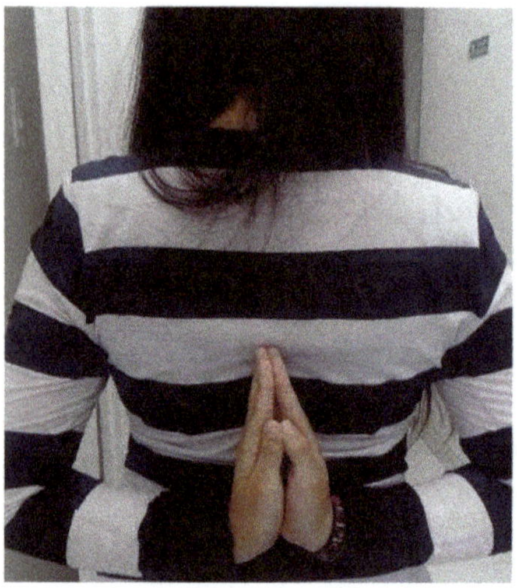

Figure 2: Hyperlaxity in the elbow.

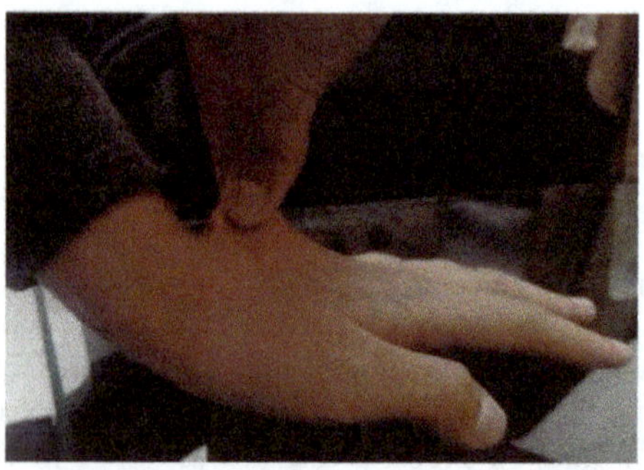

Figure 3: Cutaneous hyperlaxity.

improvement was achieved due to a decrease in the frequency of syncopal episodes.

3. Discussion

POTS was initially described in 1993 by Schondorf and Low as a disorder of the autonomic nervous system characterized mainly by orthostatic intolerance [2, 3]. It is often underdiagnosed, and therefore, quality of life can be affected. Timely diagnostic and therapeutic approach can provide sufficient

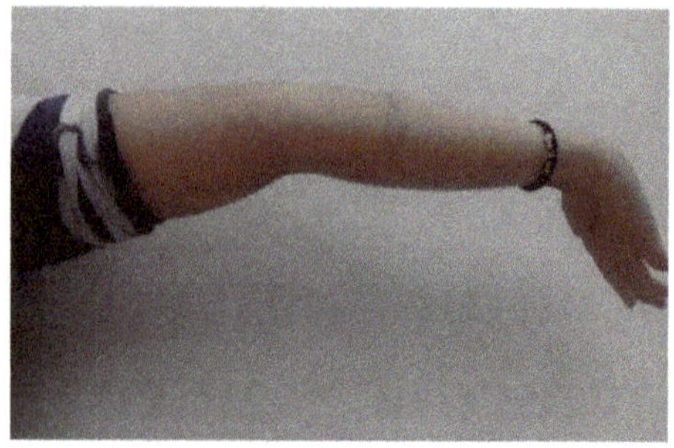

Figure 4: Hyperlaxity in the hand.

Table 1: Clinical manifestations and their relative frequencies in POTS.

Clinical manifestation	Frequency
Chronic fatigue	85-95%
Dizziness	60-80%
Palpitations	40-55%
Exercise intolerance	50-85%
Blurred vision	70%
Chest discomfort	60%
Headache	50%
Dyspnoea	40%
Syncope	40-50%

clinical control [4]. It occurs as a primary or secondary form of systemic diseases such as diabetes, joint hyperlaxity syndrome, paraneoplastic syndrome, among others [5]. POTS has a prevalence of 170 cases/100 000 inhabitants and is mainly observed in women between 20 and 40 years of age. It is caused by a failure of peripheral vascular resistance to orthostasis [6].

Although the definitions of POTS are strict, there are clinical variations in which not all the clinical findings mentioned above are observed, as in our patient's case. Some subtypes of POTS are classified considering whether the patient has a high, low, or normal flow. So, POTS can be neuropathic, hyperadrenergic, or autoimmune and may be associated with mast cell activation disorder and blood volume deregulation. None of these conditions is mutually exclusive or clearly independent [7].

Patients with POTS sometimes have a history of viral infection or a family member with similar symptoms; however, the actual association is unclear. The pathophysiology of this disease is mainly due to autonomic nervous system dysregulation, sympathetic hyperactivity, and attenuated vagal tone, resulting in hypoperfusion [8]. Clinical findings include cerebral hypoperfusion and sympathetic hyperactivity [3, 9]. Its diagnosis is based on clinical manifestations with different presentation frequencies (Table 1), such as an increase by 30 bpm compared to baseline HR vales or by 120 bpm when standing or walking within the first 10 minutes once orthostatic hypotension has been ruled out.

In the present case, although there was not a significant change in orthostasis, because there was not a decrease in systolic blood pressure (BP) of 20 mmHg or more or a decrease in diastolic BP of 10 mmHg or more, a significant variation in heart rate was indeed found when changing position. These symptoms should be present for at least six months and in the absence of another condition that could explain symptoms such as hydroelectrolytic alteration, secondary to drugs, among others. In our case, other causes were searched to explain the patient's clinical manifestations, but there were no other possible associations, and the symptoms had been present for more than 6 months.

Other findings that are not usually considered in this disease are high noradrenaline levels (600 ng/mL) and excessive response to isoproterenol. The differential diagnosis of POTS is pheochromocytoma due to sympathetic hyperreactivity, which causes neuropathies such as diabetes and vasovagal syncope [10].

Joint hyperlaxity syndrome (JHS) is characterized by joint hypermobility and other musculoskeletal manifestations in the absence of another disease. Men tend to have less hypermobility than women, and prevalence is usually inversely correlated to age, being higher in younger patients. However, there is confusion in terminology [3]. Type 3 or vascular EDS is associated with mutations in the COL3A1 allele. The main extra-articular clinical manifestations are fatigue, gastrointestinal disorders, neuropsychiatric, and cardiac manifestations, accompanied by increased skin elasticity and abnormal scarring. Musculoskeletal manifestations include polyarticular pain, enthesitis, bursitis, tenosynovitis, and mechanical lower back pain. Furthermore, a higher incidence of migraine, syncope, osteoarthritis, and osteoporosis has been found [10]. Pain is the most disabling symptom as it results from degeneration of ligaments and joint.

The association between POTS and JHS can be explained by predominant peripheral neuropathy in the autonomous system and a failure of the peripheral vascular system to maintain resistance in areas exposed to stress due to orthostasis, blood stasis in the lower limbs, or pathologies of the central nervous system [11]. The result is a functional decrease in blood volume with compensation given by increased heart rate and myocardia contractility. If compensation is not achieved in severe cases, cerebral hypoperfusion occurs with subsequent outcomes. Patients with postural orthostatic tachycardia and hypermobility syndrome present more symptoms from an early age [10].

The goal of treatment is based on nonpharmacological measures such as increased fluid intake, sodium, postural therapy, and rest, along with a multidisciplinary rehabilitative approach, which prevents muscle loss and deconditioning. Patients should perform physical activity 3 to 4 times per week for at least 45 minutes, achieving a frequency between 75 and 80% of the expected maximum heart rate with a progressive increase, mainly from aerobic exercise. Using elastic compression stockings in the lower limbs is also recommended with a pressure of at least 20 mmHg to improve venous return. Pharmacological therapy, such as the administration of fludrocortisone at doses of 0.05 to 0.2 mg per day, seeks to increase sodium retention to achieve blood volume expansion. Midodrine can also improve vascular resistance. Increased vagal tone with pyridostigmine may control postural orthostatic tachycardia, which is a similar mechanism obtained with the use of beta-blockers [3, 10, 12].

4. Conclusion

Orthostatic postural tachycardia syndrome associated with joint hypermobility is rare. The detection of patients with or susceptible to this disease becomes a challenge for clinicians to provide timely treatment that reduces complications and improves patients' quality of life.

Consent

Imaging scans are disclosed with the patient's prior consent.

Disclosure

We declare that a similar study was presented at the 21st PANLAR Congress.

References

[1] A. Fikree, Q. Aziz, and R. Grahame, "Joint hypermobility syndrome," *Rheumatic Diseases Clinics of North America*, vol. 39, no. 2, pp. 419–430, 2013.

[2] J. B. Guijarro, M. A. Ponce, A. V. Foncubierta, A. Pedrote, R. C. Barroso, and R. A. López, "Postural orthostatic tachycardia syndrome (POTS)," *Revista Espanola de Geriatria y Gerontologia*, vol. 44, no. 6, pp. 356-357, 2009.

[3] M. Mizumaki, "Postural orthostatic tachycardia syndrome (POTS)," *Journal of Arrhythmia*, vol. 27, no. 4, pp. 289–306, 2011.

[4] K. Berganzo, B. Tijero, J. J. Zarranz, and J. C. Gómez-Esteban, "Postural orthostatic tachycardia syndrome, neurally-mediated syncope, and joint hypermobility: a case report," *Neurología*, vol. 29, no. 7, pp. 447–449, 2014.

[5] R. Freeman, W. Wieling, F. B. Axelrod et al., "Consensus statement on the definition of orthostatic hypotension, neurally mediated syncope and the postural tachycardia syndrome," *Autonomic Neuroscience*, vol. 161, no. 1-2, pp. 46–48, 2011.

[6] E. E. Benarroch, "Postural tachycardia syndrome: a heterogeneous and multifactorial disorder," *Mayo Clinic Proceedings*, vol. 87, no. 12, pp. 1214–1225, 2012.

[7] M. Bryarly, L. T. Phillips, Q. Fu, S. Vernino, and B. D. Levine, "Postural orthostatic tachycardia syndrome:," *Journal of the American College of Cardiology*, vol. 73, no. 10, pp. 1207–1228, 2019.

[8] A. Fedorowski, "Postural orthostatic tachycardia syndrome: clinical presentation, aetiology, and management," *Journal of Internal Medicine*, vol. 29, 2018.

[9] V. Vykoupil, "Current look on postural tachycardia syndrome," *Cor et Vasa*, vol. 58, no. 4, pp. e426–e430, 2016.

[10] B. S. Khalil Kanjwal, B. Karabin, Y. Kanjwal, and B. P. Grubb, "Comparative clinical profile of postural orthostatic tachycardia patients with and without joint hypermobility syndrome," *Indian Pacing and Electrophysiology Journal*, vol. 10, no. 4, pp. 173–178, 2010.

[11] D. Wallman, J. Weinberg, and A. D. Hohler, "Ehlers-Danlos syndrome and postural tachycardia syndrome: a relationship study," *Journal of the Neurological Sciences*, vol. 340, no. 1-2, pp. 99–102, 2014.

[12] A. Lawrence, "Benign joint hypermobility syndrome," *Indian Journal of Rheumatology*, vol. 9, pp. S33–S36, 2014.

26

Successful Treatment of Whole Coronary Artery Spasm after Off-Pump Coronary Artery Bypass Grafting

Akihiro Kobayashi, Yoshimori Araki, Takafumi Terada, and Osamu Kawaguchi

Department of Cardiac Surgery, Toyota Kosei Hospital, Ibobara 500-1, Jousui-cho, Toyota, Aichi 470-0396, Japan

Correspondence should be addressed to Akihiro Kobayashi; ackykoba0804@gmail.com

Academic Editor: Benedetta Maria Motta

Coronary artery spasm after coronary artery bypass grafting is a rare but life-threatening condition. Herein, we report the case of a 77-year-old man who received off-pump coronary artery bypass grafting. An hour after surgery, there was a sudden hemodynamic compromise due to coronary artery spasm, prompting emergent coronary angiography with extracorporeal membrane oxygenation support. Because the angiography results showed diffuse severe spasm of the entire native coronary artery, the patient was treated with an intracoronary injection of vasodilators. The patient recovered in 7 days with mechanical support, catecholamines, and vasodilators, and he was discharged on postoperative day 30. Although coronary artery spasm after off-pump coronary artery bypass surgery is a rare condition, it must be suspected when sudden circulatory collapse occurs.

1. Introduction

Coronary artery spasm following off-pump coronary artery bypass surgery (OPCAB) is relatively rare but can lead to serious complications, including death [1]. Herein, we report a case of coronary artery spasm after OPCAB, which was successfully treated with percutaneous cardiopulmonary support, urgent coronary angiography, and intracoronary vasodilator infusion.

2. Case Presentation

A 77-year-old man had a chief complaint of chest pain at rest and was referred to our hospital with a diagnosis of unstable angina pectoris. Coronary angiography (CAG) showed 75% stenosis of the left main coronary artery and 90% stenosis of the right coronary artery. Although coronary artery bypass grafting was recommended, the patient did not agree with the operation. Instead, he opted to take medications, including aspirin, carvedilol, nicorandil, beraprost sodium, and isosorbide dinitrate. Six months later, he was admitted to our hospital because of the increasing frequency of chest pain and agreed to undergo surgery. Preoperative CAG showed 75% stenosis of the left main coronary artery and 99% stenosis of the left ascending artery (LAD), which was worse compared to the patient's condition 6 months ago (90% stenosis of the right coronary artery and 75% stenosis of the atrioventricular branch) (Figure 1). An intra-aortic balloon pump (IABP) was placed because of chest pain, ST depression on electrocardiography (ECG), and elevation of blood pressure during CAG. Following IABP placement and vasodilator infusion, the patient's symptoms disappeared. Three days later, we performed OPCAB, which was selected as the treatment method because of the highly calcified ascending aorta. Initially, the patient underwent a left internal mammary artery (LIMA) anastomosis to the LAD and a sequential great saphenous vein anastomosis to the posterior descending branch and atrioventricular branch. He returned to the intensive care unit (ICU) in a stable condition while on noradrenaline (0.07 μg/kg/min), dobutamine (2 μg/kg/minute), and nicorandil. An hour later, his heart rate and systolic blood pressure immediately decreased to 40 bpm and 40 mmHg, respectively. Moreover, his cardiac index (CI) dropped from 2.2 to 0.9, and his pulmonary artery pressure (PAP) and central venous pressure (CVP) increased. Hemodynamics improved after temporary pacing and increased administration of inotropes and volume resuscitation; however, the ECG showed no ST changes. Despite minimal bleeding from

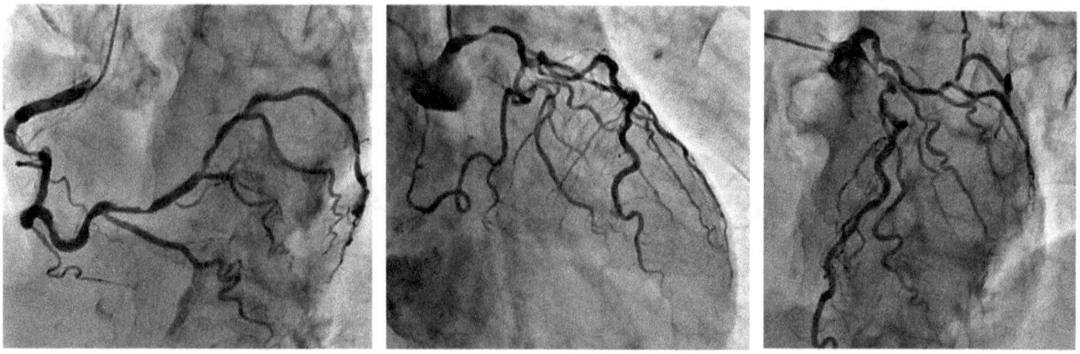

Figure 1: Coronary angiography showed a 75% stenosis of the left main coronary artery, 99% stenosis of the left ascending artery, 90% stenosis of the right coronary artery, and 75% stenosis of the atrioventricular branch.

the drain, we suspected cardiac tamponade and decided to reopen the chest. While preparing for the surgery, his heart rate suddenly decreased again and self-pulse disappeared, which prompted chest reopening in the ICU. On inspection, there was minimal hematoma, there were no signs of tamponade, and there were no signs of aortic dissection grossly or on the transesophageal echocardiogram (TEE). Hemodynamics subsequently improved, and the blood pressure increased to 90 mmHg with the administration of adrenaline; therefore, the chest was closed. At that time, his PAP was 35/25 mmHg, and his CVP was 30 mmHg. Fifteen minutes after reclosing the chest, his heart rate dropped once again, but temporary pacing was no longer responsive. Extracorporeal membrane oxygenation (ECMO) was immediately started, and the patient was transported to the cardiac catheterization laboratory. During this process, the ECG monitor showed ST elevation in lead II, and emergent CAG revealed patent grafts and diffuse severe spasms of the whole native coronary arteries (Figure 2). The right and left coronary arteries were directly infused with sodium nitroprusside hydrate, nicorandil, and isosorbide dinitrate. The ST elevation in V1–6 became clearer after the direct infusion of the drug into the right coronary artery. We also administered the aforementioned drugs into the LIMA and saphenous vein grafts. As a result, coronary flow gradually improved, and the blood pressure increased (Figure 3). Although coronary spasms of the left circumflex artery, right coronary artery, and LAD were still partially present, hemodynamics and ST elevation improved. The patient was then returned to the ICU, and nicorandil and nitroglycerin drips were continued. Peak creatinine phosphokinase and MB isozyme concentrations on postoperative day 1 were 8470 IU/L and 769 U/L, respectively. On postoperative day 3, ECMO was discontinued with dobutamine (4 μg/kg/min) and milrinone (0.2 μg/kg/min). On postoperative day 7, IABP was discontinued with dobutamine (4 μg/kg/min) and milrinone (0.25 μg/kg/min), and the patient was extubated on the next day. On postoperative day 9, his hemodynamics remained stable even without inotropes, and he was discharged from the ICU on postoperative day 30.

3. Discussion

As observed in our case, sudden hemodynamic collapse after coronary artery bypass may be due to coronary artery spasm. Although relatively rare, coronary artery spasms can lead to serious complications, including death, with a postoperative mortality of 10%–50%. The incidence of coronary artery spasm following cardiac surgery has been reported to range from 0.8% to 1.3%; however, this may be underestimated since its diagnosis requires coronary angiography [1]. From April 2002 to November 2021, a total of 1612 cardiac surgeries were performed at our institution. Among them, 936 were isolated CABG cases and 395 were OPCAB cases. Notably, there were two cases of postoperative coronary artery spasm following OPCAB, suggesting an incidence rate of 0.51%. A study reported that in a normal RCA without stenosis, coronary artery spasm commonly develops after weaning from cardiopulmonary bypass within 2 h after surgery [2]. Currently, the etiology of postoperative coronary artery spasm is unclear, but several factors have been reported to induce this condition. Smoking is a major risk factor for coronary artery spasm in the absence of significant coronary stenosis. Minato et al. reported that hypomagnesemia is one of the triggers of coronary artery spasm, which is widespread in OPCAB [3]. This is why magnesium is included in the cardioplegia solution for on-pump CABG because of its protective effect against coronary artery spasm. Preoperative use of beta-blockers and calcium blockers, trauma due to surgical manipulation, hypothermia, hyperventilation, and compression by chest tubes have also been reported as etiologic factors of postoperative coronary arterial spasm [4, 5]. This is consistent with our case, since the patient had a history of smoking and medication with preoperative beta-blockers. CAG is the gold standard for diagnosing coronary artery spasms; however, this may become apparent clinically through ECG changes, hemodynamic instability, arrhythmia, circulatory collapse, or cardiac arrest [1]. Among these, the most common manifestations are ST-segment elevation and circulatory collapse without a specific cause. In our case, ECG changes were not apparent, and the patient developed circulatory collapse. In patients with unstable hemodynamics, the use of an IABP can increase coronary flow and support the left ventricle. However, in cases of severe cardiogenic shock or cardiac arrest, an IABP is not enough to support the patient's hemodynamics. Instead, more advanced mechanical circulatory supports, such as venoarterial ECMO, should be performed. Particularly, ECMO is reported to provide full circulatory support, such that catecholamine infusions that may aggravate cardiac artery spasm by the alpha-adrenergic effect can be discontinued. Moreover, ECMO improves

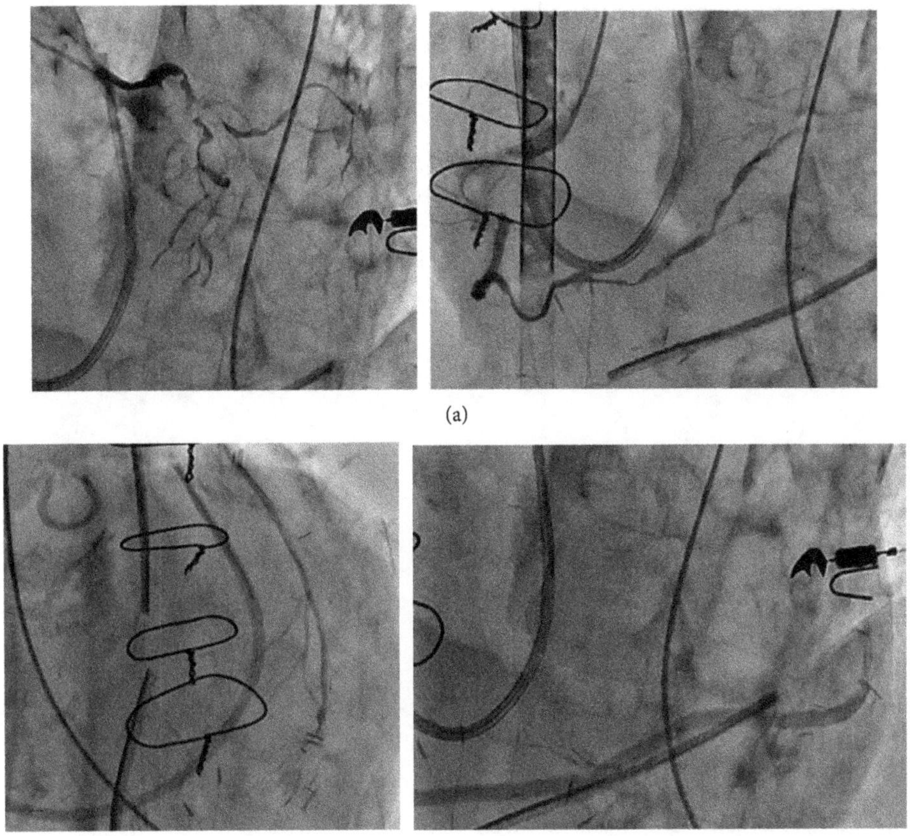

(a)

(b)

FIGURE 2: Emergent coronary angiography. Diffuse severe spasm of whole native coronary arteries (a). The internal mammary artery and great saphenous vein were patent (b).

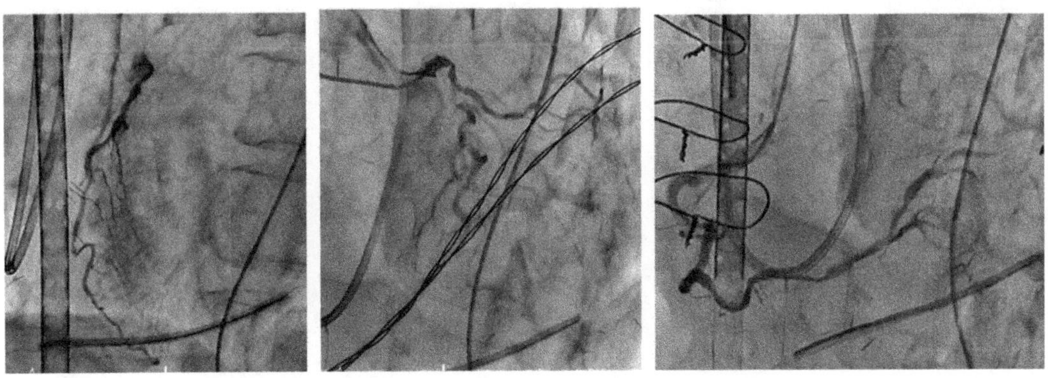

FIGURE 3: Coronary spasm was still partially present, but flow gradually improved.

oxygenation, decompresses the heart, and reduces myocardial oxygen consumption, thereby reducing any ongoing ischemia. Once stabilized on ECMO, the patient can be safely transported to the catheterization laboratory [1]. In our case, circulatory collapse suddenly occurred, making immediate diagnosis difficult. As the first priority was to stabilize the circulation, we first inserted the TEE and reopened the chest, allowing us to rule out tamponade and dissection. ECMO was then performed since the patient's hemodynamics did not improve. After the circulation was stabilized, CAG was performed, thereby allowing the diagnosis of coronary artery spasm and treatment with direct injection of vasodilators into the coronary arteries. The trigger in this case was unclear, but hypomagnesemia was noted. Specifically, the preoperative magnesium level was 1.7 mg/dL, but the postoperative level was 1.4 mg/dL. Therefore, hypomagnesemia could be considered a risk factor of coronary artery spasm in this case. Moreover, although magnesium is replenished from cardioplegia in conventional on-pump CABG, the OPCAB value of magnesium should still be monitored carefully.

In conclusion, we report a case of hemodynamically significant coronary artery spasm after OPCAB that was successfully treated with ECMO and intracoronary infusion of vasodilators. Although coronary artery spasm after OPCAB is rare, it should still be suspected when sudden circulatory collapse occurs.

Consent

The patient provided informed consent for the publication of this case report.

References

[1] S. Unai, H. Hirose, C. Gary et al., "Coronary artery spasm following off-pump coronary artery bypass surgery," *International Heart Journal*, vol. 55, no. 5, pp. 451–454, 2014.

[2] J. H. Baek, S. S. Han, and D. H. Lee, "Native coronary artery and grafted artery spasm just after coronary artery bypass grafting: a case report," *Journal of Korean Medical Science*, vol. 25, no. 4, pp. 641–643, 2010.

[3] N. Minato, Y. Katayama, M. Sakaguchi, and M. Itoh, "Perioperative coronary artery spasm in off-pump coronary artery bypass grafting and its possible relation with perioperative hypomagnesemia," *Annals of Thoracic and Cardiovascular Surgery*, vol. 12, no. 1, pp. 32–36, 2006.

[4] D. Sef, J. Szavits-Nossan, M. Predrijevac et al., "Management of perioperative myocardial ischaemia after isolated coronary artery bypass graft surgery," *Open Heart*, vol. 6, no. 1, pp. e001027–e001027, 2019.

[5] A. Fujita, H. Kurazumi, R. Suzuki, M. Takahashi, A. Mikamo, and K. Hamano, "Relief of vasospasm with fasudil after off-pump coronary artery bypass grafting: a case study," *Surgical Case Reports*, vol. 4, no. 1, p. 82, 2018.

27

Rivaroxaban as Therapy for Saphenous Venous Graft Failure due to Venous Outflow Mismatch

Matthew T. Lee,[1] Ayush Mohan,[1] Jenna E. Lee,[2] and Daniel T. Lee[2]

[1]*Central Michigan University College of Medicine, USA*
[2]*McLaren Bay City Regional Medical Center, USA*

Correspondence should be addressed to Daniel T. Lee; daniel.lee1965@gmail.com

Academic Editor: Ertugurul Ercan

Background. Recurrent angina and long-term occlusion following coronary artery bypass graft surgery is often treated with percutaneous coronary intervention, a high-risk intervention for distal embolization. Here, we present the utilization of the novel oral anticoagulant, rivaroxaban, in the treatment of saphenous vein graft thrombosis with complete resolution of the thrombus secondary to graft outflow mismatch. *Case Presentation.* A 69-year-old man with triple coronary artery bypass grafting using a saphenous vein and left internal mammary artery, performed in 2017, presented at our hospital for recurrent angina. Coronary angiography revealed a patent LIMA to LAD and a large clot burden in the venous conduit to the first OM/terminal circumflex—theorized to be due to an outflow mismatch of the large saphenous vein to the native artery resulting in stasis. Instead of percutaneous coronary intervention, he was treated with rivaroxaban 20 mg once a day. The angiography 4 weeks after starting rivaroxaban showed complete resolution of the thrombus. *Conclusion.* Rivaroxaban could become a potential treatment option in thrombus reversal due to static venous flow with subsequent long-term patency of the graft. Additionally, its use may be indicated in the generalized prevention of VGF.

1. Background

Saphenous vein grafts (SVGs) remain the most used conduit during coronary artery bypass graft (CABG) surgery. However, during the first year after bypass surgery, up to 15% of venous grafts occlude and are prone to long-term occlusion and up to 20% of patients have recurrent angina within the first year [1]. Venous graft failure (VGF) is a multifactorial process that has not been completely understood. The pathogenesis could involve accelerated atherosclerosis, inflammation, thrombosis, or any combination [2]. Graft failure, however, could be from stasis secondary to a mismatch of the venous conduit with the outflow of the native vessel [3]. Herein, we report a case report of a patient who presents NSTEMI. Angiography revealed a large SVG clot burden due to venous outflow mismatch which was subsequently resolved with four weeks of rivaroxaban.

2. Case

A 69-year-old male presents with NSTEMI, with pertinent medical history of triple coronary artery bypass grafting (CABG) from 2017. At that time, revascularization was anatomically complete and included the following grafts: left internal mammary artery (LIMA) to the left anterior descending coronary artery and saphenous vein sequential bypass graft to the first obtuse marginal coronary artery (OM) and the terminal circumflex coronary artery. There were no complications noted during the CABG procedure. Bypass angiography revealed a patent LIMA to LAD and a large clot burden in the venous conduit to the first OM/terminal circumflex (Figure 1), theorized to be due to an outflow mismatch of the large saphenous vein to the native artery resulting in stasis. With the combination of the large clot burden and poor outflow, the operator speculated high

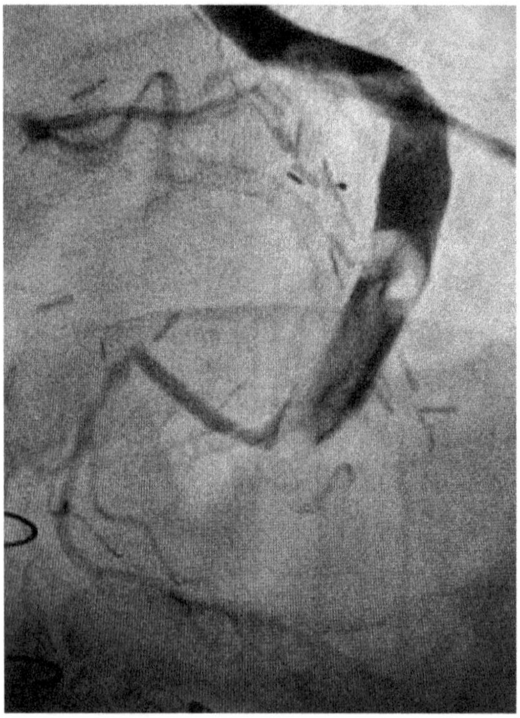

Figure 1: Initial cardiac angiogram of the first OM/terminal circumflex with high clot burden theorized to be due to venous outflow mismatch from SVG.

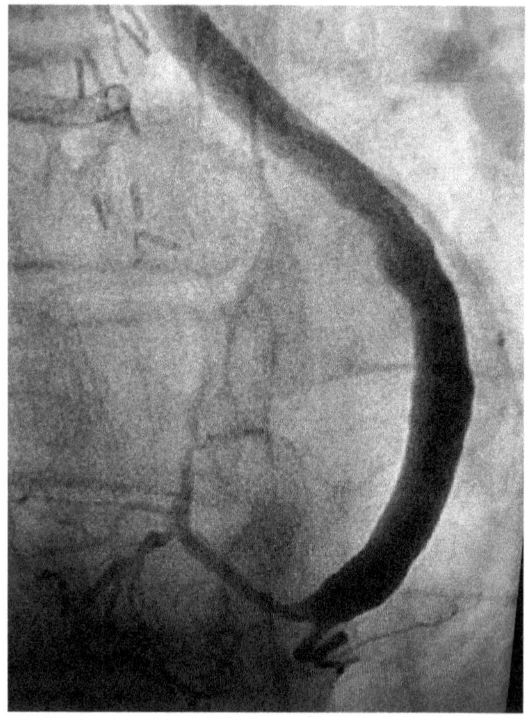

Figure 2: Postrivaroxaban therapy cardiac angiogram of the first OM/terminal circumflex with high clot burden showing complete resolution after four weeks of pharmacotherapy.

likelihood of distal embolization with SVG stenting. Subsequently, conservative management was instituted. Percutaneous intervention and repeat CABG after saphenous vein graft failure were considered but have significantly increased risks of mortality. Conservative management involving anticoagulant therapy given the cause of thrombosis was ultimately decided. Warfarin was not considered due to increased bleeding risk and delayed, unpredictable pharmacodynamic response. Instead, the patient continued aspirin 81 mg/day and added anticoagulation rivaroxaban 20 mg/day. Four weeks later, angiography of the venous conduit showed complete resolution of the thrombus (Figure 2).

3. Discussion

CABG remains an integral part of the treatment of ischemic heart disease. It is one of the most frequently performed surgical procedures in the United States, over 400,000 annually. However, the long-term patency remains at 50% degradation of the saphenous venous grafts at 10 years [4]. Standard treatment of degenerated SVG includes stent placement with or without a distal embolic protection device. These high-risk interventions lead to distal embolization with subsequent NSTEMI up to 25% of the time. Atherosclerosis is the main etiology of late VGF, occurring 12 months after the procedure [1]. Our important findings were twofold. The case clearly represented venous graft failure. The likelihood of atherosclerosis was unlikely; subsequently treating this large clot burden with stenting would have significantly increased the risk of distal embolization with subsequent postprocedure MI, with subsequent risk of in-stent restenosis and repeat thrombosis as the venous conduit to small vessel outflow mismatch would persist. This case represented thrombosis due to stasis secondary to venous outflow mismatch. As a result, rivaroxaban therapy was more appropriate to address immediate resolution of the thrombus with subsequent long-term patency of the graft.

Secondly, we have demonstrated the ability of rivaroxaban to engage in complete thrombus reversal due to static venous flow. While the anticoagulant effects of rivaroxaban are used for its improved outcomes in the treatment of many disease processes including but not limited to DVT, PE, and atrial fibrillation [5, 6], there has not been evidence of its use for complete thrombus reversal due to VGF as we have demonstrated here. This thrombus reversal was theorized to be due to rivaroxaban-induced reduction of factor Xa's inhibitor effect on fibrinolysis [7], therefore increasing the effects of endogenous plasmin.

Beyond the effects of factor Xa inhibition, rivaroxaban acts as an antiplatelet agent [8] which further decreases the rate of potential thrombus formation in the setting of SVG. Moreover, rivaroxaban induces a significant downregulation of TGF-beta [9] and other proinflammatory cytokines [10], theoretically indicating its use prophylactically to prevent fibrotic and inflammatory closure of SVGs. As a result, the use of rivaroxaban may be indicated post-SVG and serve to decrease the risk of VGF in at-risk patients.

4. Conclusion

We used rivaroxaban instead of PCI for the treatment of SVG thrombosis presented as NSTEMI. This conservative approach worked in our patient due to his high clot burden being secondary to venous graft outflow mismatch. Rivaroxaban can be used as a safer, more effective long-term therapy for VGF thrombosis secondary to stasis and potentially indicated as a preventative measure for generalized VGF. Use of rivaroxaban in VGF may also serve to decrease the overuse of PCI in its treatment.

References

[1] J. G. Motwani and E. J. Topol, "Aortocoronary saphenous vein graft disease," *Circulation*, vol. 97, no. 9, pp. 916–931, 1998.

[2] F. Y. Kim, G. Marhefka, N. J. Ruggiero, S. Adams, and D. J. Whellan, "Saphenous vein graft disease," *Cardiology in Review*, vol. 21, no. 2, pp. 101–109, 2013.

[3] C. N. Hess, R. D. Lopes, C. M. Gibson et al., "Saphenous vein graft failure after coronary artery bypass surgery," *Circulation*, vol. 130, no. 17, pp. 1445–1451, 2014.

[4] S. F. Aranki and A. J. Tatooles, "Disconnect between vein graft failure and clinical events after coronary artery bypass graft surgery," *Circulation*, vol. 130, no. 17, pp. 1439–1441, 2014.

[5] S. K. Kakkos, G. I. Kirkilesis, and I. A. Tsolakis, "Efficacy and safety of the new oral anticoagulants dabigatran, rivaroxaban, apixaban, and edoxaban in the treatment and secondary prevention of venous thromboembolism: a systematic review and meta-analysis of phase III trials," *Journal of Vascular Surgery*, vol. 60, no. 5, p. 1397, 2014.

[6] A. G. G. Turpie, "Advances in oral anticoagulation treatment: the safety and efficacy of rivaroxaban in the prevention and treatment of thromboembolism," *Therapeutic Advances in Hematology.*, vol. 3, no. 5, pp. 309–323, 2012.

[7] R. L. Carter, K. Talbot, W. S. Hur et al., "Rivaroxaban and apixaban induce clotting factor xa fibrinolytic activity," *Journal of Thrombosis and Haemostasis*, vol. 16, no. 11, pp. 2276–2288, 2018.

[8] T. Petzold, M. Thienel, L. Dannenberg et al., "Letter by Violi et al. Regarding Article, "Rivaroxaban reduces arterial thrombosis by inhibition of FXA-driven platelet activation via protease activated Receptor-1"," *Circulation Research*, vol. 126, no. 10, pp. 486–500, 2020.

[9] L. Di Lullo, C. Lavalle, M. Magnocavallo et al., "New evidence of direct oral anticoagulation therapy on cardiac valve calcifications, renal preservation and inflammatory modulation," *International Journal of Cardiology*, vol. 345, pp. 90–97, 2021.

[10] M. Laurent, U. Joimel, R. Varin et al., "Comparative study of the effect of rivaroxaban and fondaparinux on monocyte's coagulant activity and cytokine release," *Experimental Hematology & Oncology*, vol. 3, no. 1, p. 30, 2014.

28

Branch Retinal Artery Occlusion after Percutaneous Coronary Intervention

Tommaso La Macchia,[1] Remo Albiero,[2] Tommaso Invernizzi,[3] Giorgia Ceravolo,[4] and Ida Ceravolo[5]

[1]*Department of Clinical and Experimental Medicine, Unit of Cardiology, University of Messina, Via C. Valeria, 98125 Messina, Italy*
[2]*Interventional Cardiology Unit-Sondrio Hospital, Via Stelvio, 25, 23100 Sondrio, Italy*
[3]*Ophthalmology Unit-Sondrio Hospital, Via Stelvio, 25, 23100 Sondrio, Italy*
[4]*Department of Human Pathology and Evolutive Age "Gaetano Barresi", University of Messina, Via C. Valeria, 98125 Messina, Italy*
[5]*Department of Clinical and Experimental Medicine, University of Messina, Via C. Valeria, 98125 Messina, Italy*

Correspondence should be addressed to Remo Albiero; albiero@panvascular.com

Academic Editor: Expedito E. Ribeiro

We report a case of branch retinal artery occlusion (BRAO) that occurred after percutaneous coronary intervention (PCI). A 59-year-old man with no other previous diseases presented visual acuity deterioration in the left eye 24 hours after PCI. Fundus examination revealed ischemia at the temporal branch of the retinal artery associated with inner layer edema. Prompt treatment was performed with ocular digital massage and paracentesis of the anterior chamber. However, at discharge, the patient had a persistent visual loss with a central scotoma that persisted at 35-day follow-up without improvement of the visual acuity. The patient did not suffer from any other systemic complications. Retinal infarction should be considered a potential complication of PCI. Patients and health care providers should be aware of any visual signs. Permanent visual disability can be prevented by immediate diagnosis and prompt intervention.

1. Introduction

Percutaneous coronary intervention (PCI) is currently indicated for the management of patients presenting with coronary artery disease (CAD). Advances in technology, development of more potent and effective antiplatelet therapy, and judicious use of PCI are increasing the safety of the procedure. However, major complications during and after PCI still occur that can be related to the access site, intubation of the coronary artery ostia, or the intervention itself. The most common problems occur in the context of coronary intubation and target vessel or site intervention [1]. However, different organs including renal, brain, eye, and gastrointestinal systems could be targets of thromboembolic events during PCI or cardiac catheterization [2]. In particular, the association with some retinal alterations has been occasionally reported [3–9]. We report a case of branch retinal artery occlusion (BRAO) that occurred 24 hours after PCI.

2. Case Report

In November 2020, a 59-year-old man, an ex-smoker with negative previous medical history of heart disease, was admitted to the emergency department of Sondrio Hospital (Sondrio, Italy), 48 hours after the onset of episodes of rest angina associated with atypical angina symptoms (jaw pain in the dental arches).

Admission ECG showed a heart rate of 95 bpm and a slight ST segment depression in the lateral leads. Measurement of cardiac biomarkers showed a rise in high-sensitivity troponin I (hs-cTnI, 142 ng/L). Double antiplatelet

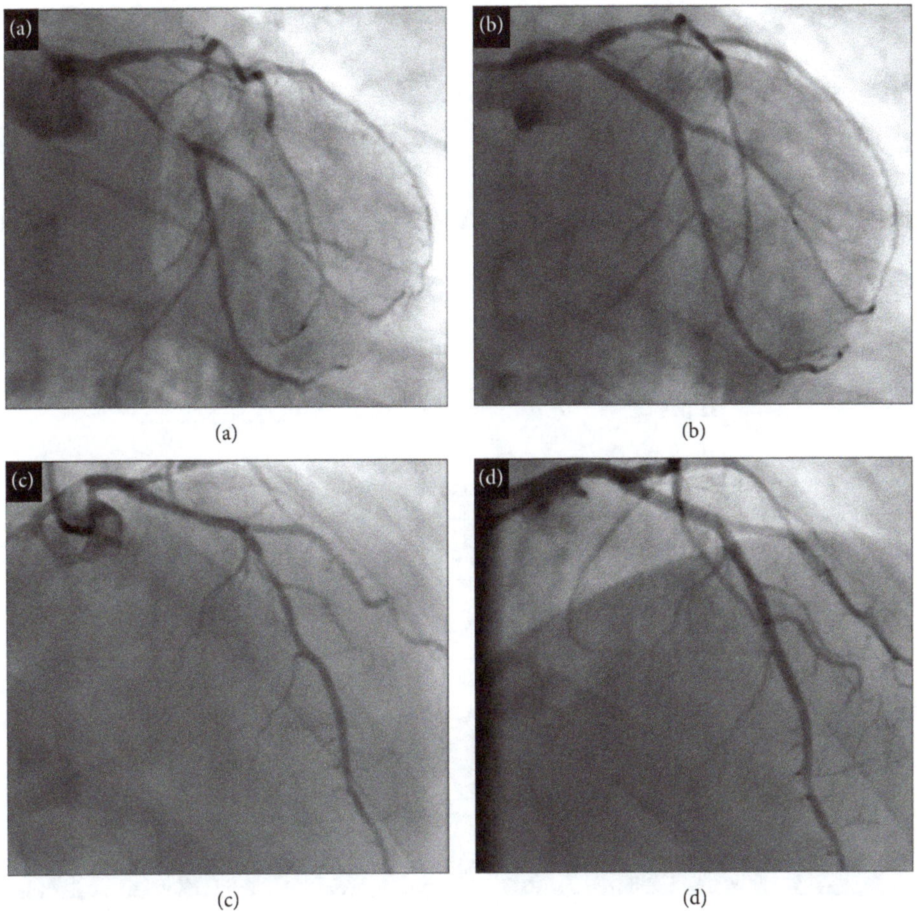

FIGURE 1: The angiogram shows 2-vessel CAD (coronary artery disease) with subocclusion of the proximal circumflex coronary artery (LCx) (a) and critical stenosis of the proximal and middle anterior descending coronary artery (LAD) (c). Good final result after PCI with implantation of a DES (drug-eluting stent) in the proximal-middle LCx at the bifurcation with the MO1 branch (b) and two contiguous DES on the proximal-middle LAD (d).

therapy (DAPT) with aspirin 100 mg/day and clopidogrel 75 mg/day was started on admission, and the same day, the patient underwent coronary angiography by right transradial access. The angiogram showed 2-vessel CAD (coronary artery disease) with subocclusion of the proximal circumflex coronary artery (LCx) and critical stenosis of the proximal and middle anterior descending coronary artery (LAD) (Figures 1(a) and 1(c)). After administration of heparin 100 U/kg, ad hoc PCI was performed with implantation of a drug-eluting stent (DES) in the proximal-middle LCx at the bifurcation with the MO1 branch and two contiguous stents on the proximal-middle LAD, with a good final angiographic result on both vessels (Figures 1(b) and 1(d)).

Twenty-four hours after PCI, the patient reported the onset of a left central scotoma and an ophthalmological evaluation was requested. The left visual acuity was reduced to 0.7 logMAR with a central scotoma. There was no alteration in the anterior segment. Intraocular pressure (IOP) was 10 mmHg. Fundus examination revealed a white embolus in the temporal branch of the central retinal artery (Figure 2). A computerized visual field (Humphrey II 740 Visual Field, Carl Zeiss Meditec AG, Jena, Germany) revealed a paracentral visual defect (Figure 3(a)). Moreover,

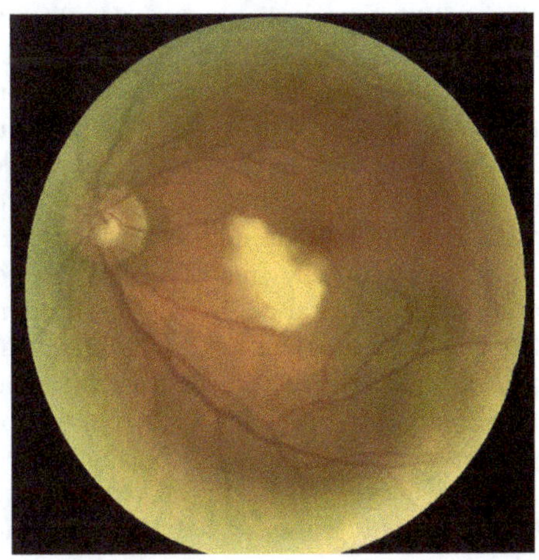

FIGURE 2: Fundus photograph of the left eye branch retinal artery occlusion (BRAO) showing white pallor at the inferior temporal branch of the central retinal artery.

spectral domain-optical coherence tomography (SD-OCT) (RS-3000 Nidek, Gamagori, Japan) was performed which showed inner layer edema in the temporal sector (Figure 3(b)). The right eye was normal. The diagnosis was

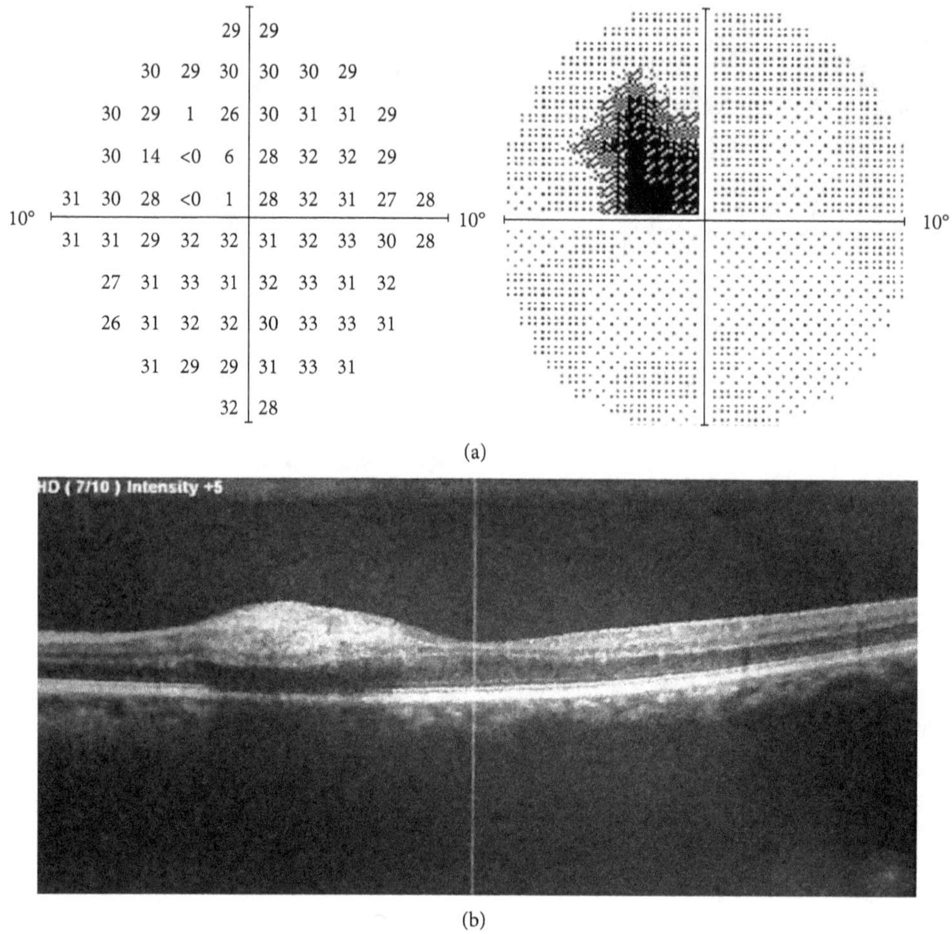

FIGURE 3: (a) Visual field examination demonstrating defects in the 5° temporal in the left eye. (b) Optical coherence tomography (OCT) images of the left eye showing temporal inner layer edema.

consistent with BRAO. Immediate conventional treatment of BRAO was performed, with ocular digital massage and paracentesis of the anterior chamber. Complete neurological examination was normal. The patient underwent supra-aortic trunks echo-color Doppler (TSA) which showed bilaterally diffuse hyperplasia affecting the common carotid, the carotid bulb, and the internal and external carotid in the absence of hemodynamically significant flow accelerations. It showed no morphological alterations of the supra-aortic vessels. No other systemic complications occurred during hospitalization. At discharge, the patient had a persistent visual loss with a central scotoma that persisted at 35-day follow-up. In addition, follow-up OCT showed persistent macular edema. This study followed the tenets of the Declaration of Helsinki, and written consent was obtained from the patient.

3. Discussion

Branch retinal artery occlusion (BRAO) is one common cause of retinal vascular disease; it is caused by a reduction in arterial blood flow, resulting in retinal ischemia which can lead to severe vision loss and visual field defects despite therapy. Commonly, it is associated with systemic risk factors including hypertension, diabetes, carotid artery disease, and atherosclerosis. Few studies suggest that different retinal complications could be observed after coronary angiography procedures. Eye involvement includes central retinal artery occlusion (CRAO) [3, 4], branch retinal artery occlusion (BRAO) [5–7], or cilioretinal artery occlusion [8]. In addition, retinal embolisms following coronary catheterization can be clinically silent with any visual impairment. Moreover, it has been found that the risk factor for retinal emboli can be significantly associated with patient age, hypertension, and operator expertise [9]. Our patient had no additional risk factors. In the current case, the concomitance between the onset of eye disease and the coronary procedure suggests a correlation between the two conditions.

An immediate treatment is required if the occlusion occurs within 24 hours from the procedure. Conventional therapy consists in the reduction of intraocular pressure with hypotensive drugs, digital massage of the eyelid, and anterior chamber paracentesis. In some cases, thrombolytics can be infused into the carotid artery, or a laser embolectomy can be performed. The goal of the treatment is reperfusion of the blocked retinal vessels particularly when it is done within 6 h, because retinal ischemic damage after 240 min is normally permanent [10]. However, treatments rarely improve visual acuity, and in BRAO, the visual field damage is typically permanent. Furthermore, in rare case, the condition could be complicated with retinal or iris neovascularization leading to glaucoma or vitreous hemorrhage.

4. Conclusion

With the growing occurrence of PCI, all physicians involved in patient care should be worried in keeping special attention towards ocular signs. Visual symptoms and retinal artery occlusions caused by embolization in patients after PCI could occur even 24 hours after catheterization. Prompt diagnosis and early treatment may help improve the outcome and preserve vision deterioration.

Additional Points

Learning Objective. Retinal infarction should be considered a potential complication of PCI with the risk of permanent visual disability that can be prevented by immediate diagnosis and prompt intervention. Patients and health care providers should be aware of any visual signs after PCI.

References

[1] Y. R. Manda and K. M. Baradhi, *Cardiac Catheterization Risks and Complications*, StatPearls Publishing LLC, Treasure Island, FL, USA, 2021.

[2] M. Tavakol, S. Ashraf, and S. J. Brener, "Risks and complications of coronary angiography: a comprehensive review," *Global Journal of Health Science*, vol. 4, no. 1, pp. 65–93, 2012.

[3] P. Kraśnicki, E. Proniewska-Skretek, Z. Mariak, A. Dubicki, G. Mezyński, and S. Dobrzycki, "Embolic central retinal artery occlusion as a complication of percutaneous coronary angioplasty–case report," *Klinika Oczna*, vol. 110, no. 1-3, pp. 64–66, 2008.

[4] J. Selton, T. Maalouf, A. Olivier, R. Anxionnat, M. Angioi, and K. Angioi, "Central retinal artery occlusion following coronary angiography: a case report," *Journal Français d'Ophtalmologie*, vol. 34, no. 3, pp. 181–185, 2011.

[5] G. D. Kymionis, M. K. Tsilimbaris, E. B. Christodoulakis, and I. G. Pallikaris, "Late onset branch retinal artery occlusion following coronary angiography," *Acta Ophthalmologica Scandinavica*, vol. 83, no. 1, pp. 122-123, 2005.

[6] K. C. Chan, D. J. Wu, K. C. Ueng et al., "Branch retinal artery occlusion after diagnostic cardiac catheterization," *Japanese Heart Journal*, vol. 43, no. 2, pp. 193–196, 2002.

[7] M. D. O'Neill, T. Akerele, and M. Dancy, "Branch retinal artery occlusion during coronary angiography," *Postgraduate Medical Journal*, vol. 81, no. 961, p. 710, 2005.

[8] A. Loewenstein, M. Goldstein, A. Roth, and M. Lazar, "Cilioretinal artery occlusion during coronary catheterization," *Acta Ophthalmologica Scandinavica*, vol. 77, no. 6, pp. 717-718, 1999.

[9] J. Kojuri, M. Mehdizadeh, H. Rostami, and D. Shahidian, "Clinical significance of retinal emboli during diagnostic and therapeutic cardiac catheterization in patients with coronary artery disease," *BMC Cardiovascular Disorders*, vol. 11, no. 1, p. 5, 2011.

[10] Y. M. Hsien, M. Mustapha, J. C. Hamzah, O. Maskon, C. C. Ken, and C. H. Hamdi, "Why can't I see after my heart is fixed: a case series of ocular complications after cardiac intervention," *BMC Ophthalmology*, vol. 16, no. 1, p. 32, 2016.

29

Life-Saving Emergency Adrenalectomy in a Pheochromocytoma Crisis with Cardiogenic Shock

Thalia Bekelaar,[1] Gervais Nougon,[2] Marc Peters,[2] Frederic De Roeck,[1] Steven Haine,[1] Dirk Ysebaert,[3] Maarten Spinhoven,[4] Philippe G. Jorens,[5] Rudi De Paep,[5] and Frederik Lahaye[5]

[1]*Department of Cardiology, Antwerp University Hospital, University of Antwerp, Edegem, Belgium*
[2]*Department of Emergency Medicine, Sint-Jozef Hospital, Malle, Belgium*
[3]*Department of Hepatobiliary-Transplantation-Endocrine Surgery, Antwerp University Hospital, University of Antwerp, Edegem, Belgium*
[4]*Department of Radiology, Antwerp University Hospital, University of Antwerp, Edegem, Belgium*
[5]*Intensive Care Medicine, Antwerp University Hospital, University of Antwerp, Edegem, Belgium*

Correspondence should be addressed to Philippe G. Jorens; philippe.jorens@uza.be

Academic Editor: Ertugrul Ercan

Cardiogenic shock during a pheochromocytoma crisis is a life-threatening disorder. This case report illustrates a 49-year-old male with profound cardiogenic shock, extreme hemodynamic instability (systolic blood pressure ranging from 45 up to 290 mmHg in a cyclic pattern), and progressive multiple organ failure in the presence of a unilateral adrenal mass. Emergency adrenalectomy led to rapid hemodynamic stabilization. Histological investigation confirmed the diagnosis of pheochromocytoma. This case indicates that emergency adrenalectomy, although usually not considered first choice, is a valid option in cardiogenic shock and extremely fluctuating hemodynamics due to a pheochromcytoma-induced catecholamine storm.

1. Introduction

A pheochromocytoma crisis is an acute, life-threatening condition [1–3]. Excessive catecholamine release can cause hemodynamic instability, multiple organ failure, and cardiogenic shock. The primary underlying mechanism is activation of alpha-adrenergic receptors, which induces arterial vasoconstriction, reduced end-organ perfusion, and tissue ischemia [1]. The best treatment strategy during an acute crisis is still unclear, but hemodynamic stabilization prior to intervention is considered most appropriate. We present a case in whom emergency adrenalectomy of a (presumed) pheochromocytoma during cardiogenic shock led to a quick recovery.

2. Case Presentation

A 49-year-old male patient presented at the emergency room of the referring hospital with hematemesis and abdominal pain. The previous medical history included active smoking, epileptic seizures treated with lamotrigine, and an ischemic stroke treated with aspirin and simvastatin.

Clinical examination showed a tender abdomen. His vital signs at initial evaluation were an oxygen saturation of 85% on room air, a blood pressure of 177/125 mmHg, pulse rate 127 bpm, body temperature 37.3°C, and Glasgow coma scale of 15/15. Arterial blood gas analysis revealed a pH of 7.25, with a paO_2 of 52 mmHg, $paCO_2$ of 33 mmHg, a marked elevated serum lactate 7.2 mmol/L (normal value < 2.2 mmol/L), and a low bicarbonate level 14 mmol/L (normal range 21–26 mmol/L). Due to progressive respiratory failure with hypoxemia and hypercapnia, the patient was intubated in the emergency room. Laboratory data showed an increased hemoglobin level of 18.8 g/dL (normal range 13.5-17.0 g/dL) and leukocytosis of 30.6×10^9/L (normal range $4.3–9.6 \times 10^9$/L) with a normal CRP (<5 mg/L). Acute renal failure with a creatinine of 2.5 mg/dL (normal range

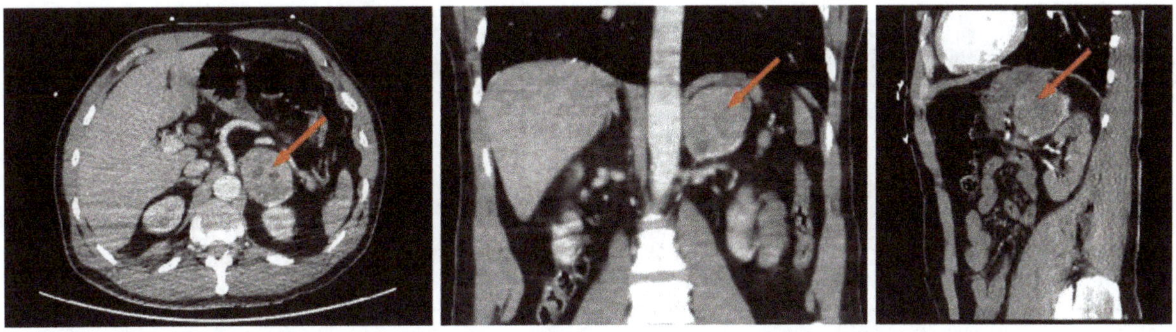

Figure 1: Abdominal computed tomography scan showed a left-sided adrenal mass of 5.7 cm (arrow).

0.7-1.3 mg/dL) was seen albeit normal electrolyte serum levels, accompanied by mildly deranged liver function tests, mildly elevated NT-pro-BNP (399 pg/mL; normal range 20-125 pg/mL), and markedly elevated high-sensitive troponin I level (2.490 ng/mL; normal range < 0.4 ng/mL). The electrocardiogram displayed sinus tachycardia with normal repolarization. Chest X-ray was compatible with pulmonary edema. Echocardiography showed a severe left ventricular dysfunction (ejection fraction of 25%) due to hypokinesia of the mid and basal segments, with preserved apical contractility. A Takotsubo syndrome was suspected. On the abdominal computerized tomography (CT) scan, which was performed because of the tender abdomen, a left-sided adrenal mass of 5.7 cm was seen (Figure 1).

The patient was referred to our tertiary intensive care unit (ICU) for hemodynamic stabilization and further (cardiac) investigation. Urgent coronary angiography revealed triple vessel disease with significant stenoses in the midleft anterior descending coronary artery (LAD) and proximal left circumflex coronary artery (LCX) and a chronic total occlusion of the proximal RCA with collaterals from the left-sided coronary artery. Ventriculography was suggestive for a basal (reverse or inverted) Takotsubo syndrome, with severe hypokinetic midventricular segments (Figure 2, Svideo). Revascularization was not performed at that stage because of the inconsistency between the coronary lesions and the regional wall abnormalities and the severe hemodynamic instability, due to a suspected pheochromocytoma, possible requiring surgery in the future.

The patient was deeply sedated and treated with the alpha-blocking agent phenoxybenzamine at high dose (20 mg b.i.d.) and an intra-aortic balloon pump. Nevertheless, he remained profoundly unstable with extreme blood pressure fluctuations (systolic blood pressure ranging from 45 mmHg to 290 mmHg) (Figure 3). Biochemically, progressive multiple organ failure was documented, with deterioration of the kidney and liver functions and a further rise in high-sensitive troponin I level to 49.821 ng/L (normal value < 45 ng/L). The placement of an extracorporeal life support (ECLS) was seriously considered, though not executed in view of the extreme hemodynamic instability.

As a catecholamine crisis was the most likely reason for the persistent hemodynamic instability, cardiogenic shock, and progressive multiple organ failure, an urgent open adrenalectomy was performed 21 hours after admission in the

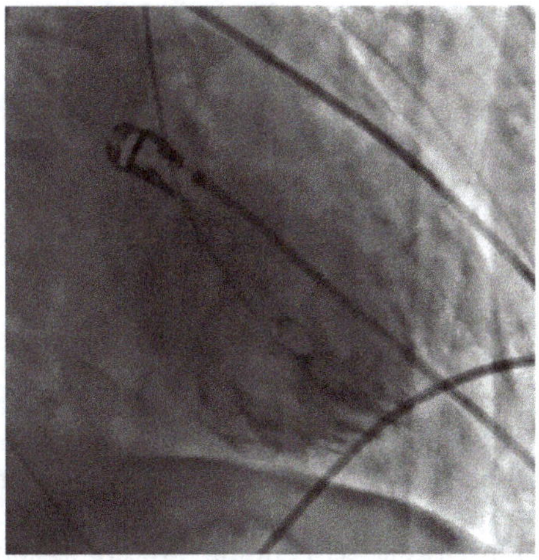

Figure 2: Left ventricular angiography during systole (RAO 24°/CRAN 8°). Severe hypokinetic midventricular segments compatible with an inverted Takotsubo syndrome (see also Supplementary Material: S1 video).

ICU; in the presence of board certified anesthesiologists, ICU physicians, and a skilled abdominal surgeon. Intraoperative rigorous fluid resuscitation was needed. After clamping of the adrenal vein and initiation of vasoactive drugs (adrenaline, noradrenaline, vasopressin, and phenylephrine), hemodynamic stabilization was rapidly achieved. Postoperatively, inotropes and vasopressors were continued. The IABP could be removed after 4 days. Due to further deterioration of the renal function, the patient received continuous venovenous hemofiltration during 7 days.

A 24-hour urine collection at admission showed extremely elevated levels of adrenaline (3001 μg/g, normal value 1–44 μg/g), noradrenaline (1600 μg/g, normal value 9–112 μg/g), metanephrine (3796 μg/g, normal value 20–174 μg/g), dopamine (435 μg/g, normal value 30–350 μg/g), and normetanephine (1210 μg/g, normal value 48–452 μg/g), compatible with massive catecholamine release by a pheochromocytoma. Histological investigation confirmed the presumed diagnosis of pheochromocytoma. A control echocardiography 7 days postoperatively showed a left ventricular ejection fraction recovery to 50%, further confirming the suspicion of left ventricular systolic dysfunction due to Takotsubo. Three weeks after surgery, coronary artery

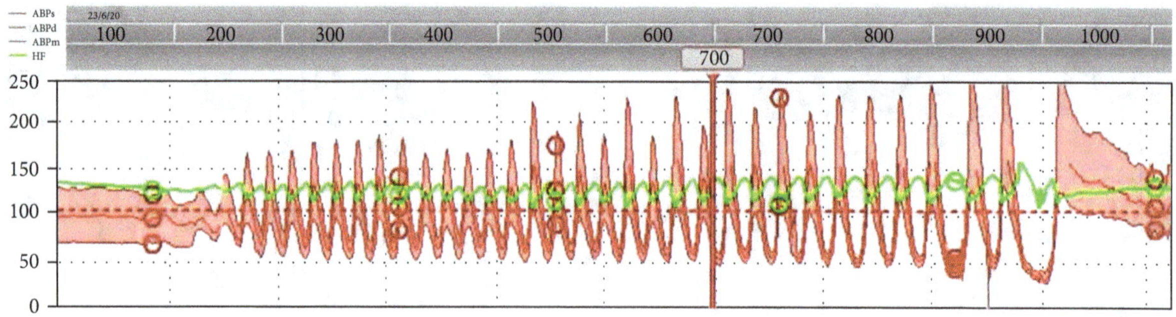

FIGURE 3: Invasive blood pressure monitoring. Cyclic fluctuations of blood pressure and heart rate with systolic blood pressures ranging from 45 mmHg up to 290 mmHg despite administration of alpha-blocking agent Phenoxybenzamine. Stabilization after emergency adrenalectomy. ABPs: arterial blood pressure systolic; ABPd: arterial blood pressure diastolic; ABPm: arterial blood pressure mean; HF: heart frequency.

revascularization was performed with implantation of drug-eluting stents in the mid-LAD and proximal LCX stenosis. The patient was discharged from the ICU 16 days after admission and from the hospital after 24 days. At a follow up visit 2 weeks after discharge and now 3 months after the acute event, the patient was doing fine.

3. Discussion

The pathophysiological mechanism of cardiac dysfunction in a pheochromocytoma crisis is not fully understood but is mainly attributed to coronary artery vasospasm provoking myocardial ischemia and a direct toxic effect of the catecholamines on myocardial cells causing myocarditis and cardiomyopathy [3]. In most cases, left ventricular dysfunction presents as a typical or 'inverted' Takotsubo cardiomyopathy [4], as was observed in our case. However, other left ventricular segments can also be affected due to individual differences in cardiac sympathetic innervation or distribution of adrenoreceptors [3]. In most patients, the cardiac dysfunction is fully reversible within a few days or weeks [5, 6]. This suggests that myocardial dysfunction is probably caused by myocardial stunning or metabolic anomaly rather than myocardial necrosis [7].

Mortality during a pheochromocytoma crisis remains high and is estimated at 15-30% [1, 2, 5]. Early diagnosis and appropriate management, including curative surgical resection, are considered essential. Based on retrospective studies, preoperative stabilization with medical treatment and fluid resuscitation is recommended, as it is believed to reduce morbidity and mortality due to hemodynamic stabilization [8, 9]. Pretreatment for 7 to 14 days before surgery is advised [9]. However, in case of an acute catecholaminergic crisis, optimal timing of surgery remains controversial as evidence from randomized controlled clinical trials is lacking [10].

Alpha-blocking agents, e.g., phenoxybenzamine or phentolamin, are the first choice therapy but not always instantly available [1]. Alternatively, calcium channel blockers can be administered, although profound hypotension in cardiogenic shock might be a limiting factor. Since beta-blockade could induce worsening of the hemodynamic status, it should only be used after prior initiation of alpha-blockade [1]. Add-on treatment with metyrosine to inhibit catecholamine synthesis can be considered [9].

In patients with a catecholaminergic crisis and cardiogenic shock, initiation of medical therapy can be challenging and organ-specific mechanical support is often needed. As represented in a multicenter retrospective study by Sauneuf et al., patients often require mechanical ventilation (85%), circulatory support (vasoactive drugs in 68% and extracorporeal membrane oxygenation (ECMO) in 41%), and renal replacement therapy (24%) [5]. Out of a pathophysiological perspective, circulatory support with inotropes or vasopressors could be associated with adverse effects on the heart and other end organs. Therefore, mechanical circulatory support, including ECLS, is increasingly used in patients with cardiogenic shock or refractory arrest to ensure adequate organ perfusion [11]. Unfortunately, ECLS-related complications (such as bleeding, infection, ischemic stroke, or lower limb ischemia) are frequent [5]. Furthermore, mechanical support systems might experience technical difficulties in patients with extreme fluctuating blood pressure, as was observed in our case.

In order to break the vicious circle of catecholamine excess and progressive organ failure, early surgical resection of a pheochromocytoma can be considered. Although a cohort study and review literature by Scholten et al. suggest that urgent surgery is associated with increased morbidity [8], these findings were biased since patients undergoing elective surgery were more stable at baseline. Also, when limiting their literature review to cases after 1990, mortality was only 1 in 18 cases (6%), which compares to the expected mortality for any severe crisis. More recent case reports and cohort studies showed no increased mortality in patients treated with emergency surgery [2, 5, 12, 13]. In a German cohort study by Riester et al., 2 out of 15 patients with life-threatening catecholamine crisis needed emergency resection because of cardiorespiratory instability and both patients survived [2]. In a French cohort study by Sauneuf et al., 5 of 34 patients underwent urgent surgery and all five were discharged alive [5].

In selected patients with extreme hemodynamic fluctuations, urgent adrenalectomy is the only option to achieve (rapid) hemodynamic stabilization, as is illustrated by our case [1, 2]. Of course, this delicate operation needs to be performed by a skilled multidisciplinary team with rigorous blood pressure monitoring and careful surgical handling of the tissue to prevent massive catecholamine release during surgical manipulation [10].

4. Conclusion

The first presentation of a pheochromocytoma can be a severe catecholaminergic crisis with hemodynamic instability, Takotsubo syndrome, cardiogenic shock, and multiple organ failure, as is illustrated in this case. Curative treatment consists of complete surgical resection. Preoperative medical management using alpha-blocking agents is recommended. Nevertheless, in persistently unstable patients with rapid deterioration, emergency resection with complete removal of the pheochromocytoma might be life-saving.

Consent

The patient granted permission for publication of his case report anonymously and had full access to the final version of the manuscript.

References

[1] B. C. Whitelaw, J. K. Prague, O. G. Mustafa et al., "Phaeochromocytoma crisis," *Clinical Endocrinology*, vol. 80, no. 1, pp. 13–22, 2014.

[2] A. Riester, D. Weismann, M. Quinkler et al., "Life-threatening events in patients with pheochromocytoma," *European Journal of Endocrinology*, vol. 173, no. 6, pp. 757–764, 2015.

[3] A. Prejbisz, J. W. M. Lenders, G. Eisenhofer, and A. Januszewicz, "Cardiovascular manifestations of phaeochromocytoma," *Journal of Hypertension*, vol. 29, no. 11, pp. 2049–2060, 2011.

[4] J. H. Park, K. S. Kim, J. Y. Sul et al., "Prevalence and patterns of left ventricular dysfunction in patients with pheochromocytoma," *Journal of Cardiovascular Ultrasound*, vol. 19, no. 2, pp. 76–82, 2011.

[5] B. Sauneuf, N. Chudeau, B. Champigneulle et al., "Pheochromocytoma crisis in the ICU: a French multicenter cohort study with emphasis on rescue extracorporeal membrane oxygenation," *Critical Care Medicine*, vol. 45, no. 7, pp. e657–e665, 2017.

[6] G. Sojod, M. Diana, J. Wall, J. D'Agostino, D. Mutter, and J. Marescaux, "Successful extracorporeal membrane oxygenation treatment for pheochromocytoma- induced acute cardiac failure," *The American Journal of Emergency Medicine*, vol. 30, no. 6, pp. 1017.e1–1017.e3, 2012.

[7] G. Hekimian, F. Kharcha, N. Bréchot et al., "Extracorporeal membrane oxygenation for pheochromocytoma-induced cardiogenic shock," *Annals of Intensive Care*, vol. 6, no. 1, p. 117, 2016.

[8] A. Scholten, R. M. Cisco, M. R. Vriens et al., "Pheochromocytoma crisis is not a surgical emergency," *The Journal of Clinical Endocrinology and Metabolism*, vol. 98, no. 2, pp. 581–591, 2013.

[9] J. W. Lenders, Q. Y. Duh, G. Eisenhofer et al., "Pheochromocytoma and paraganglioma: an endocrine society clinical practice guideline," *The Journal of Clinical Endocrinology and Metabolism*, vol. 99, no. 6, pp. 1915–1942, 2014.

[10] C. Lentschener, S. Gaujoux, A. Tesniere, and B. Dousset, "Point of controversy: perioperative care of patients undergoing pheochromocytoma removal-time for a reappraisal?," *European Journal of Endocrinology*, vol. 165, no. 3, pp. 365–373, 2011.

[11] T. Aziz, M. F. Khazi, Y. Karaly et al., "Extracorporeal membrane oxygenation (ECMO) - A lifesaving modality for treatment of pheochromocytoma-induced inverted Takotsubo-like cardiomyopathy," *The Egyptian Journal of Critical Care Medicine*, vol. 6, no. 3, pp. 133–136, 2018.

[12] K. Kakoki, Y. Shida, T. Hakariya et al., "Pheochromocytoma multisystem crisis treated with emergency surgery: a case report and literature review," *BMC Research Notes*, vol. 8, no. 1, p. 758, 2015.

[13] N. Uchida, K. Ishiguro, T. Suda, and M. Nishimura, "Pheochromocytoma multisystem crisis successfully treated by emergency surgery: report of a case," *Surgery Today*, vol. 40, no. 10, pp. 990–996, 2010.

30

Otherwise Unexplained Transient QTc Prolongation in a Patient Admitted with COVID Disease

Mark Coyle, Mark Wilkinson, and Mark Sheehy

Department of Medicine, Midlands Regional Hospital Mullingar, Longford Road, Robinstown, Mullingar, Westmeath, Ireland

Correspondence should be addressed to Mark Coyle; markcoyle95@gmail.com

Academic Editor: Assad Movahed

Background. Several cardiovascular manifestations of coronavirus disease 2019 (COVID-19) have been previously described. QT prolongation has been reported in COVID-19 infection in association with medications such as azithromycin, hydroxychloroquine, and chloroquine but has not previously been reported as a direct result of COVID-19 infection. *Case summary.* We report the case of a 65-year-old female who developed a prolonged corrected QT interval (QTc) during a hospital admission with COVID-19. This patient was not on any QT prolonging treatment, serum electrolytes were normal, and there was no identifiable reversible cause for the QTc lengthening. Daily serial ECGs during admission showed resolution of the ventricular repolarization abnormality in synchronization with resolution of her COVID-19 viral illness. *Discussions.* Although there have been reports of QTc prolongation in COVID-19 patients, previous reports of this are for patients receiving medication that causes QT prolongation. This case uniquely demonstrates the development and resolution of this temporary ventricular repolarization abnormality in a patient with a structurally normal heart with no evidence of myocardial fibrosis or edema on cardiac MRI, that is unexplained by other confounding factors, such as medication. This suggests there may be a direct association between COVID-19 and temporary QTc prolongation.

1. Introduction

Prolonged QTc is a potentially dangerous ventricular repolarization disorder that can lead to adverse events including torsades de pointes, ventricular fibrillation cardiac arrest, and sudden cardiac death. Causes include both congenital prolongation and acquired causes. Acquired causes include medication, acute electrolyte disturbances, systemic inflammation, and hypoxia [1–3]. There is increasing evidence that inflammatory cytokines, in particular, interleukin 6 (IL-6), can have a direct effect on ventricular cardiomyocyte ion channels, prolonging the action potential and hence the QTc [4–7]. There are few existing case reports of QTc prolongation in patients with COVID in the absence of conventional risk factors [8, 9]. This case suggests there may be an association with the severe acute respiratory syndrome coronavirus 2 (SARS-CoV-2) virus and temporary QTc prolongation.

2. Case Presentation

We report the case of a 65-year-old Caucasian female referred to hospital by her general practitioner with dyspnoea, chest pain, and general malaise, following a recent diagnosis of COVID-19 in the community two days prior to presenting. She had a 5-day history of dyspnoea on exertion and orthopnoea. This was associated with intermittent pleuritic chest pain and fevers. Her medical history included breast cancer treated with a lumpectomy, chemotherapy, and radiotherapy. There was no family history of sudden cardiac death or sudden adult death syndrome, no family history of long QT syndrome, and no family history of congenital deafness. She was not on any QT-prolonging treatment or any rate-limiting therapy, and her only regular medication was rosuvastatin. Her physical examination on presentation was unremarkable. Laboratory investigations revealed a mildly elevated troponin I of 0.06 ng/mL (normal range 0–0.04 ng/mL)

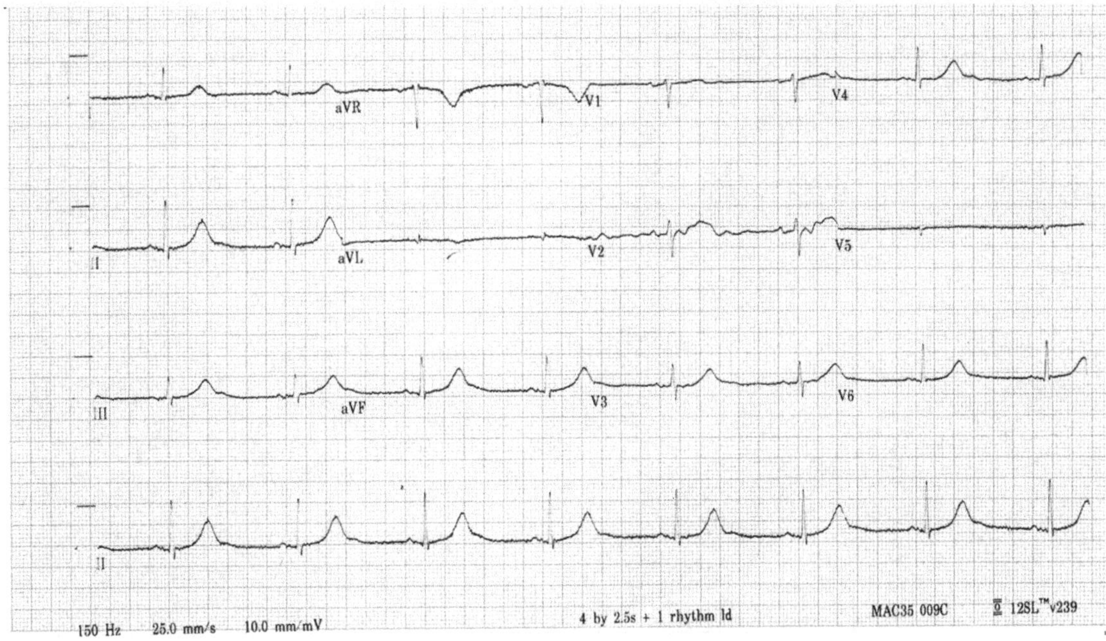

FIGURE 1: Shows day 1 ECG with a QTc of 495 ms.

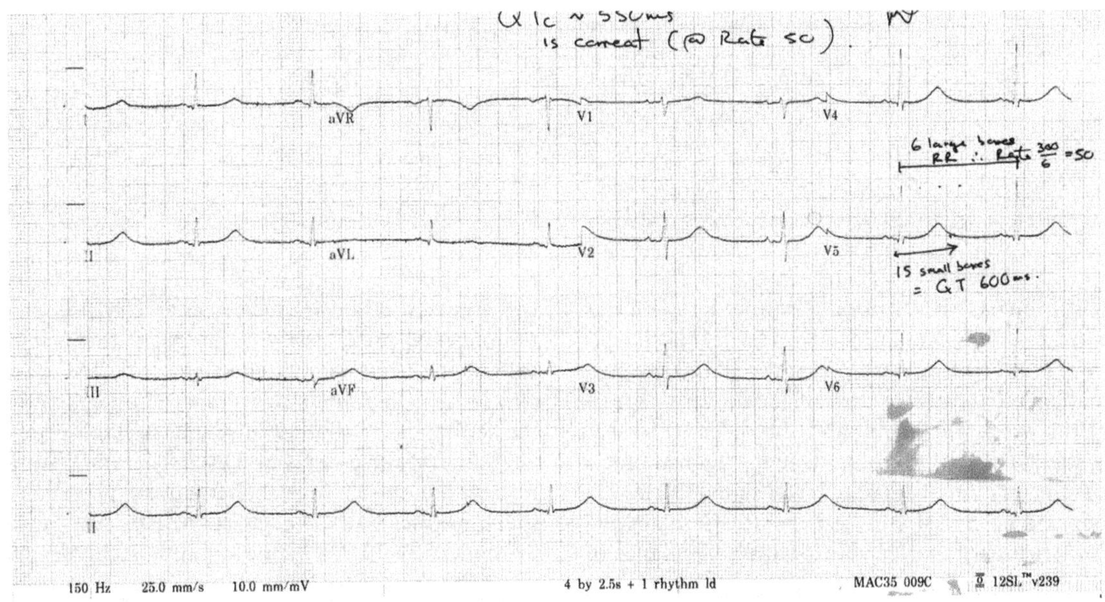

FIGURE 2: Shows day 2 ECG with a QTc of 621 ms.

which remained at 0.06 ng/mL on serial checking and a D-dimer of 624 ng/mL. Inflammatory markers were normal on admission with a C-reactive protein (CRP) of 7 mg/L (reference range 0.1–5 mg/L) and a white cell count (WCC) of 3×10^9/L. Her lymphocyte count was 1.25×10^9/L. IL-6 levels were not measured. Radiological investigations on admission revealed a normal chest X-ray, and a CT pulmonary angiogram showed patchy peripheral pulmonary infiltrates with no pulmonary embolus. Her admission ECG showed sinus bradycardia with a heart rate of 47 beats per minute and a QTc of 495 ms, shown in Figure 1. QT intervals and RR intervals were measured manually for the calculation of the QTc using Bazett's method; the calculated values were consistent with the automatic machine measurements.

A repeat ECG one day postadmission showed a QTc of 621 ms, shown in Figure 2. She was commenced on telemetry with daily monitoring of electrolytes and ECGs. Her serum electrolytes were within normal limits throughout the course of the admission. Medications used throughout the admission included enoxaparin and rosuvastatin regularly and paracetamol, lactulose, and cyclizine as required. Cetirizine was subsequently prescribed after the first week of admission. A cardiac MRI was booked in an external centre, and the patient remained in our hospital until she became

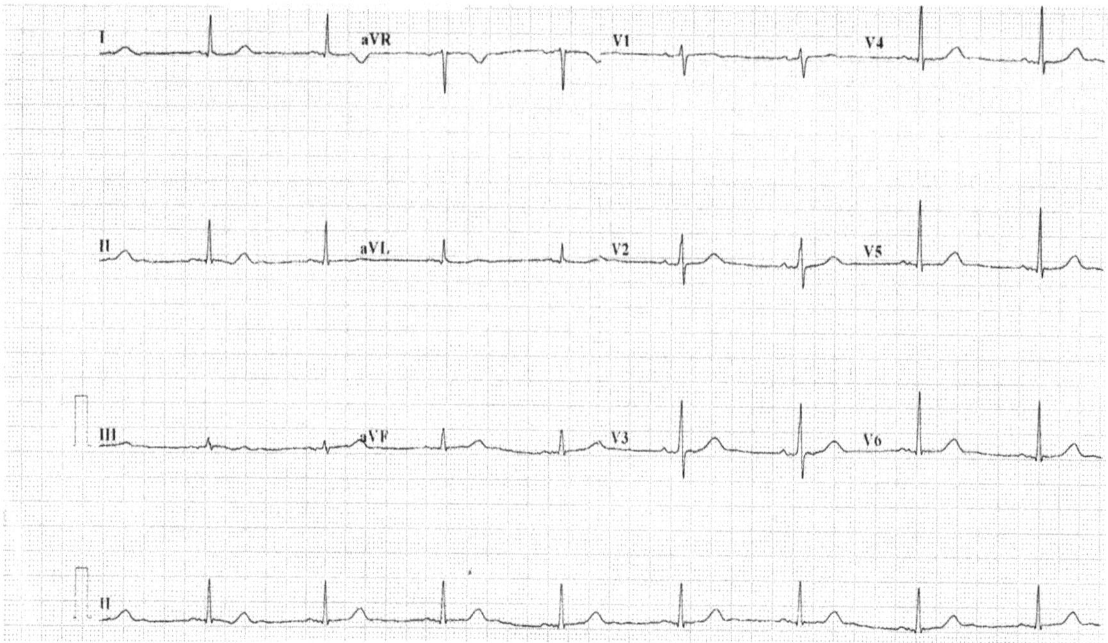

Figure 3: Shows day 24 ECG with a QTc of 445 ms.

Table 1: Association between inflammatory markers and corrected QT interval.

	Day 1	Day 2	Day 3	Day 5	Day 6	Day 7	Day 8	Day 10	Day 13	Day 20	Day 24
CRP (mg/L)	7.3	7.4	6.2	9.2	10.4	11	12	15.5	8.2	5.5	Not recorded
WCC ($\times 10^9$/L)	3.57	4.11	2.85	2.97	3.21	2.77	3.7	3.5	5.52	5.44	
QTc (ms)	495	621	561	516	502	479	Not recorded		465	465	445

CRP: C-reactive protein; mg/L: milligrams per liter; WCC: white cell count, QTc: QT interval corrected; ms: milliseconds.

noninfectious from COVID-19 prior to transfer for MRI. Her QTc decreased gradually over the course of her 24-day hospital admission. From a respiratory perspective, she remained well, her peripheral oxygen saturation levels were normal throughout the entire admission, and she did not develop any supplementary oxygen requirement. Transthoracic echocardiogram was unremarkable, revealing a structurally normal heart and no evidence of heart failure. Cardiac MRI confirmed a structurally normal heart with no evidence of myocardial fibrosis or edema. A trivial pericardial effusion was present. Her QTc resolved to a normal level of 445 ms, shown in Figure 3. She remained clinically well and was discharged.

3. Discussion

The average QTc in healthy persons after puberty is 420 ± 20 milliseconds. Generally, the 99th percentile QTc values are 470 milliseconds in postpubertal males and 480 milliseconds in postpubertal females [10]. A QTc > 500 milliseconds is considered highly abnormal for both males and females. Several manifestations of cardiovascular disease have been previously described in COVID-19 [11]. Existing literature regarding QTc prolongation in COVID-19 focuses on predictable pharmacodynamic effects of offlicense pharmacotherapeutic strategies such as antimalarial drugs [12]. The prolongation previously seen has been attributable to medications with this known effect [13, 14]. This case demonstrates an acute ventricular repolarization abnormality in the setting of COVID-19 infection, that self-resolved as the viral illness course resolved. This self-limiting temporary disturbance, in the absence of alternative explanations, suggests that there may be a direct effect on ventricular repolarization from COVID-19. Cetirizine, an anti-H1 histamine receptor drug, was prescribed following a week of admission, which is recognized to have QT-prolonging potential [15]. It is possible that the effects of COVID-associated systemic inflammation on the QTc may have been enhanced by the concomitant cetirizine treatment.

The relationship between COVID-19 and ventricular repolarization is an area of worldwide interest with an ongoing trial in critically unwell patients to determine the effect of COVID-19 (and its treatments) on ventricular repolarization as measured by the QTc [16]. Systemic inflammation rapidly induces cytokine-mediated ventricular electrical remodeling and significant QTc prolongation [17, 18]. It is possible that an important factor involved in QTc prolongation in COVID-19 is the systemic inflammation characterizing the disease, often described as a "cytokine storm" in which IL-6 seems to play a central role. This systemic inflammation via elevated IL-6 is itself an independent risk factor for QTc prolongation, by modulating cardiomyocyte ion channel expression [18]. Other viral illnesses have been reported to exhibit this effect—HIV seropositivity is associated with a prolonged QT [19]. Physiological changes in acute illness can also lead to a temporary ventricular repolarization abnormality—core body temperature can impact QT duration with moderate hypothermia causing temporary prolongation of the QTc as well as fever [20, 21]. However, in this case, our patient remained normothermic throughout the admission, and her CRP and WCC were only very mildly elevated while these electrocardiographic changes occurred, as shown in Table 1. Although CRP synthesis is largely dependent on direct hepatocyte stimulation by IL-6, it is possible for a mismatch to exist (for example, in patients with abnormal liver function) between circulating levels of IL-6 and CRP. Despite this patient having a normal liver function, it cannot be excluded that the blood concentration of IL-6 (which is the actual mediator of the electrophysiologic effects of systemic inflammation on the cardiomyocyte) was higher than expected based on the CRP levels. However, this case suggests that there may be a novel COVID-19 infection-specific mechanism for QT prolongation not previously described.

Consent

Written informed consent was obtained from the patient.

References

[1] E. Vandael, B. Vandenberk, J. Vandenberghe, R. Willems, and V. Foulon, "Risk factors for QTc-prolongation: systematic review of the evidence," *International Journal of Clinical Pharmacy*, vol. 39, no. 1, pp. 16–25, 2017.

[2] P. E. Lazzerini, M. Boutjdir, and P. L. Capecchi, "COVID-19, arrhythmic risk, and inflammation," *Circulation*, vol. 142, no. 1, pp. 7–9, 2020.

[3] P. Dherange, J. Lang, P. Qian et al., "Arrhythmias and COVID-19: a review," *JACC: Clinical Electrophysiology*, vol. 6, no. 9, pp. 1193–1204, 2020.

[4] P. E. Lazzerini, F. Laghi-Pasini, M. Boutjdir, and P. L. Capecchi, "Cardioimmunology of arrhythmias: the role of autoimmune and inflammatory cardiac channelopathies," *Nature Reviews Immunology*, vol. 19, no. 1, pp. 63-64, 2019.

[5] A. S. Aromolaran, U. Srivastava, A. Alí et al., "Interleukin-6 inhibition of hERG underlies risk for acquired long QT in cardiac and systemic inflammation," *PLoS One*, vol. 13, no. 12, article e0208321, 2018.

[6] P. E. Lazzerini, F. Laghi-Pasini, I. Bertolozzi et al., "Systemic inflammation as a novel QT-prolonging risk factor in patients with torsades de pointes," *Heart*, vol. 103, no. 22, pp. 1821–1829, 2017.

[7] P. E. Lazzerini, P. L. Capecchi, N. El-Sherif, F. Laghi-Pasini, and M. Boutjdir, "Emerging arrhythmic risk of autoimmune and inflammatory cardiac channelopathies," *Journal of the American Heart Association*, vol. 7, no. 22, article e010595, 2018.

[8] B. K. Anupama, S. Adhikari, and D. Chaudhuri, "Prolonged QT interval in a patient with Coronavirus disease-2019: beyond hydroxychloroquine and azithromycin," *Journal of Investigative Medicine High Impact Case Reports*, vol. 8, 2020.

[9] O. Elsaid, P. A. McCullough, K. M. Tecson, R. S. Williams, and A. Yoon, "Ventricular fibrillation storm in coronavirus 2019," *The American Journal of Cardiology*, vol. 135, pp. 177–180, 2020.

[10] J. R. Giudicessi, P. A. Noseworthy, P. A. Friedman, and M. J. Ackerman, "Urgent Guidance for Navigating and Circumventing the QTc-Prolonging and Torsadogenic Potential of Possible Pharmacotherapies for Coronavirus Disease 19 (COVID-19)," in *Mayo Clinic Proceedings*, pp. 1213–1221, Elsevier, 2020.

[11] M. Nishiga, D. W. Wang, Y. Han, D. B. Lewis, and J. C. Wu, "COVID-19 and cardiovascular disease: from basic mechanisms to clinical perspectives," *Nature Reviews Cardiology*, vol. 17, no. 9, pp. 543–558, 2020.

[12] F. Bessière, H. Roccia, A. Delinière et al., "Assessment of QT intervals in a case series of patients with coronavirus disease 2019 (COVID-19) infection treated with hydroxychloroquine alone or in combination with azithromycin in an intensive care unit," *JAMA Cardiology*, vol. 5, no. 9, pp. 1067–1069, 2020.

[13] N. J. Mercuro, C. F. Yen, D. J. Shim et al., "Risk of QT interval prolongation associated with use of hydroxychloroquine with or without concomitant azithromycin among hospitalized patients testing positive for coronavirus disease 2019 (COVID-19)," *JAMA Cardiology*, vol. 5, no. 9, pp. 1036–1041, 2020.

[14] S. Agstam, A. Yadav, M. P. Kumar, and A. Gupta, "Hydroxychloroquine and QTc prolongation in patients with COVID-19: a systematic review and meta-analysis," *Indian Pacing and Electrophysiology Journal*, vol. 21, no. 1, pp. 36–43, 2021.

[15] E. Poluzzi, E. Raschi, B. Godman et al., "Pro-arrhythmic potential of oral antihistamines (H1): combining adverse event reports with drug utilization data across Europe," *PLoS One*, vol. 10, no. 3, article e0119551, 2015.

[16] M. Zaballos, "Effects on the Qt interval of COVID-19 coronavirus infection (QT-COVID-19)," https://clinicaltrials.gov/ct2/show/study/NCT04422535.

[17] P. E. Lazzerini, M. Acampa, F. Laghi-Pasini et al., "Cardiac arrest risk during acute infections: systemic inflammation directly prolongs QTc interval via cytokine-mediated effects on potassium channel expression," *Circulation. Arrhythmia and Electrophysiology*, vol. 13, no. 8, article e008627, 2020.

[18] K. C. Wu, L. Zhang, S. A. Haberlen et al., "Predictors of electrocardiographic QT interval prolongation in men with HIV," *Heart*, vol. 105, no. 7, pp. 559–565, 2019.

[19] D. B. Chastain, M. P. Veve, and J. L. Wagner, "Abnormal QTc syndrome in HIV-infected patients: a systematic review of prevalence and risk factors," *Antiviral Therapy*, vol. 24, no. 6, pp. 459–465, 2019.

[20] E. S. Dietrichs, T. Tveita, and G. Smith, "Hypothermia and cardiac electrophysiology: a systematic review of clinical and experimental data," *Cardiovascular Research*, vol. 115, no. 3, pp. 501–509, 2019.

[21] A. Burashnikov, W. Shimizu, and C. Antzelevitch, "Fever accentuates transmural dispersion of repolarization and facilitates development of early afterdepolarizations and torsade de pointes under long-QT conditions," *Circulation: Arrhythmia and Electrophysiology*, vol. 1, no. 3, pp. 202–208, 2008.

31

A Case of Asymptomatic Pulmonary Artery Aneurysm with Review of Management Strategies

Muhammad Talha Ayub,[1] Allison Zimmerman,[2] Wajeeha Rasool,[3] Dinesh Kalra,[1] Melissa Tracy,[1] and Anupama K. Rao[1]

[1]*Division of Cardiovascular Medicine, RUSH University Medical Center, Chicago IL, USA*
[2]*Department of Medicine, RUSH University Medical Center, Chicago IL, USA*
[3]*Department of Medicine, Amita Health Presence St Francis Hospital, Evanston IL, USA*

Correspondence should be addressed to Muhammad Talha Ayub; talhaayubmd@gmail.com

Academic Editor: Takatoshi Kasai

Pulmonary artery aneurysm (PAA) is defined as pulmonary artery diameter greater than 4 cm. With advances in cardiac imaging, the detection rate has increased but the natural history remains unknown. We present the case of a large, incidentally identified PAA in a patient with a history of congenital pulmonic stenosis.

1. History of Presentation

A 57-year-old Caucasian female presented to the cardiology clinic for evaluation of an incidentally diagnosed pulmonary artery aneurysm that was previously identified during workup of epigastric pain. Her epigastric pain was responsive to a trial of proton pump inhibitors. The patient was asymptomatic when she presented to the clinic. Vital signs on presentation were remarkable for blood pressure of 118/70 mmHg, temperature 98.2 F, heart rate 66/min, and respiratory rate 16/min. Her cardiopulmonary physical exam was unremarkable, with a normal S1 and S2 and without an audible murmur.

2. Past Medical History

(i) Moderate to severe congenital pulmonic stenosis (PS) diagnosed at 2 years of age based on right heart catheterization (RHC) findings; right ventricular (RV) systolic pressure 70 mmHg, mean pulmonary artery (PA) pressure 30 mmHg, and transvalvular systolic pressure gradient of 50 mmHg. Repeat RHC at the age of 5 years showed spontaneous regression to mild pulmonic stenosis; RV pressure of 50 mmHg, mean PA pressure 16 mmHg, with a transvalvular systolic pressure gradient of 30 mmHg

(ii) Idiopathic ventricular tachycardia status post right ventricular outflow tract (RVOT) ablation at age 52

3. Differential Diagnosis and Etiology of PAA

(i) Congenital structural cardiac anomalies that alter hemodynamics and increase stress on the pulmonary artery: pulmonary valve stenosis, persistent ductus arteriosus, ventricular septal defects, atrial septal defects, hypoplastic aortic valve, and bicuspid aortic valve

(ii) Pulmonary hypertension

(iii) Trauma (iatrogenic from previous right heart catheterization)

(iv) Infections: tuberculosis and syphilis

(v) Connective tissue diseases: Marfan syndrome, Ehlers-Danlos syndrome, and cystic medial necrosis

(vi) Vasculitides: Bechet disease and giant cell arteritis

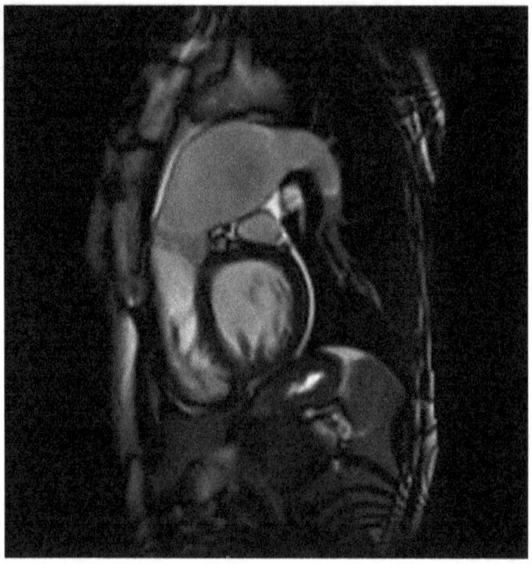

FIGURE 1: Cardiac MR RVOT view showing large PAA.

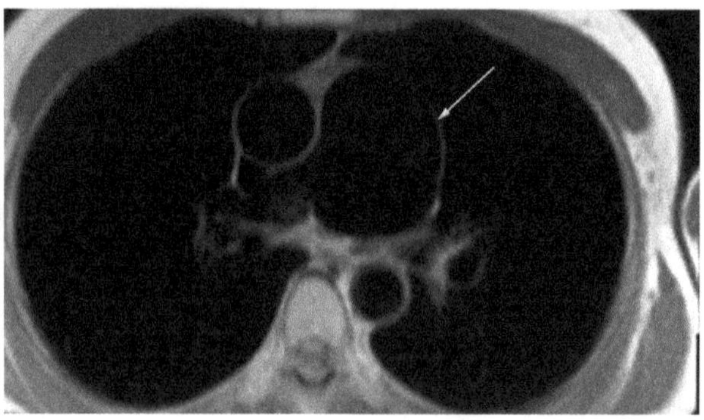

FIGURE 2: Cardiac MR axial localizer image showing PAA.

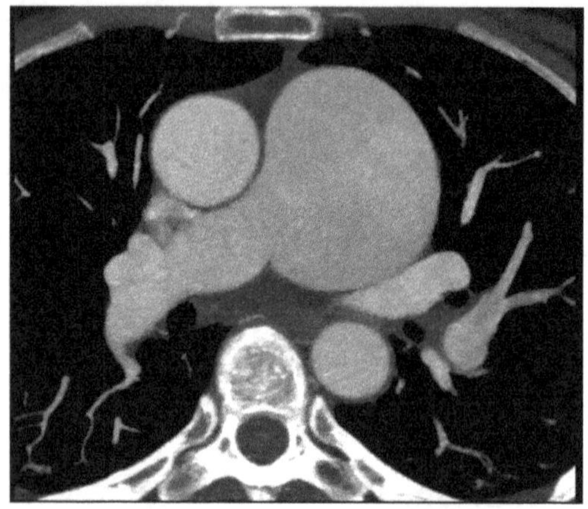

FIGURE 3: Cardiac CT axial images showing a 6.2 × 6.1 cm PAA.

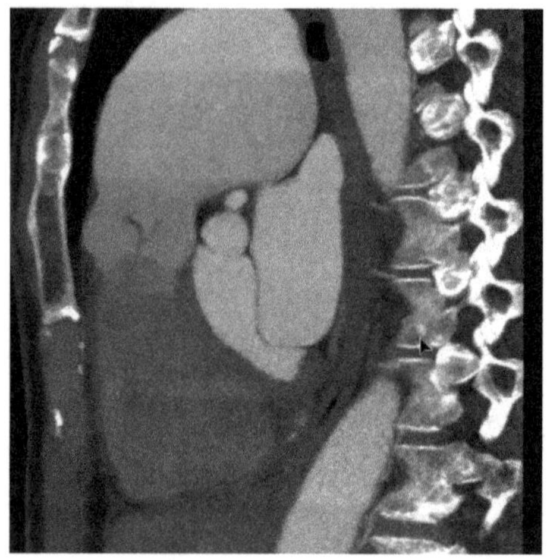

FIGURE 4: Cardiac CT sagittal section with PAA and pulmonic valve anatomy.

4. Investigations

Routine laboratory testing did not reveal any abnormalities. Electrocardiogram was revealing of normal sinus rhythm with left bundle branch block morphology of QRS complex. Transthoracic echocardiogram was remarkable for normal left ventricular systolic function. Right atrium and ventricle were mildly dilated with normal systolic function. Pulmonic valve was not visualized. Cardiac MRI performed, at our facility, prior to her clinic visit demonstrated a large 58 × 57 mm aneurysm of the PA and mild pulmonic valve thickening (Figures 1 and 2) with mild PS by velocity encoded phase contrast imaging (peak velocity 1.6 m/s and peak gradient 10 mmHg).

5. Management

Given the large size of the PAA, the patient was evaluated by an adult congenital heart specialist as well as by the cardiovascular surgery service. She underwent right and left heart catheterization that demonstrated a normal peak gradient (8 mmHg) across the pulmonic valve, normal right- and left-sided pressures, and angiographically normal coronary arteries. Cardiac CT was performed for additional anatomic assessment with a PAA of 62.6 × 61.7 mm without thrombus within the aneurysm sac (Figures 3, 4 and 5). The pulmonic root and RVOT were normal in size; there was no evidence of compression of adjacent structures (Figures 3 and 5). Surgical intervention was ultimately deferred due to her asymptomatic status and absence of high-risk features such as pulmonary hypertension, sac thrombus, compressive effect on the surrounding structures, and insufficient evidence for rate of growth of the aneurysm. Multidisciplinary cardiovascular team discussion concluded medical management with close follow-up was the best strategy. The patient is scheduled for serial imaging to monitor for growth in the size of the aneurysm and clinical surveillance for development of resultant complications. She will undergo annual transthoracic echocardiogram to monitor for development of pulmonary regurgitation and pulmonary hypertension. Strict blood pressure control was also recommended. She was instructed to avoid heavy lifting and high intensity workouts.

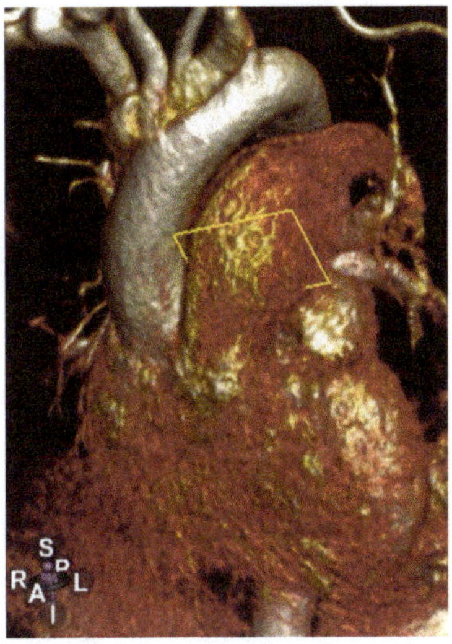

Figure 5: Cardiac CT 3D reconstruction.

6. Discussion

Our patient had a large PAA presumably due to poststenotic dilatation from congenital, self-resolving, moderate to severe PS. Pulmonic stenosis has frequently been described as an isolated cause of PAA formation (1). PAAs were believed to be exceedingly rare but are increasingly recognized in the era of modern imaging. In a review of 109,571 autopsy cases over 100 years, only 8 cases of PAAs were identified (incidence rate 0.0073%) (2). Currently, there is no consensus regarding treatment of PAA based on size criteria; additionally, there are no clear guidelines delineating the roles of medical or surgical/percutaneous therapies for PAA. Treatment strategies include conservative management, endovascular repair, and surgical repair via aneurysmorrhaphy or PA replacement with allogeneic/synthetic grafts.

Conservative management is reasonable in the absence of pH, PAA thrombus, compression of adjacent structures, ≥5 mm increase in PAA diameter in 6 months, absolute PA diameter>5.5 cm, evidence of valvular pathology or shunt flow, and/or signs of rupture/dissection. Conservative management is focused on the treatment of underlying cause, especially in cases of infectious and vasculitis mediated etiologies. Favorable hemodynamic effects of beta blockers and diuretics (which decrease PA pressure and shear stress on the vessel wall) appear to be key features in the medical management of idiopathic PAAs (3).

While the size of the PAA (>5.5 cm) in this case could be considered large enough to necessitate surgical repair, the patient was asymptomatic and had evidence of low pressures within the PA system, with absence of high risk features on imaging. A conservative approach was deemed reasonable after a detailed multidisciplinary team and patient discussion considering the high risk to benefit ratio for surgical correction. Elevated PA pressure, due to medial necrosis, is by far the most important determinant favoring surgical intervention (4). A systematic review by Duijnhouwer et al. showed that the presence and duration of elevated intravascular pressure is the most important predictive factor for complications in PAA associated with congenital diseases (5). In patients who have low pressure systems, as in our patient, there appears to be a low incidence of PAA dissection (6).

Reisenauer et al. have recommended a management strategy by classifying patients into three groups. Those with "giant" aneurysm (greater than 8 cm) should undergo surgical intervention. PAAs between 5 and 8 cm are candidates for surgical intervention if symptomatic have evidence of serial growth or a high-pressure PA system. Those with PAAs less than 5 cm should be monitored with serial imaging (4).

In cases where intervention is needed, there are several surgical approaches described in the literature. Aneurysmorrhaphy is recommended in patients with an area of focal dilatation of the pulmonary artery. It involves excision and repair of the most dilated part of the aneurysm. Although there are no specific guidelines for endovascular vs. surgical repair of PAA, most of the literature suggests that endovascular treatment be offered when feasible as there is less morbidity and mortality. Other endovascular options that have been described include the use of coil embolization, vascular plugs, stent-assisted coil embolization, and stent grafting of the pulmonary arteries (7) {Park, 2018 #254}. While endovascular treatments carry less risk compared to surgery, they maintain similar risks to other endovascular embolization procedures elsewhere in the body including nontarget embolization, arterial thrombosis, arterial dissection, contrast-induced nephropathy, and end-organ damage. More invasive options involve complete replacement of the entire pulmonary trunk with a synthetic graft. This approach is typically used for PAAs secondary to infectious and inflammatory diseases (3). In cases where the pulmonic valve is involved, repair or replacement should be considered for the relief of right ventricular volume overload and vessel wall burden. In fact, aneurysmorrhaphy alone without pulmonic valve replacement was associated with recurrence of PA dilatation, possibly as a result of hemodynamic stress on the vessel wall (8). Treatment of distal PAAs is more complex and may require lung resection and combined heart-lung transplantation, particularly in patients with PAH (1). There is a lack of data regarding morbidity and mortality in relation to surgery, because no large series of PAA patients have been studied; however, it has been suggested that perioperative morbidity is comparable to that of aortic aneurysm repair (1). Given the lack of consensus on guidelines for treatment, a multidisciplinary approach between specialists is necessary to increase survival and minimize the risk of procedure-related complications.

7. Conclusions

(1) PAAs are a rare albeit important clinical entity with an increase in the incidence due to the advent of multimodality cardiac imaging

(2) Careful management is crucial because of the fatal complications including rupture, dissection, pulmonary embolism, and heart failure

(3) An absolute diameter threshold for intervention does not exist. We believe that there should be a higher threshold for surgical management of PAA than for aneurysms of the aorta, especially when the PA pressure is normal

(4) Pulmonary artery pressure, aneurysm size, symptoms, and etiology of PAA are the important determinants of treatment strategy

7.1. Take-Home Messages/Learning Objectives

(1) Definite thresholds for surgical correction of PAA do not exist. Studies aiming at describing the natural history of PAAs, risk of complications, and optimal management strategy are needed

(2) Patients with PAAs should be closely monitored for signs and symptoms of heart failure, pulmonary insufficiency, pulmonary hypertension, and/or rapid increase in the size in which case surgical correction should not be delayed

References

[1] M. Kreibich, M. Siepe, J. Kroll, R. Hohn, J. Grohmann, and F. Beyersdorf, "Aneurysms of the pulmonary artery," *Circulation*, vol. 131, no. 3, pp. 310–316, 2015.

[2] R. A. Deterling Jr. and O. T. Clagett, "Aneurysm of the pulmonary artery; review of the literature and report of a case," *American Heart Journal*, vol. 34, no. 4, pp. 471–499, 1947.

[3] R. Hou, G. T. Ma, X. R. Liu et al., "Surgical treatment of pulmonary artery aneurysm: an institutional experience and literature review," *Interactive Cardiovascular and Thoracic Surgery*, vol. 23, no. 3, pp. 438–442, 2016.

[4] J. S. Reisenauer, S. M. Said, H. V. Schaff, H. M. Connolly, J. J. Maleszewski, and J. A. Dearani, "Outcome of surgical repair of pulmonary artery aneurysms: a single-center experience with 38 patients," *The Annals of Thoracic Surgery*, vol. 104, no. 5, pp. 1605–1610, 2017.

[5] A. L. Duijnhouwer, E. P. Navarese, A. P. J. van Dijk, B. Loeys, J. W. Roos-Hesselink, and M. J. de Boer, "Aneurysm of the pulmonary artery, a systematic review and critical analysis of current literature," *Congenital Heart Disease*, vol. 11, no. 2, pp. 102–109, 2016.

[6] S. Ercan, A. Dogan, G. Altunbas, and V. Davutoglu, "Giant pulmonary artery aneurysm: 12 years of follow-up. Case report and review of the literature," *The Thoracic and Cardiovascular Surgeon*, vol. 62, no. 5, pp. 450–452, 2014.

32

Acute Coronary Artery Occlusion during Transcatheter Aortic Valve Replacement in a Patient with an Anomalous Left Circumflex Coronary Artery

Rongfeng Xu, Jiandong Ding, Lijuan Chen, Yi Feng, and Genshan Ma

Department of Cardiology, Zhongda Hospital, Medical School of Southeast University, Nanjing, 210009 Jiangsu, China

Correspondence should be addressed to Genshan Ma; magenshan@hotmail.com

Academic Editor: Yigit Canga

Background. Acute coronary artery occlusion (CAO) during transcatheter aortic valve replacement (TAVR) is a rare but life-threatening complication during the procedure; there were a few case reports about an anomalous LCX during perioperative period. We report a case of successful coronary protection using the chimney stenting technique in a patient with a severely calcified aortic valve and an anomalous LCX. *Case Summary.* A 75-year-old man was found an anomalous left circumflex coronary artery (LCX) originating from the right coronary cusp with severely calcified aortic valve stenosis requiring TAVR. When a self-expanding aortic valve was deployed, we found flow compromise in the right coronary system and circumflex to TIMI-0 flow. By using the chimney stenting technique, we rapidly planted 2 stents from the proximal CX branch to the sinotubular junction and the coronary flow was maintained. *Conclusion.* Chimney stenting protection as a bailout technique is safe and feasible and should be considered in patients deemed to be at high risk of coronary flow compromise, especially with an anomalous LCX.

1. Introduction

Although traditional surgical aortic valve replacement (SAVR) has been the mainstream treatment method for symptomatic severe aortic stenosis, transcatheter aortic valve replacement (TAVR) is becoming a standard-of-care procedure for those patients who would be at high or intermediate risk for cardiac surgery. Acute coronary artery occlusion (CAO) during TAVR is a rare (<1%) but life-threatening complication in contemporary practice, and specific subsets of patients remain at risk [1]. Displacement of the calcified native valve leaflet over the coronary ostium and direct occlusion of the coronary ostium by the covered skirt of the transcatheter aortic prosthesis are the usual causes of CAO. This phenomenon is associated with anatomical factors, including lower-lying coronary ostia and shallow sinuses of Valsalva (SOVs), and especially valve-in-valve (VIV) for surgical bioprostheses [2]. Furthermore, an anomalous coronary artery may be an unusual cause of CAO [3]. There are only a few reports of TAVR in the context of an anomalous LCX [4]. Coronary protection during TAVR is a preemptive technique recommended in certain cases to avoid this complication. As an important bailout technique, the "chimney" stenting technique is performed during or after TAVR if coronary blood flow is compromised [5]. We report a case of successful coronary protection by using the chimney stenting technique in a patient with a severely calcified aortic valve and an anomalous LCX.

2. Case Presentation

A 75-year-old man was admitted to our hospital with a history of active dyspnea for 1 year and no coronary heart disease, hypertension, or diabetes. He had been smoking for 40 years, with 10 cigarettes per day. Physical exam revealed a grade 5 crescendo-decrescendo murmur without elevated JVP and lower extremity edema. Laboratory findings were pertinent for creatinine NT pro-BNP of 2320 pg/ml and TNI 0.023 ng/ml. The rest of his physical exam and laboratory was normal. Electrocardiogram showed a normal sinus

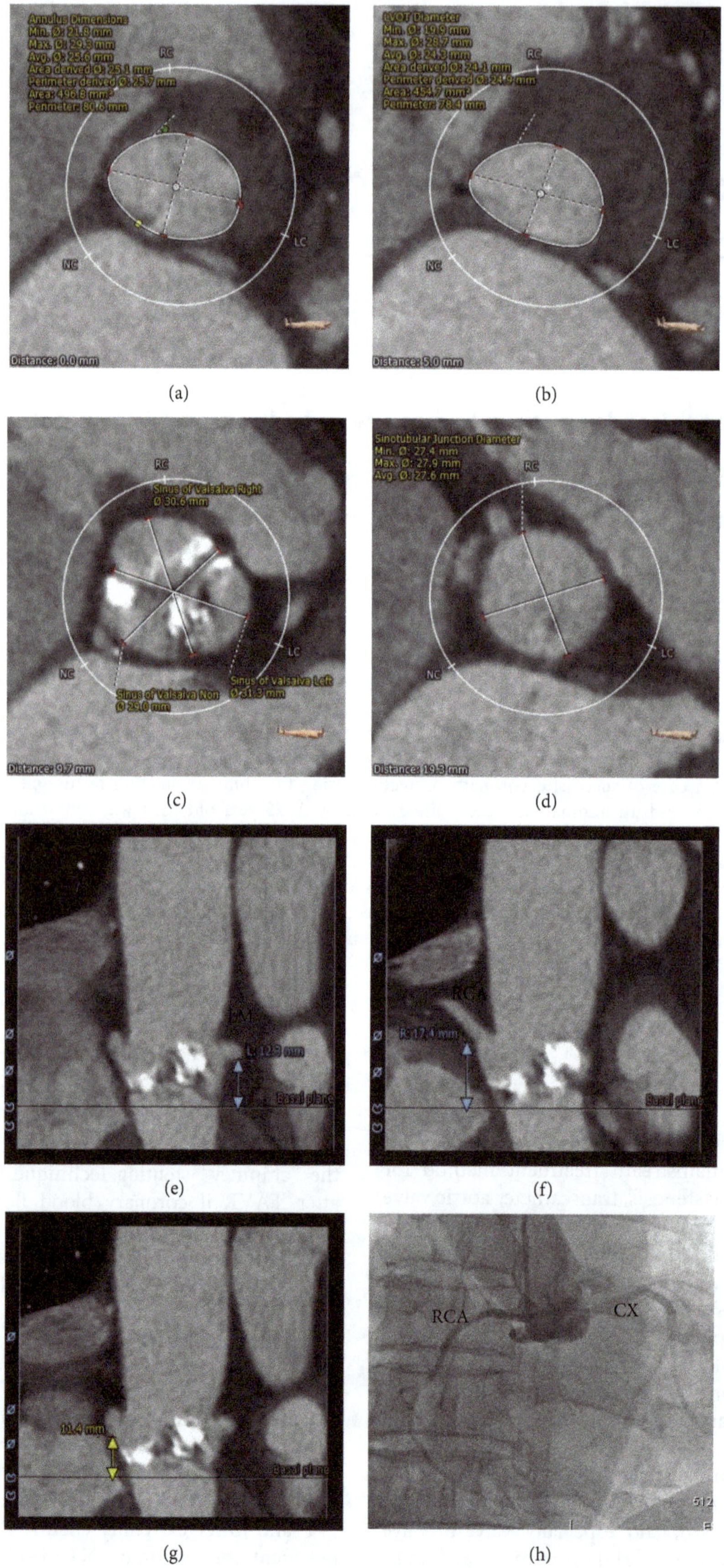

Figure 1: Cardiac computed tomography angiography showed severely calcified aortic leaflets with anatomical abnormalities of the right coronary system, which revealed a circumflex branch originating from the right coronary sinus, as shown by CAG.

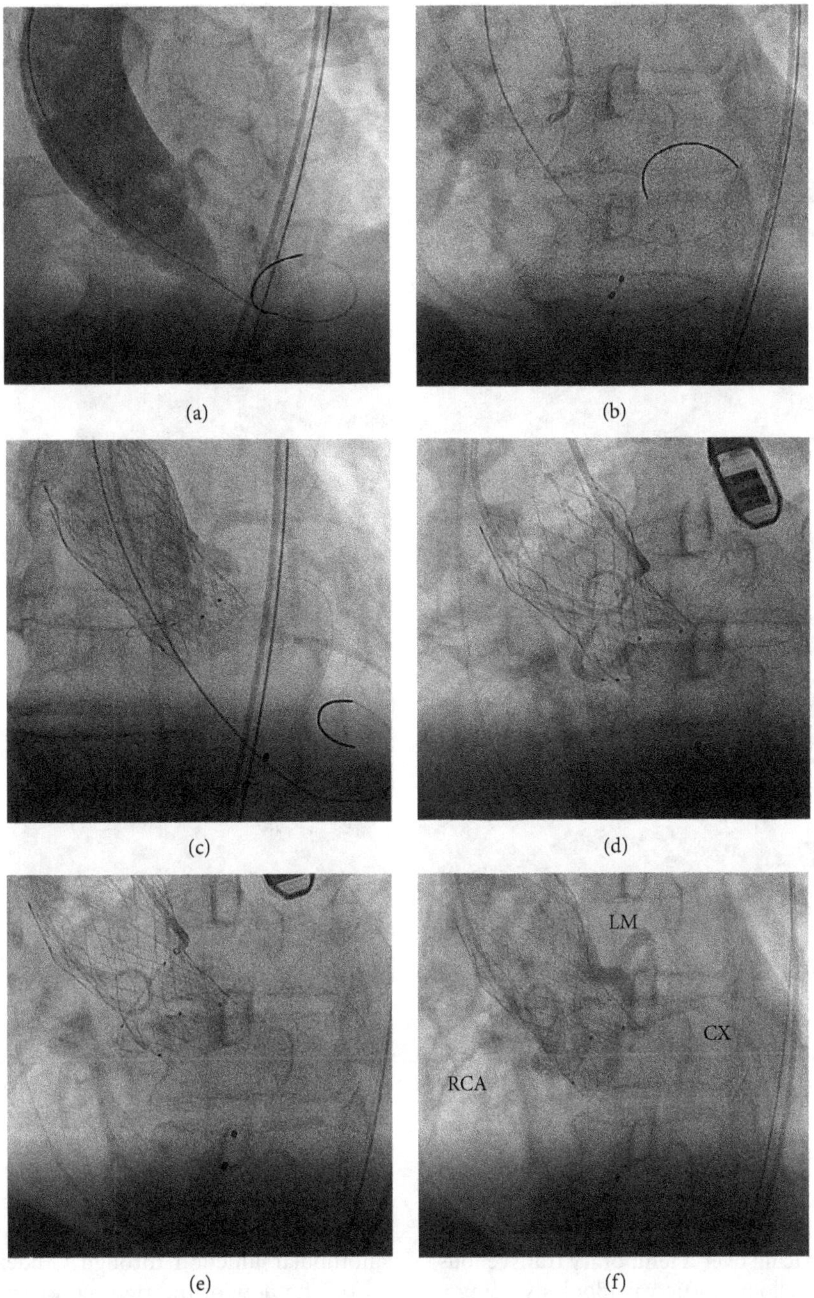

Figure 2: Balloon aortic valvuloplasty and simultaneous aortic root injection showing decreased coronary flow to TIMI-0 in the RCA and CX. One guidewire was advanced to the RCA and CX with a 2.0 * 20 mm semicompliant balloon. There was flow compromise in the right coronary system and CX to TIMI-0 flow after TAVR, followed by deployment of two stents from the proximal CX branch to the sinotubular junction. The flow of the right coronary artery and CX was retained, and the elevated ST segment in the EKG was reversed.

rhythm with a known right bundle branch block. Echocardiogram demonstrated severe aortic stenosis with a mean aortic valve pressure gradient of 100.5 mmHg and peak velocity of 5.60 m/s, with preserved systolic function. The patient received intravenous diuretics with some clinical improvement. He was seen and evaluated by a cardiothoracic surgeon for evaluation of aortic valve replacement but deemed intermediate risk for SAVR, with an estimated surgical mortality risk of 4.15% according to the Society of Thoracic Surgeons score. Cardiac computed tomography angiography was performed as part of the TAVR evaluation (Figures 1(a)–1(d)) and showed severely calcified aortic leaflets with an anomalous LCX, which revealed a circumflex branch originating from the right SOV. The ostial heights of the left and right coronaries were 12.3 mm and 17.4 mm, respectively (Figures 1(e) and 1(f)), while the ostial height of the circumflex artery was 11.4 mm (Figure 1(g)). Coronary angiography revealed normal left and right coronary arteries and an anomalous circumflex coronary artery without stenosis (Figure 1(h)). Special attention was given to right coronary leaflet calcification and anatomical abnormalities of the circumflex. The decision was then made to

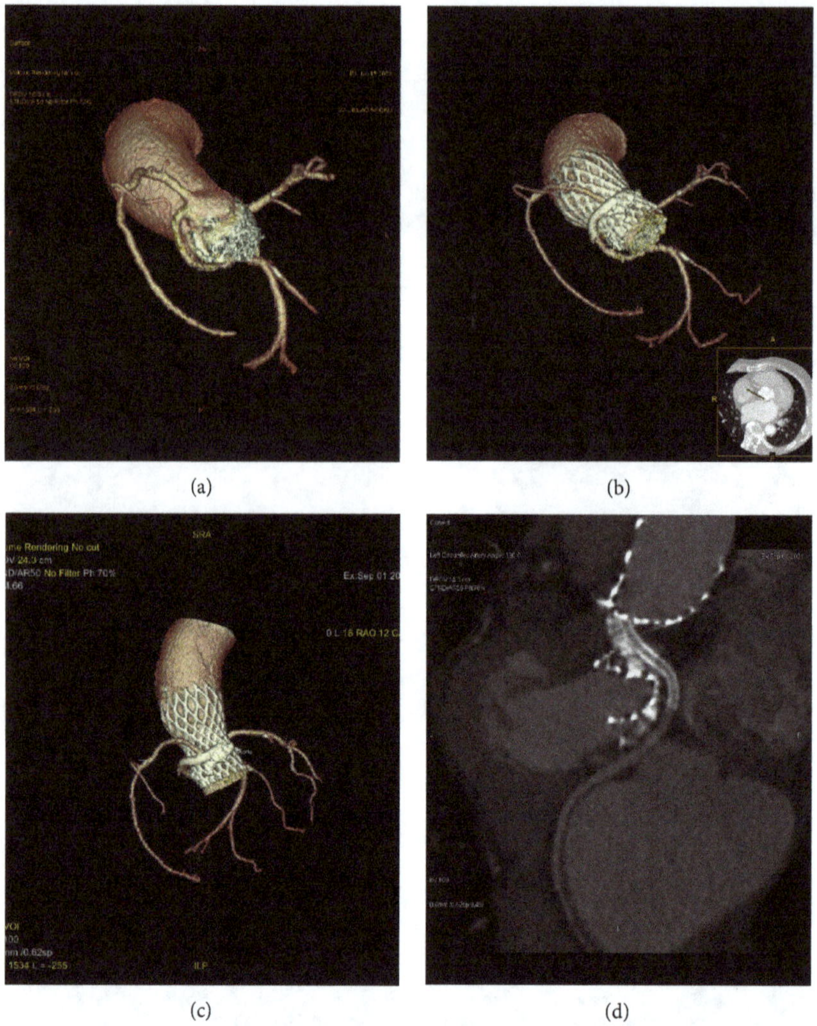

Figure 3: Six-month follow-up results after TAVR. (a) Cardiac computed tomography angiography showed a circumflex branch originating from right coronary sinus before TAVR. (b–d) Six-month follow-up after TAVR. CTA of the aortic and coronary regions suggested unobstructed coronary flow of the CX.

proceed with TAVR utilizing the coronary protection technique during the procedure. TAVR was then undertaken from the right femoral artery through a 19F arterial sheath. With rapid ventricular pacing over a temporary transvenous pacing wire (180 bpm), balloon aortic valvuloplasty using a 22 × 40 mm balloon (VENUS MEDTECH, Hangzhou, China) with simultaneous root aortography was performed. There was flow compromise in the right coronary artery and circumflex to TIMI-0 flow (Figure 2(a)). To perform the coronary protection technique to avoid CAO, a 6F JR-4 guide catheter inserted through a transradial access was used to engage the anomalous LCX, and a guiding wire of 0.014 inches was advanced to the CX arteries with a 2.0 × 20 mm semicompliant balloon (Figure 2(b)). A 26 mm Venus-A self-expanding valve (VENUS MEDTECH, Hangzhou, China) with rapid ventricular pacing was then deployed. The position of the valve and function were confirmed by aortography and transesophageal echocardiography (TEE). We found flow compromise in the right coronary system and circumflex to TIMI-0 flow (Figure 2(c)), and the ST segments in the EKG were elevated. One drug-eluting stent (2.75 × 23 mm) was deployed from the proximal CX branch to the ostium, followed by deployment of another drug-eluting stent (3.0 × 18 mm) from the ostium of CX to the sinotubular junction through Guidezilla (Figures 2(d) and 2(e)). The flow of the right coronary artery and circumflex was retained, and the elevated ST segment in the EKG was reversed (Figure 2(f)). The patient tolerated the procedure well without complications, recovered uneventfully, and was discharged 7 days after the procedure without complications. At the 30-day follow-up, he had notable improvement of symptoms and physical activity, with a change to NYHA class I from class III. Six months after being discharged from our hospital, CTA of coronary artery suggested unobstructed coronary flow of the CX (Figures 3(b)–3(d)).

3. Discussion

TAVR is an acceptable and effective alternative to SAVR in high-risk or intermediate-risk patients. However, a rare but devastating complication is coronary ostial obstruction during the TAVR procedure. There are some key predictors of

CAO, including low coronary ostia, inadequate SOV width, and, in the context of VIV procedures, surgical bioprostheses with externally mounted leaflets or a short virtual transcatheter valve-to-coronary ostium (VTC) distance [6, 7]. An anomalous coronary artery can be a predictor of CAO. In some special patients at high risk of CAO during TAVR procedure, upfront coronary artery protection can be provided by positioning a coronary guidewire, balloon, undeployed stent, or guide extension in the artery [8, 9]. Recent research has reported that chimney stenting is infrequently performed in modern TAVR practice (approximately 0.5% of overall TAVR cases), and this technique is not only performed for the acute treatment of total occlusion of coronary flow but also applied when imaging reveals partial obstruction of the coronary ostium or reduced coronary blood flow and an evolution to complete CAO is anticipated [5]. Thorough evaluation of each case prior to TAVR using coronary angiography, CT scanning, and echocardiography enabled us to identify patients we believed to be at increased risk for coronary compromise during the TAVR procedure. The utilization of the chimney stenting protection method helped in the early diagnosis and efficient treatment of coronary compromise during TAVR. The stent is retracted to extend from the proximal portion of the coronary artery cranially, exteriorly, and parallel to the transcatheter heart valve and is deployed to create a channel for coronary perfusion between the displaced leaflets and the aortic wall. In this case, we successfully performed coronary protection by using the chimney stenting technique in anatomical abnormalities of the circumflex system, which originated from the right SOV. When the ostium of the right coronary artery and circumflex artery were occluded by calcified valve cusps, we rapidly planted 2 stents from the proximal CX branch to the sinotubular junction and created a channel for coronary perfusion between the displaced leaflets and the aortic wall; hence, the coronary flow was maintained. Bioprosthetic or native aortic scallop intentional laceration to prevent iatrogenic coronary artery obstruction during TAVR (BASILICA) is a transcatheter procedure performed immediately before TAVR at high risk of coronary artery obstruction, in which the target aortic native or bioprosthetic leaflets are split using focused radiofrequency energy directed by catheters and guide wires [10]. One-year outcome of the BASILICA trial reveals that there was no late stroke, myocardial infarction, or death related to BASILICA, and the mitigation of coronary obstruction remained intact at 1 year, thereby, the BASILICA technique could avoid the long-term complications related to snorkel stenting [11]. In our case, pre-TAVR cardiac CT imaging suggested a relatively high risk for coronary obstruction in right SOV; therefore, it could be a good alternative to perform BASILICA technique before TAVR.

4. Conclusions

Chimney stenting protection as a bailout technique is safe and feasible and should be considered in patients deemed to be at high risk of coronary flow compromise, especially with an anomalous LCX.

Consent

The authors confirm that written consent for submission and publication of this case report including images and associated text has been obtained from the patient in line with COPE guidance.

Acknowledgments

The authors thank everyone who was involved directly and indirectly in the data collection and writing process of this case report. This work was financially supported by the National Natural Science Foundation of China (No. 82070295).

References

[1] H. B. Ribeiro, L. Nombela-Franco, M. Urena et al., "Coronary obstruction following transcatheter aortic valve implantation: a systematic review," *JACC: Cardiovascular Interventions*, vol. 6, no. 5, pp. 452–461, 2013.

[2] D. Dvir, J. Webb, S. Brecker et al., "Transcatheter aortic valve replacement for degenerative bioprosthetic surgical valves: results from the global valve-in-valve registry," *Circulation*, vol. 126, no. 19, pp. 2335–2344, 2012.

[3] J. G. Acosta-Vélez, B. García del Blanco, J. Guindo et al., "Acute artery occlusion during transcatheter aortic valve replacement in a patient with an anomalous origin of the circumflex artery," *JACC. Cardiovascular Interventions*, vol. 7, no. 11, pp. 1324-1325, 2014.

[4] M. Mbai, A. Sharma, B. Oestreich et al., "Transcatheter aortic valve implantation in the presence of an anomalous left circumflex coronary artery: a case report," *Cardiovascular Diagnosis and Therapy*, vol. 10, no. 2, pp. 223–226, 2020.

[5] F. Mercanti, L. Rosseel, A. Neylon et al., "Chimney stenting for coronary occlusion during TAVR: insights from the Chimney Registry," *JACC. Cardiovascular Interventions*, vol. 13, no. 6, pp. 751–761, 2020.

[6] H. B. Ribeiro, J. Rodes-Cabau, P. Blanke et al., "Incidence, predictors, and clinical outcomes of coronary obstruction following transcatheter aortic valve replacement for degenerative bioprosthetic surgical valves: insights from the VIVID registry," *European Heart Journal*, vol. 39, no. 8, pp. 687–695, 2018.

[7] D. Dvir, J. Leipsic, P. Blanke et al., "Coronary obstruction in transcatheter aortic valve-in-valve Implantation," *Circulation. Cardiovascular Interventions*, vol. 8, no. 1, article e002079, 2015.

[8] Y. Abramowitz, T. Chakravarty, H. Jilaihawi et al., "Clinical impact of coronary protection during transcatheter aortic valve implantation: first reported series of patients," *EuroIntervention*, vol. 11, no. 5, pp. 572–581, 2015.

[9] M. Yamamoto, T. Shimura, S. Kano et al., "Impact of preparatory coronary protection in patients at high anatomical risk of acute coronary obstruction during transcatheter aortic valve implantation," *International Journal of Cardiology*, vol. 217, pp. 58–63, 2016.

[10] J. M. Khan, A. B. Greenbaum, V. C. Babaliaros et al., "The BASILICA trial: prospective multicenter investigation of intentional leaflet laceration to prevent TAVR coronary

obstruction," *JACC. Cardiovascular Interventions*, vol. 12, no. 13, pp. 1240–1252, 2019.

[11] J. M. Khan, A. B. Greenbaum, V. C. Babaliaros et al., "The BASILICA trial: one-year outcomes of transcatheter electrosurgical leaflet laceration to prevent TAVR coronary obstruction," *Circulation. Cardiovascular Interventions*, vol. 14, no. 5, article e010238, 2021.

33

An Incidental Diagnosis of Rheumatic Mitral Stenosis and Secundum Atrial Septal Defect (Lutembacher's Syndrome) in a Young Woman

Md Mashiul Alam[1] **and Md Fakhrul Islam Khaled**[2]

[1]*Jahurul Islam Medical College Hospital, Bhagalpur, Bajitpur, Kishoregonj, Bangladesh*
[2]*University Cardiac Center, Bangabandhu Sheikh Mujib Medical University, Room No-418, D Block, Dhaka, Bangladesh*

Correspondence should be addressed to Md Mashiul Alam; mashiull@gmail.com

Academic Editor: Kathleen Ngu

Lutembacher's syndrome is a rare cardiovascular defect comprising of mitral stenosis and atrial septal defect. A combination of acquired mitral stenosis and congenital atrial septal defect is the most well-recognized pattern. As atrial septal defect acts as a pressure relieving gateway, signs and symptoms of mitral stenosis may be attenuated and/or delayed in such patients. We have presented a case with Lutembacher's syndrome that was incidentally diagnosed as having such defect during outpatient check-up for upper respiratory infection.

1. Introduction

Lutembacher's syndrome (LS) is a rare cardiovascular anomaly defined as any combination of congenital or iatrogenic atrial septal defect (ASD) with congenital or acquired mitral stenosis (MS) [1]. As mentioned, it can happen rarely, and according to the American Heart Journal, a lone person with this combination of syndrome can be found out of 1 billion people [2]. People with mitral stenosis has 0.6% to 0.7% chance of having congenital ASD while congenital MS is a rare entity accounting for only 0.6% of congenital heart disease [3]. Hence, Lutembacher's syndrome is common in the form of congenital ASD with acquired MS due to rheumatic heart disease. However, in the current era of percutaneous transluminal mitral commissurotomy (PTMC) in a patient with rheumatic MS, iatrogenic ASD due to transseptal puncture is more common than congenital ASD, where it is named as iatrogenic Lutembacher's syndrome [3]. Assuming uniform incidence of ASD, worldwide incidence of LS is more like in the region where incidence of rheumatic mitral stenosis is more such as in Southeast Asia or sub-Saharan Africa, and at the same time, this combination is rare in the western world where rheumatic mitral stenosis is uncommon. In 1916, French physician Rene Lutembacher first described the comprehensive account of these two defects in a 61-year-old woman. We have presented a case of a 25-year-old woman who was seen in the outpatient department due to simple flu-like illness and eventually diagnosed as having Lutembacher's syndrome.

2. Case Report

A 25-year-old young woman presented to the outpatient medicine department with the complaints of dry cough which was relentless for 1 month provisionally diagnosed as upper respiratory tract infection. On enquiry, the patient revealed that she had shortness of breath during cold seasons suggestive of bronchial asthma. She had no childhood illness indicating rheumatic heart disease. There was no significant past medical or surgical illness. She was married for two years but did not conceive yet. Her immunization history cannot be elicited as she could not remember them all. Her family members were in good health, and there was no worth mentioning illness that runs in the family. The patients' menstrual cycle was regular with an average menstrual flow. She was of a lower middle class socioeconomic status family.

No family member had been suffering from any significant illness.

General examination revealed she was ill looking with mild tachypnea. Her heart rate was 90 beats per minute which was regular in rhythm; blood pressure was 80/60 mmHg; JVP was not raised. There was no anemia or edema. Her nasal mucosa was congested indicating upper airway infection.

Precordial examination showed normal apex beat in the left 5th intercostal space with little bit lateral displacement. There was palpable p2 with left parasternal heave but no palpable thrill. Intensity of the 1st heart sound was normal. The second heart sound was loud over the pulmonary area but not definitely splitted. There was an ejection systolic murmur over the pulmonary area with no radiation or respiratory variation.

Respiratory system examination revealed a respiratory rate of 22 breaths per minute. There was no crepitation or rhonchi.

As our patient was being investigated for her illness, her chest X-ray revealed cardiomegaly with RV type apex, pulmonary conus was full and bulged, and right pulmonary artery was dilated (Figure 1). ECG showed right bundle branch block with right axis deviation.

Subsequently, her echocardiogram was done which depicted hugely dilated right atrium (RA) and right ventricle (RV) with restricted opening of the mitral valve (Figure 2).

Mitral valve planimetry showed the mitral valve area (MVA) was 1.24 cm^2 with thickened calcified mitral valves and mild subvalvular changes (Figure 3). But the mean pressure gradient across the MV was 5 mmHg, and the MVA according to the pressure half time (PHT) method was 3.77 cm^2. Left atrial (LA) diameter in M mode echo was 32.73 mm.

There was an atrial septal defect measuring 17.38 mm in the apical 4 chamber view (A4CV) (Figure 4) and 13.43 mm in the subcostal view. RV was dilated with a diameter of 55 to 60 mm at the base in the A4CV. Trabecula in RV was prominent. All rims of ASD were adequate (more than 5 mm).

The main pulmonary artery (PA) and right ventricular outflow tract (RVOT) just before the pulmonary valve (PV) were mildly dilated with 29 mm and 33 mm in diameter, respectively.

Color Doppler echocardiogram showed a mosaic flow across the mitral valve (MV) towards the LV apex during LV diastole but no regurgitation during systole. There was a butterfly-like laminar flow across the intra-atrial septum (IAS) in subcostal and A4C views.

Continuous wave Doppler across the tricuspid valve (TV) that revealed a maximum velocity through TV was 3.65 m/s. Hence, measured PASP according to the Bernoulli equation was 53.31 + 5 mm Hg = 58.31 mmHg.

A thorough study with transesophageal echo and cardiac cath could not be done due to unavailability in our center. So the patient was properly counselled about her disease condition, and she was treated with rheumatic heart disease prophylaxis, low dose of diuretics along with treatment for her presenting ailment. Furthermore, she was referred to a tertiary level hospital where all the facilities for subsequent evaluation and treatment were available. Eventually, she was undergone mitral valve replacement with metallic prosthetic valve and patch closure of ASD at a higher center. The patient had severe mitral stenosis and ASD secundum; therefore, intervention is required to prevent rising pulmonary artery pressure by increased flow through the right-sided heart, and she had occasional shortness of breath as well which she thought might be due to bronchial asthma.

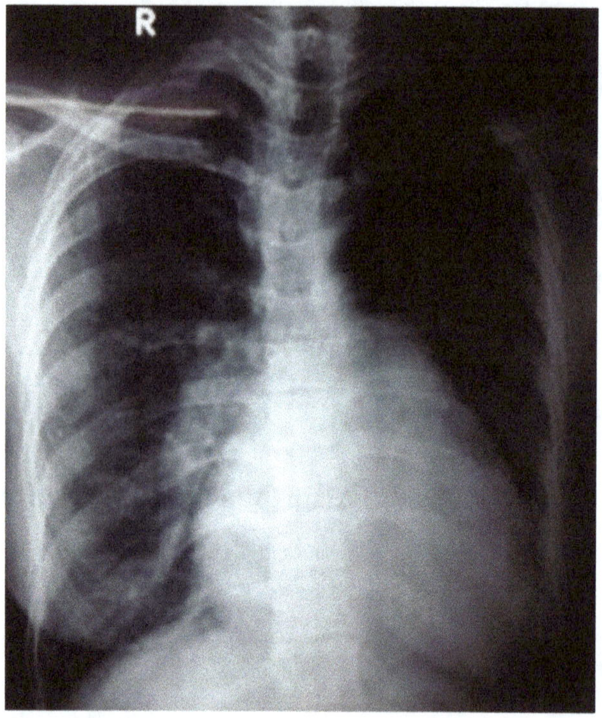

FIGURE 1: Chest X-ray P/A view showing bulged pulmonary conus, cardiomegaly, and prominent right pulmonary artery.

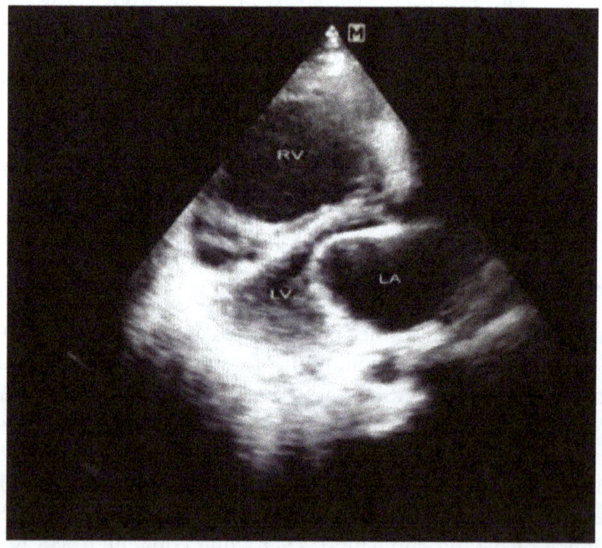

FIGURE 2: PLAX view 2D echocardiogram picture showing dilated RV and restricted MV opening.

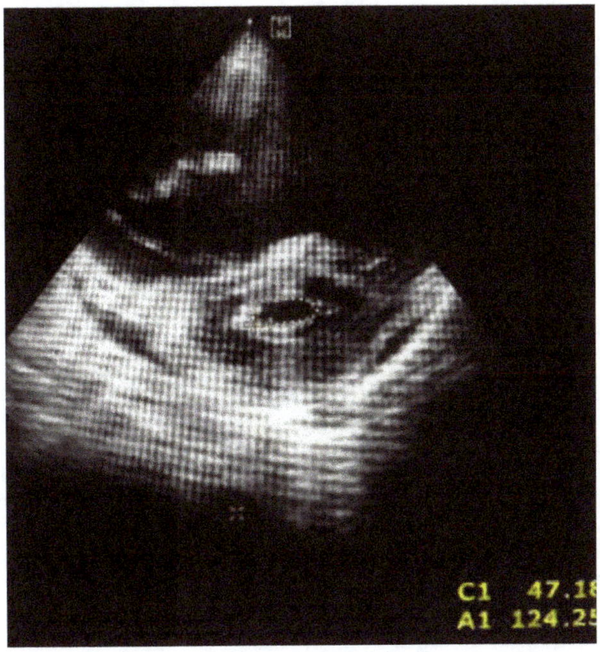

Figure 3: 2D echocardiogram-guided planimetry showing MVA is $1.24\,cm^2$.

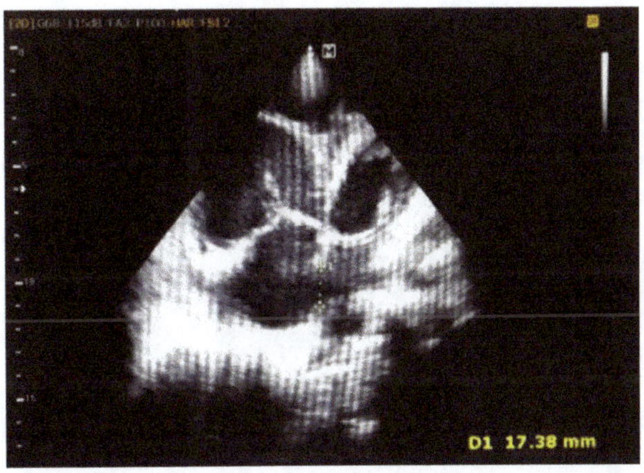

Figure 4: The A4CV showing RA and RV dilated compromising a left-sided heart view and ASD measuring 17.38 mm.

Though interventional treatment of LS is an option nowadays, our patient had undergone surgical repair as experience regarding percutaneous treatment is inadequate in our centers.

3. Discussion

Lutembacher's syndrome is one of the rare cardiovascular syndrome more commonly presents as acquired MS with congenital ASD [2]. As both ASD and MS are more frequent among female patients, this syndrome is also commonly found in female population [4]. There are several reports of familial cases of Lutembacher's syndrome, but they are isolated observations [5, 6].

Initially, it was postulated that high LA pressure due to mitral stenosis stretches open the patent foramen ovale causing left to right shunt or atrial septal defect [7]. But according to the current definition of this syndrome ASD could be acquired or congenital. High LA pressure causing ASD is further supported by some observations by Ansari and Maron [8] in 1997 when they published a case of mitral valve replacement in a 49-year-old woman. After the valve replacement, left to right shunt was no longer detectable. Similar observation was reported by Ananthasubramaniam et al. in 2001 [9].

As MS and ASD occur together, hemodynamic expression and clinical features depend on the interplay of several conditions, namely, size of ASD, severity of MS, and distensibility of RV [4]. Increased LA pressure due to mitral stenosis in Lutembacher's syndrome finds ASD as a second exit for LA blood as a result severity of MS abates by shunting of blood from LA to RA and size of ASD can regulate blood shunt consequently deleterious effect of rising LA pressure. In case there is no ASD, increased atrial pressure due to MS causes blood to find its way to pulmonary veins and hence causes pulmonary congestion more frequently and easily. In Lutembacher's syndrome, ASD prevents back pressure to pulmonary vasculature and congestion. Likewise, features related to lung congestion such as orthopnea, paroxysmal nocturnal dyspnea, hemoptysis, and pulmonary edema are delayed or attenuated. In contrast, these symptoms are substituted by features of low cardiac output, namely, fatigue, low blood pressure.

The ameliorating effect of atrial septal defect in Lutembacher's syndrome was reported by Lutembacher's original article in 1916; a 61-year-old female patient had been pregnant for seven times despite this cardiovascular anomaly [10]. Perloff revealed a case of 74-year-old woman who had gone through 11 pregnancies and survived until advance age in spite of Lutembacher's syndrome [11].

Though ASD ameliorate the severity features of MS, increased blood flow through ASD due to stenosis in mitral valve causes more blood shunted to right-sided heart predisposing atrial fibrillation and right ventricular failure [12]. In late advanced stage, such patients develop pulmonary hypertension and heart failure with poor prognosis [13]. Nevertheless, correcting this dual problem by surgical closure of ASD and mitral valve replacement bears a good prognosis and prolongs life. In recent days, an interventional technique is frequently judged to be implemented if feasible by doing percutaneous transluminal mitral commissurotomy (PTMC) and closing ASD by the Amplatzer device [14].

Hemodynamic decompression of LA pressure builds up by mitral stenosis has a considerable effect on the physical examination of a patient with Lutembacher's syndrome. The clinical examination finding of pure MS are attenuated or may be absent. Loud first heart sound, opening snap, and middiastolic murmur with presystolic accentuations are usually not heard. Generally, a continuous murmur is heard because of high LA to low RA pressure difference across ASD which persist during the entire cycle [15]. As more blood is shunted in contrast to isolated ASD, increased pulmonary blood flow across the pulmonary valve produces loud ejection systolic murmur over the pulmonary area. A holosystolic murmur over the left lower sternal edge may accompany as a finding, while pulmonary hypertension may cause a regurgitant tricuspid lesion.

References

[1] P. Vaideeswar and S. Marathe, "Lutembacher's syndrome: is the mitral pathology always rheumatic?," *Indian Heart Journal*, vol. 69, no. 1, pp. 20–23, 2017.

[2] S. Y. Ali, M. Rahman, M. Islam, R. C. Barman, M. Y. Ali, and M. M. S. U. Islam, ""Lutembacher's syndrome"-a case report," *Faridpur Medical College Journal*, vol. 6, no. 1, pp. 59-60, 2011.

[3] K. Mahajan and T. I. Oliver, "Lutembacher syndrome," in *StatPearls*StatPearls Publishing, Treasure Island (FL), USAJan 2019, https://www.ncbi.nlm.nih.gov/books/NBK470307/.

[4] A. Olivare-Reyes and A. Al-Kamme, "Lutembacher's syndrome with small atrial septal defect diagnosed by transthoracic and transesophageal echocardiography that underwent mitral valve replacement," *Journal of the American Society of Echocardiography*, vol. 18, no. 10, pp. 1105.e1–1105.e3, 2005.

[5] S. R. Courter, B. Felson, and J. McGuire, "Familial interauricular septal defect with mitral stenosis (Lutembacher's syndrome)," *The American Journal of the Medical Sciences*, vol. 216, no. 5, pp. 501–508, 1948.

[6] C. V. Patil, M. Vijaykumar, A. V. Pande, and L. S. Shah, "Familial Lutembacher's syndrome in mother and daughter," *Indian Heart Journal*, vol. 49, no. 4, pp. 415–417, 1997.

[7] J. K. Perloff, *The clinical recognition of congenital heart disease*, WB Saunders, Philadelphia, 4th ed edition, 1994.

[8] A. Ansari and B. J. Maron, "Lutembacher's syndrome," *Texas Heart Institute Journal*, vol. 24, no. 3, pp. 230-231, 1997.

[9] K. Ananthasubramaniam, G. Iyer, and V. Karthikeyan, "Giant left atrium secondary to tight mitral stenosis leading to acquired Lutembacher syndrome: a case report with emphasis on role of echocardiography in assessment of Lutembacher syndrome," *Journal of the American Society of Echocardiography*, vol. 14, no. 10, pp. 1033–1035, 2001.

[10] R. Lutmenbacher, "De la sténose mitrale avec communication interauriculaire," *Archives des Maladies du Coeur et des Vaisseaux*, vol. 9, pp. 237–260, 1916.

[11] L. Rostenthal, "Atrial septal defect with mitral stenosis in a woman of 81," *British Medical Journal*, vol. 2, p. 1351, 1956.

[12] T. O. Cheng, "Coexistent atrial septal defect and mitral stenosis (Lutembacher syndrome): an ideal combination for percutaneous treatment," *Catheterization and Cardiovascular Interventions*, vol. 48, no. 2, pp. 205-206, 1999.

[13] A. R. Levin, M. S. Spach, J. P. Boineau, R. V. Canent, M. P. Capp, and P. H. Jewett, "Atrial pressure flow dynamics and atrial septal defects (secundum type)," *Circulation*, vol. 37, no. 4, pp. 476–488, 1968.

[14] Q. T. Phan, H. L. Nguyen, T. D. Le et al., "Combined percutaneous procedure in patient with Lutembacher syndrome: a case report and real-world experience review," *Cardiology Research*, vol. 9, no. 6, pp. 385–391, 2018.

[15] J. Ross Jr., E. Braunwald, D. T. Mason, N. S. Braunwald, and A. G. Morrow, "Interatrial communication and left atrial hypertension: a cause of continuous murmur," *Circulation*, vol. 28, no. 5, pp. 853–860, 1963.

34

Perioperative Application of Transesophageal Echocardiography in Left Atrial Appendage Occlusion in an Elderly Patient with Mirror-Image Dextrocardia and Atrial Fibrillation

Lu Zhang,[1,2,3] Ming Bai,[1,2,3] Ji-zhe Xu,[1,2,3] Ga-xue Jiang,[1,2,3] Ai-yun Deng,[1,2,3] and Zheng Zhang[1,2,3]

[1]*Department of Cardiology, The First Hospital of Lanzhou University, China*
[2]*Gansu Provincial Clinical Research Center for Cardiovascular Diseases and Gansu Provincial Key Laboratory of Cardiovascular Disease, China*
[3]*National Project of Improving the Diagnosis and Treatment Ability of Cardiovascular and Cerebrovascular Diseases, The First Hospital of Lanzhou University, China*

Correspondence should be addressed to Ming Bai; baiminglzu@gmail.com and Zheng Zhang; zhangccu@163.com

Academic Editor: Yigit Canga

Mirror-image dextrocardia is non-life-threatening but not commonly diagnosed in the clinic. With the internal organs reversed, most of the patients with mirror-image dextrocardia have no clinical symptoms if the dextrocardia is not combined with other intracardiac malformations. Mirror-image dextrocardia is often discovered during other physical check or performing other examinations. In the present study, we reported a successful closure of a left atrial appendage in an 84-year-old patient with mirror-image dextrocardia with atrial fibrillation under the guidance of transesophageal echocardiography (TEE). Detailed perioperative steps of patient procedure description and TEE monitoring were described in this report.

1. Introduction

Mirror-image dextrocardia, the most common form of cardiac malposition, refers to the dextrocardia with situs inversus, L-loop ventricles, and inverted great arteries resulting from situs inversus with a concordant L-bulboventricular loop [1]. As the mirror view of a normal heart, its visceral position is opposite to the normal. While some studies reported that about 40-50% of mirror-image dextrocardia patients have other cardiac malformations [2], other patients have normal cardiac structures.

Atrial fibrillation is the most common type of tachyarrhythmia. Thromboembolism is one of the most severe complications of atrial fibrillation; the most clinically evident thromboembolic event is ischemic stroke. Although long-term administration of oral anticoagulants can prevent embolism, some patients are still facing the risk of bleeding, anticoagulation taboo, and thromboembolism even under the anticoagulation treatment, which is the major indication for left atrial appendage occlusion [3].

2. Case Report

The 84-year-old female patient had a history of hypertension for 10 years. The patient was diagnosed with cerebral infarction and atrial fibrillation 2 years ago, with the symptoms of dizziness, palpitations, and chest tightness followed by loss of speaking and fatigue. Treatments including antiarrhythmia and hypertension treatment (β-blocker, calcium channel blocker), anticoagulation (aspirin and warfarin), cholesterol treatment (atorvastatin), and neuronutrition supplementation (vitamin B) were prescribed to the patient before administration, and the symptoms were partially relieved after treatment. One year ago, the patient went to the outpatient office claiming for lower left limb fatigue and repeatedly falling and then diagnosed as cerebral infarction, constant atrial

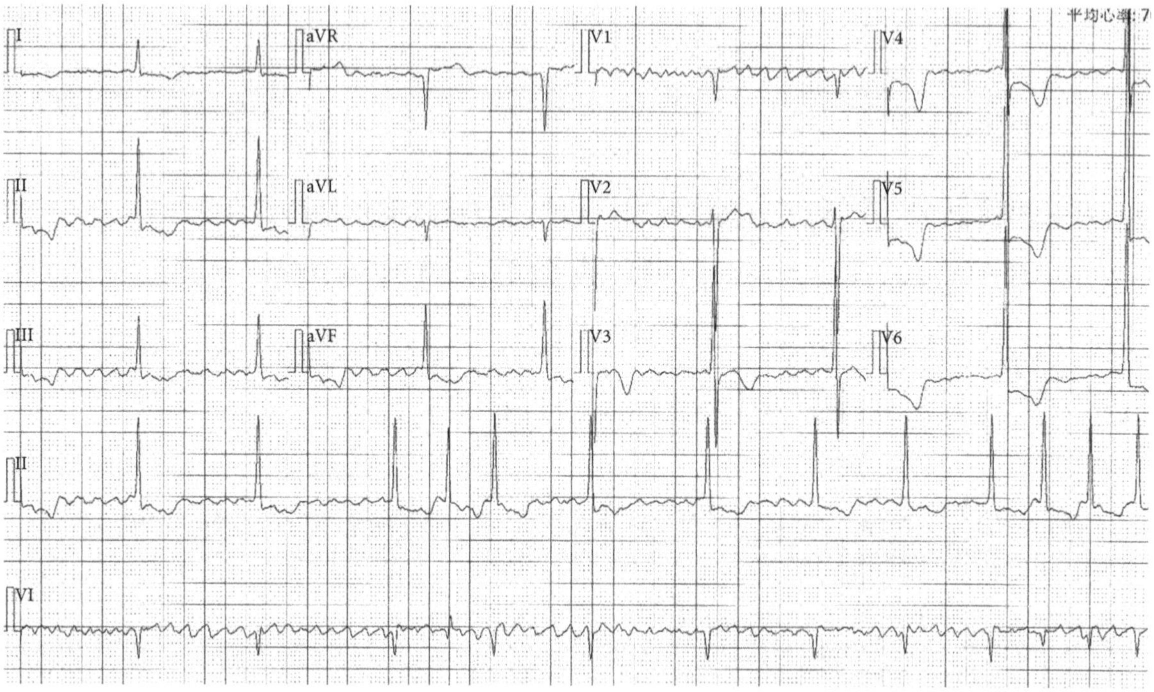

Figure 1: Electrocardiogram. No visible P waves and an irregularly irregular QRS complex showed atrial fibrillation.

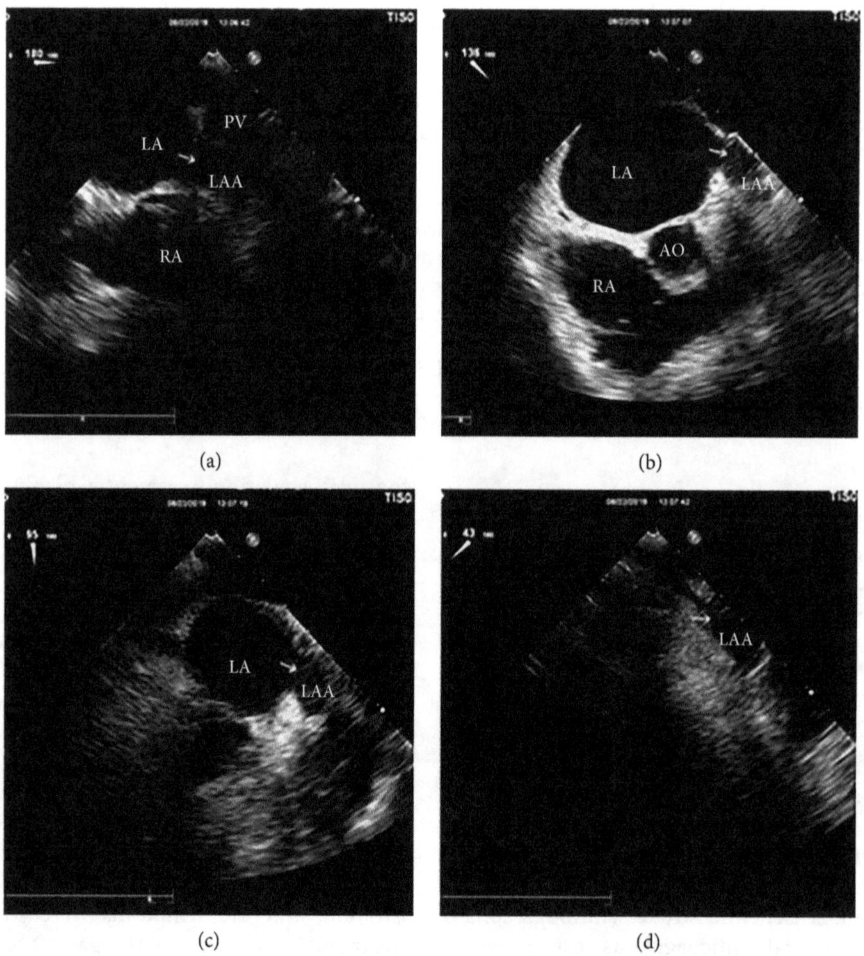

Figure 2: Transesophageal echocardiography (TEE) images before the operation. Transesophageal echocardiography images demonstrated no existing thrombus in the left atrial appendage before the operation.

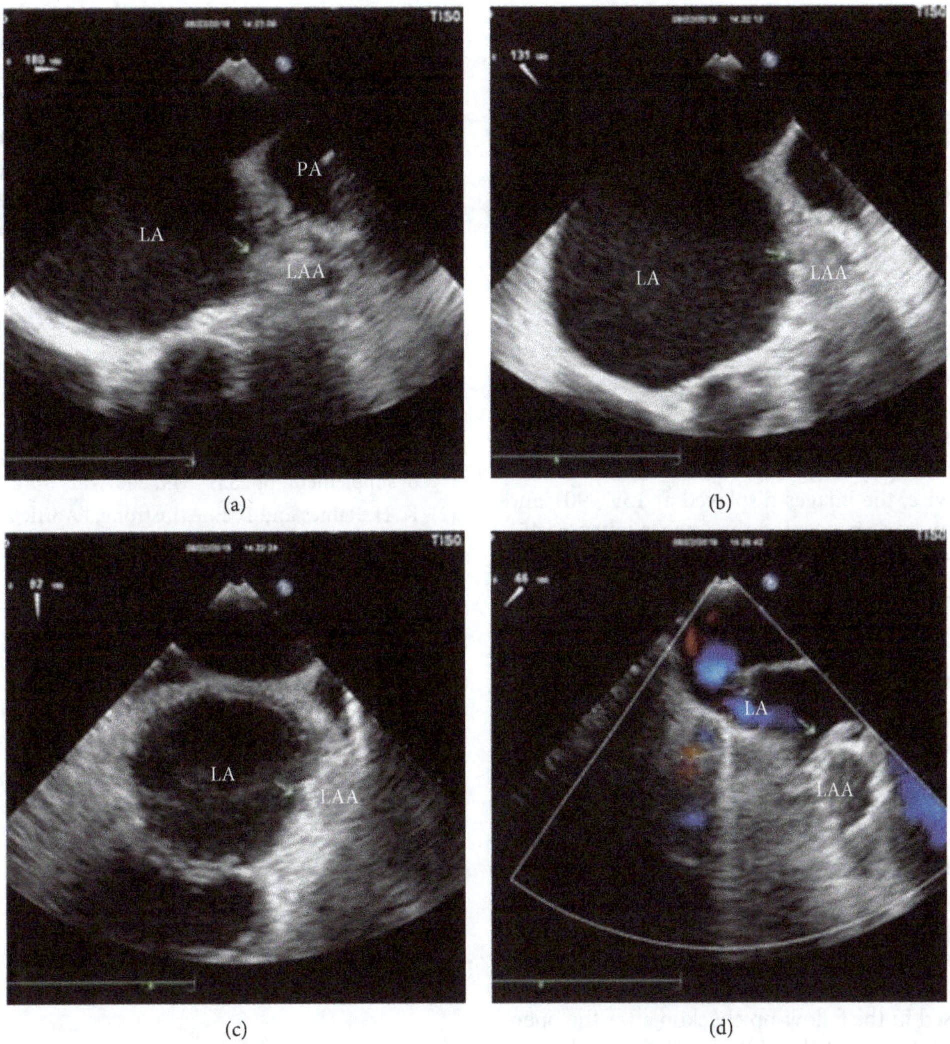

FIGURE 3: Transesophageal echocardiography (TEE) images after the operation. TEE showed the left atrial appendage from four different angles (the green arrow points to the ostium of the left atrial appendage).

fibrillation, hypertension, and lower left limb deep vein thrombosis. The patient continued taking the prescribed medication during the long-term treatment before this time of hospitalization. Holter monitoring and electrocardiogram (EKG) results showed atrial fibrillation (Figure 1). Transthoracic echocardiography (TTE) suggested a diagnosis of mirror-image dextrocardia. The diameters of the patient's left atrium and right atrium were significantly enlarged; the CHA2DS2-VAS score was 6, and the HAS-BLED score was 4. All the test results indicate a left atrial appendage occlusion.

Therefore, after evaluating the risk and potential benefit, we decided to perform left atrial appendage occlusion in the patient. Before the operation, a TEE examination was conducted to determine whether thrombus had developed in the left atrial appendage. It is noted that during the examination, it should be kept in mind that the TEE images of this patient are completely mirror symmetrical to the corresponding images of a normal person. The TEE result demonstrated that no thrombus existed in the left atrial appendage before the operation (Figure 2).

During the operation, general anesthesia was given to the patient. The TEE probe was inserted smoothly through the esophagus, and the diameter of the ostium and the depth of the left atrial appendage were measured from four different angles. The measurement was the following: 19×20 mm at the 180° angle, 14×20 mm at the 135° angle, 14×16 mm at the 90° angle, and 15×19 mm at the 45° angle. After that, the positions of interatrial paracentesis were located at 120° and 70° under the guidance of TEE, respectively. After the successful paracentesis of the atrial septum, angiography imaging showed that the left atrial appendage was cauliflower type. Then, a 21 mm watchman occluder was selected to occlude the left atrial appendage successfully. No residual shunt was left shown by angiography. After the placement of the occluder, TEE was used to observe the location of the occluder two-dimensionally and three-dimensionally. The result showed that the occluder was well embedded. The compression ratio of the occluder was measured from four different angles separately and the positioning (Figure 3). No residual shunt was observed from all angles by color Doppler ultrasound.

3. Discussion

During the examination, the TEE probe should be rotated slightly to the right side of the patient since the patient had mirror-image dextrocardia. Keeping in mind that the TEE images of this patient were completely mirrored symmetrical to the TEE images of a normal person, the angles at which the left atrial appendage was observed by TEE should also be axisymmetric to the angles that apply to a normal person. Therefore, when observing the internal structure of the left atrial appendage, in this case, the angle pointer of the probe chip should be rotated clockwise, from 180° to 45°, and the internal structure of the left atrial appendage should be scanned continuously and meticulously. Consequently, the TEE images displayed at the 180° angle, in this case, mirror represented the corresponding images at 0° angle for a normal person. Likewise, the images displayed at 135°, 90°, and 45°, in this case, mirror represented the images taken at 45°, 90°, and 135°, respectively. When guiding the paracentesis of the atrial septum during the operation, the TEE angle to the long axis of the atrial septum was about 70°, and it is also axisymmetric to the corresponding angle for a normal person. Furthermore, the images of the short axis of the atrial septum were taken at 120° approximately.

4. Conclusion

In routine clinical practice, TEE is not only used to determine the existence of thrombus in the left atrium and left atrial appendage before left atrial appendage occlusion but also used to screen if the patient's condition meets the indications for left atrial appendage occlusion. Furthermore, TEE could also be used to guide and monitor the procedures during the operation and to be used in the follow-up checkup after the operation. Thus, it is obvious that the TEE examination plays an important role in managing patients before, during, and after surgeries [4]. During the operation, TEE could provide clinicians and surgeons with reliable measurements of the left atrial appendage such as diameter and depth, guide the paracentesis of atrial septum during operation, observe the position of the placed occlude, and calculate the compression ratio, through which to guarantee the success of the surgery. For some special patients, including patients with mirror-image dextrocardia, a higher level of sonographer's technique and experience is required to perform the TEE due to the differences of the operational method and observation compared to those of a normal person, even if the position and the internal structure of the patient's heart have been determined in advance.

Abbreviations

TEE: Transesophageal echocardiography
EKG: Electrocardiogram.

Consent

The patient signed an informed consent prior to image collection. All the authors and the institution consented to publish.

Authors' Contributions

We confirm that the manuscript has been read and approved by all named authors and that there are no other persons who satisfied the criteria for authorship but are not listed. We further confirm that the order of authors listed in the manuscript has been approved by all of us. L.Z. and M.B. carried out the study; L.Z. wrote the manuscript with support from M.B.; Z.Z., A.D., J.X., and G.J. fabricated the analysis; M.B., Z.Z., and A.D. helped supervise the project.

References

[1] D. H. Pierre and S. Muhamed, "Approach to dextrocardia in adults: review," *American Journal of Roentgenology*, vol. 188, 6_supplement, pp. S39–S49, 2007.

[2] K. H. Raines and B. E. Armstrong, "Aortic atresia with visceral situs inversus with mirror-image dextrocardia," *Pediatric Cardiology*, vol. 10, no. 4, pp. 232–235, 1989.

[3] Authors/Task Force Members, A. J. Camm, G. Y. H. Lip et al., "2012 focused update of the ESC Guidelines for the management of atrial fibrillation," *European Heart Journal*, vol. 33, no. 21, pp. 2719–2747, 2012.

[4] B. Goebel, S. Wieg, A. Hamadanchi et al., "Interventional left atrial appendage occlusion: added value of 3D transesophageal echocardiography for device sizing," *The International Journal of Cardiovascular Imaging*, vol. 32, no. 9, pp. 1363–1370, 2016.

An Extremely Rare Presentation of Four Coronary Anomaly Patterns Originating from the Right Coronary Sinus

Nabil Braiteh,[1] **Wajeeh Rehman**,[2] **Wajiha Ali**,[3] **and Owais Ahmed**[4]

[1]*United Health Services Hospitals, Wilson Medical Center, Department of Cardiology, 30 Harrison St, Johnson City, NY, USA*
[2]*United Health Services Hospitals, Wilson Medical Center, Department of Internal Medicine, 33-57 Harrison St, Johnson City, NY, USA*
[3]*American University of Antigua College of Medicine, USA*
[4]*United Health Services Hospitals (Heart & Vascular Institute), Wilson Medical Center, Department of Cardiology, 30 Harrison St, Johnson City, NY 13790, USA*

Correspondence should be addressed to Nabil Braiteh; nab.braiteh@gmail.com

Academic Editor: Luigi Sciarra

Background. "Coronary anomaly" is defined as the coronary feature or pattern seen in <1% of the population. The most common CAAs are anomalies of origin, specifically having a separate LCX and LAD origin with an incidence of 0.41%. The second most common anomaly is the LCX arising from the RCA (0.37%). Treatment options include CABG, coronary unroofing, reimplantation, or medical therapy. *Case Presentation.* We present the case of an 85-year-old male who presents with an acute coronary syndrome who was found to have an extremely rare combination of different coronary anomaly patterns including left main coronary artery (LMCA) atresia, small LAD arising posteriorly from the right coronary cusp, anomalous left circumflex artery arising from the RCA, and an anomalous LAD arising from the left circumflex artery which is originating from the RCA. *Conclusions.* To the best of our knowledge, this is the first case report to describe four coronary anomalies in a single patient. When CAAs are diagnosed, it is of utmost importance for cardiologists to do further imaging and workup that might include a stress test to be able to offer patients the best management options.

1. Introduction

Is it a coronary anomaly or a normal variant? This has been a challenging question to answer in the literature and between experts. Villa et al. proposed to define "normal variants" as any coronary pattern that is observed in >1% in the general population, and a "coronary anomaly" is the coronary feature or pattern seen in <1% of the population [1].

Normal variants include coronary codominance, inferior wall supply, AV nodal supply, ramus intermedius, separate origin of the conus branch, myocardial bridging, acute take-off of LCX, high take-off of the coronary ostium, and shepherd's crook RCA.

Coronary anomalies are classified based on anatomical features, and they include anomalies of the ostium, of origin, of anatomy, and of termination; congenital absence; and hypoplasia.

The most common CAAs are anomalies of origin, specifically having a separate LCX and LAD origin with an incidence of 0.41%. The second most common anomaly is the LCX arising from the RCA (0.37%) [1, 2].

In concept, if a coronary arises from the contralateral side, it has 4 possible paths: (A) interarterial (between the aorta and pulmonary artery), (B) transeptal (subpulmonic); (C) prepulmonic (anterior to the right ventricular outflow tract), and (D) retroaortic (posterior to the aortic root). The first (interarterial) is considered malignant and is at higher risk for SCD especially when it is associated with an intramural segment (proximal part of the artery is contained within the aortic wall), while the latter three (transseptal, retroaortic, and prepulmonic) are benign with low risk for adverse events [1, 2].

Herein, we report an 85-year-old man who presented with an acute coronary syndrome and heart failure, who was found to have an extremely rare combination of different coronary anomaly patterns.

2. Case Presentation

We present an 85-year-old Caucasian male who presented to the emergency department (ED) with complaints of dyspnea and a productive cough. His past medical history is significant for dyslipidemia, hypertension, diabetes mellitus type 2, chronic kidney stage 3b, obesity, and obstructive sleep apnea. He denied tobacco use but did report occasional alcohol use. His family history was unremarkable. At baseline, the patient was able to ambulate and perform daily activities without functional limitations.

Physical examination showed an ill-appearing elderly male, in mild respiratory distress. Vital signs on admission noted blood pressure 124/93 mmHg, heart rate 120 beats per minute, respiratory rate of 24 breaths per minute, and oxygen saturation of 91% on room air initially. The patient was alert and oriented. Heart sounds revealed normal S1 and S2, breath sounds were rhonchorous and diminished bilaterally with evidence of bilateral lower extremity edema. EKG revealed an accelerated ventricular rate of 131 beats per minute and idioventricular rhythm with a right bundle branch block. Anterior posterior chest radiograph revealed cardiomegaly with evidence of mild bilateral hilar congestion. Troponin I level was 0.171 ng/mL.

The patient was diagnosed with mild decompensated heart failure in the setting of non-ST elevated myocardial infarction. Oral clopidogrel 300 mg was administered along with heparin drip per ACS protocol. He was then transferred to the cardiovascular intensive care unit for close monitoring. Transthoracic echocardiogram revealed severely increased left ventricular thickness, normal left ventricular size with ejection fraction of 40-45%, and no wall regional wall motion abnormalities or significant valvular disease. After effective diuresis, the patient underwent cardiac catheterization which revealed anomalous coronary anatomy. The patient had no left coronary system and a large ectatic right coronary artery (RCA) with evidence of 2 left anterior descending arteries. The first was originating posteriorly from the right cusp (Figure 1, blue arrows) and the second (Figure 2, blue arrows) was originating from the anomalous left circumflex artery (Figures 1 and 2, white arrows). Additionally, he had an extremely ectatic large caliber right coronary artery (RCA) with multiple lesions (Figure 1, green arrows). The most significant was a 80-90% mid to distal calcified eccentric lesion (Figure 1, green arrow with asterixis). There was also evidence of a filling defect representing a thrombotic occlusion in the distal RCA (Figure 1, red arrow), and this gives rise to the anomalous left circumflex artery (LCX) (Figures 1 and 2, white arrows).

The above findings were confirmed by CT coronary, where it shows the absence of a left coronary system (Figure 3, blue arrow), large calcified RCA originating posteriorly from the right coronary cusp (Figure 3, yellow arrow, Figure 4; green arrow), and a small LAD artery originating from the right coronary cusp and into the interventricular groove (Figure 3, red arrows; Figure 4, green arrow with asterixis) which is also represented in Figure 1 by the blue arrows.

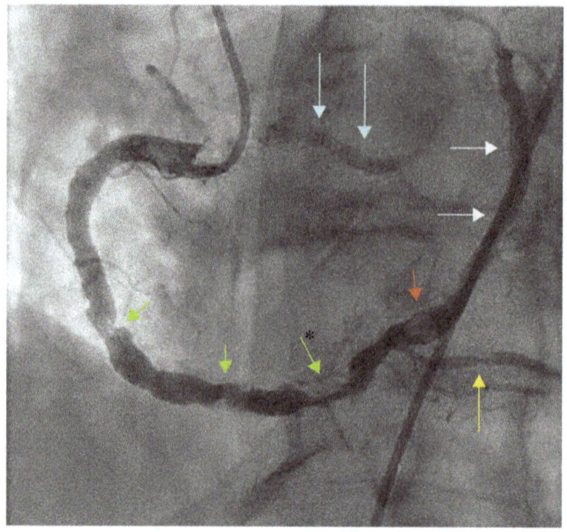

FIGURE 1: Right coronary angiogram (left anterior oblique 30°/cranial 30°) revealing a small anomalous LAD artery (blue arrows), a large ectatic RCA giving rise to the LCx (white arrows), multiple RCA lesions (green arrows) with an 80-90% mid to distal calcified eccentric lesion (green arrow with asterixis), a filling defect representing a thrombotic occlusion in the distal RCA (red arrow), and a 70% mid right posterior descending artery concentric lesion (yellow arrow).

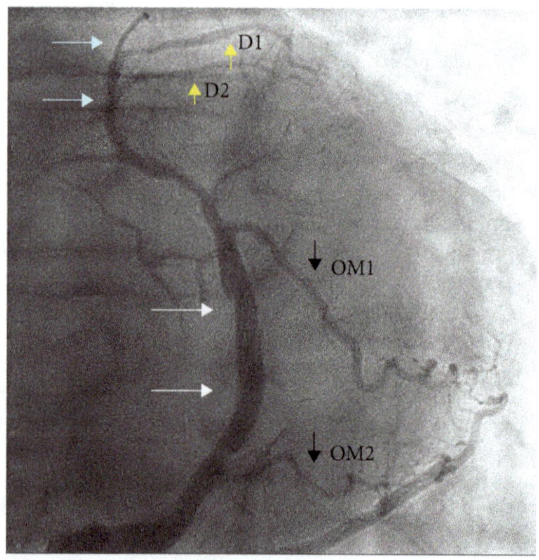

FIGURE 2: Right coronary angiogram (left anterior oblique 30°/cranial 30°) revealing an anomalous LCx artery (white arrows), the second small LAD artery (blue arrows), 1st and second diagonal arteries (yellow arrows), and 1st and second obtuse marginal arteries (blue arrows).

The patient had an episode of asymptomatic nonsustained idioventricular tachycardia followed by supraventricular tachycardia. As such, CT heart and coronary artery angiogram was done which confirmed the left coronary artery to arise from the aortic cusp making its course in front

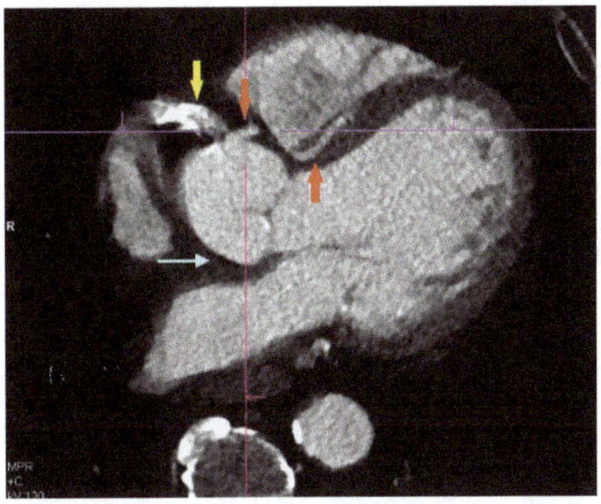

Figure 3: Coronary CT showed the absence of a left coronary system (blue arrow), a large calcified RCA originating posteriorly from the right coronary cusp (yellow arrow), and a small LAD artery originating from the right coronary cusp into the interventricular groove (red arrows).

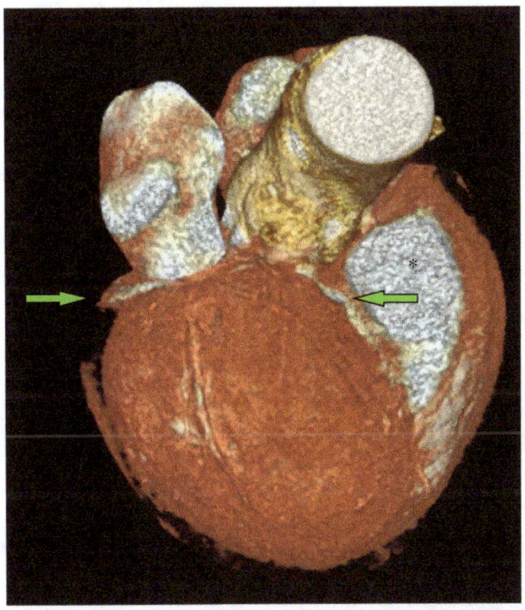

Figure 4: CT coronary showing a large calcified RCA originating posteriorly from the right coronary cusp (green arrow) and a small LAD artery originating from the right coronary cusp into the interventricular groove (green arrow with asterixis).

of the right ventricle between the great vessels thereby giving rise to a small caliber LAD. Likewise, the patient's circumflex artery appeared to also arise from the right coronary artery.

CABG was offered to the patient; unfortunately, he declined the intervention. He was medically optimized and discharged to rehab due to deconditioning. Three months after discharge, the patient suffered a cardiac arrest and passed after 25 minutes of unsuccessful CPR.

3. Discussion

Incidence of coronary arterial anomalies (CAAs) has been reported to range from 0.78% to 1.3% by invasive angiography and 0.99%-5.8% by coronary computed tomographic (CT) imaging [3, 4]. The wide range of incidence is likely due to the variability in defining "normal variants" and "anomalous" arteries. The most common CAA is having a separate LCX and LAD origins with an incidence of 0.41%. The second most common anomaly is the LCX arising from the RCA (0.37%) [1, 2].

Most CAAs do not have clinical significance or complications, but some (transseptal and interarterial) anomalies can lead to significant manifestations including heart failure, myocardial infarction, angina, and arrhythmias [5]. The pathophysiology is not completely understood, but several mechanisms have been proposed that include interarterial coronaries coursing intramurally through the wall of the aorta resulting in their compression due to aortic pulsation, angulation of the anomalous vessel acting like a valve-like ostial ridge, spasm of the anomalous artery due to ischemia or endothelial injury caused by its long distance, acute angle of take-off that can kink or occlude during exercise causing coronary hypoperfusion, and the fact that an artery has abnormal origin and take-off makes it more prone for atherosclerosis [1, 3, 6].

Spasm of the anomalous artery due to ischemia or endothelial injury is caused by its long distance, acute angle of take-off that can kink or occlude during exercise, and the fact that an artery has abnormal origin and take-off makes it more prone for atherosclerosis[1, 3, 6]CAAs are the second most common cause of sudden cardiac death accounting for 17% after hypertrophic cardiomyopathy (36%) reported by the U.S national registry of competitive athletes [7].

Diagnosis of CAAs can be done by noninvasive imaging techniques such as echocardiography, coronary CT angiography, and MR imaging. Alternatively, they can also be diagnosed invasively by coronary angiography.

While echocardiography has a limited role in adults, it has a good diagnostic benefit in children and adolescents (0-21 years of age) [7] Previously, coronary angiography was the standard test to diagnose CAAs, but with advancement in imaging, ECG-gated coronary CT angiography was shown to be more sensitive in multiple studies [8, 9]. While MRI has less radiation exposure, it has a similar diagnostic accuracy in comparison with CT [4].

Treatment of CAAs is complex and can be challenging specifically with the anomalous origin of the coronary artery from the opposite sinus (ACAOS). Decision to treat is mainly made for ACAOS with an interarterial course. While some experts recommend treatment for left ACAOS for asymptomatic patients, others take into account results of stress testing and age to decide on treatment. Ischemic symptoms will definitely warrant treatment. Options include CABG, coronary unroofing, reimplantation, or medical therapy [1, 4].

Our patient had four coronary anomalies detected: left main coronary artery (LMCA) atresia, small LAD arising posteriorly from the right coronary cusp, anomalous left circumflex artery arising from the RCA, and an anomalous LAD arising from the left circumflex artery which is originating from the RCA (Figures 1–4). To the best of our knowledge, this is the first case report to describe the above combination of coronary anomalies in a single patient.

It was an interesting finding to see a late presentation in a patient with the above 4 anomalies described. Survival until the age of 85 is most likely explained by the presence of large caliber RCA to supply the whole right and left side and the absence of an interarterial course. Another explanation is that he was more sedentary and was never involved in competitive sports. The Italian cardiological guidelines for competitive sport eligibility in athletes with heart disease [10] do recommend further workup that may include a CTA in symptomatic athletes. Had he been involved in sports, his coronary anomaly could have been diagnosed at an earlier time and could have been corrected with surgery.

4. Conclusion

Although CAA is a rare entity, when diagnosed, it is of utmost importance for cardiologists to do further imaging in order to differentiate between benign and high-risk anomalies. Moreover, a heart team approach and further workup might be required, including a stress test in order to offer patients the best management options.

Disclosure

We declare that this manuscript is original and is not currently being considered for publication elsewhere.

References

[1] A. D. Villa, E. Sammut, A. Nair, R. Rajani, R. Bonamini, and A. Chiribiri, "Coronary artery anomalies overview: the normal and the abnormal," *World Journal of Radiology*, vol. 8, no. 6, pp. 537–555, 2016.

[2] P. M. Young, T. C. Gerber, E. E. Williamson, P. R. Julsrud, and R. J. Herfkens, "Cardiac imaging: part 2, normal, variant, and anomalous configurations of the coronary vasculature," *American Journal of Roentgenology*, vol. 197, no. 4, pp. 816–826, 2011.

[3] J. C. Lim, A. Beale, and S. Ramcharitar, "Anomalous origination of a coronary artery from the opposite sinus," *Nature Reviews. Cardiology*, vol. 8, no. 12, pp. 706–719, 2011.

[4] P. P. Agarwal, C. Dennie, E. Pena et al., "Anomalous coronary arteries that need intervention: review of pre- and postoperative imaging appearances," *Radiographics*, vol. 37, no. 3, pp. 740–757, 2017.

[5] R. M. Reul, D. A. Cooley, G. L. Hallman, and G. J. Reul, "Surgical treatment of coronary artery anomalies: report of a 37 1/2-year experience at the Texas Heart Institute," *Texas Heart Institute Journal*, vol. 29, no. 4, pp. 299–307, 2002.

[6] P. Angelini, "Coronary artery anomalies: an entity in search of an identity," *Circulation*, vol. 115, pp. 1296–1305, 2007.

[7] B. J. Maron, J. J. Doerer, T. S. Haas, D. M. Tierney, and F. O. Mueller, "Sudden deaths in young competitive athletes," *Circulation*, vol. 119, no. 8, pp. 1085–1092, 2009.

[8] Z. Cheng, X. Wang, Y. Duan et al., "Detection of coronary artery anomalies by dual-source CT coronary angiography," *Clinical Radiology*, vol. 65, no. 10, pp. 815–822, 2010.

[9] R. Schmitt, S. Froehner, J. Brunn et al., "Congenital anomalies of the coronary arteries: imaging with contrast-enhanced, multidetector computed tomography," *European Radiology*, vol. 15, no. 6, pp. 1110–1121, 2005.

[10] P. Delise, L. Mos, L. Sciarra et al., "Italian Cardiological Guidelines (COCIS) for Competitive Sport Eligibility in athletes with heart disease," *Journal of Cardiovascular Medicine*, vol. 22, no. 12, pp. 874–891, 2021.

An Unusual Case of an Acquired Aortopulmonary Fistula after Surgical Replacement of a Bicuspid Aortic Valve

Y. Khalid,[1] **N. Dasu**,[2] **M. Daneshvar**,[3] **P. Jang**,[3] **A. Patel**,[4] **K. Dasu**,[5] **and A. Shah**[6]

[1]*Department of Cardiology, The Wright Center for Graduate Medical Education, Scranton, PA, USA*
[2]*Department of Gastroenterology, Jefferson Health New Jersey, Cherry Hill, NJ, USA*
[3]*Department of Internal Medicine, Jefferson Heath New Jersey, Stratford, NJ, USA*
[4]*Department of Internal Medicine, St. Mary's Medical Center, Langhorne, PA, USA*
[5]*Department of Biomedical Sciences and Professional Studies, Drexel University, Philadelphia, PA, USA*
[6]*Department of Cardiology, University of Pittsburgh Medical Center, Pittsburgh, PA, USA*

Correspondence should be addressed to N. Dasu; dasu@rowan.edu

Academic Editor: Ertugurul Ercan

Aortopulmonary fistulas are extremely rare and often occur as a result of long-standing aortic aneurysms. They are most frequently due to the erosion of a false aneurysm of the ascending or descending thoracic aorta into the pulmonary artery. Patients generally present with symptoms of acute decompensated heart failure due to a sudden formation of a left-to-right shunt. Here, we present the case of a 63-year-old male who acquired an aortopulmonary fistula four months after undergoing successful bioprosthetic aortic valve replacement.

1. Introduction

Infective endocarditis (IE) is a commonly seen diagnosis that is often managed with antimicrobial therapy. It can require surgical intervention in certain complicated cases. There are a number of indications for early surgical intervention including signs of heart failure, paravalvular extension of the infection with the development of an annular or aortic abscess, destructive penetrating lesions (i.e., fistula), persistent infection 5-7 days after starting antibiotic therapy, and difficult-to-treat infections [1]. Postoperative complications commonly include acute renal failure, prolonged mechanical ventilation, and tamponade. More rarely, there can be fistula formation not just between cardiac chambers, but also between the aorta and pulmonary artery leading to the formation of an aortopulmonary fistula.

Furthermore, an acquired aortopulmonary fistula is an extremely rare, but often fatal complication that requires prompt recognition and urgent surgical intervention. It can rapidly lead to cardiac tamponade or hemorrhagic shock. The majority of aortopulmonary fistula cases have been diagnosed post mortem and extremely rarely in patients who are alive [2]. Case studies have shown its associations with infective endocarditis (IE) and valvular surgery as a result of thoracic aortic aneurysm formation [3–5]. In the following case report, we discuss the rare, but important, complication of an aortopulmonary fistula formation following a bioprosthetic surgical aortic valve replacement (SAVR) for treatment of an aortic valve endocarditis with aortic root abscess.

2. Case Presentation

A 63-year-old male with a past medical history of hypertension, hyperlipidemia, and obstructive sleep apnea initially presented with altered mental status and was admitted for septic shock secondary to methicillin-sensitive *Staphylococcus aureus* bacteremia and NSTEMI with troponin level up

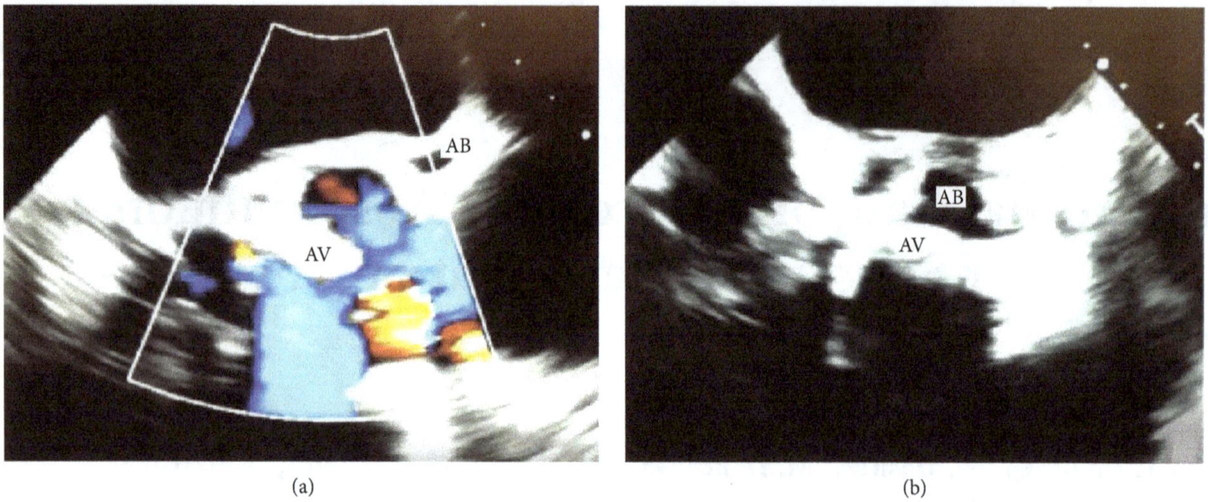

Figure 1: (a, b) Transesophageal echocardiogram showing aortic valve endocarditis (AV) and associated aortic root thickness and abscess. View in (a): color Doppler, apical long axis. View in (b): short-axis.

to 40 ng/mL. His cardiopulmonary exam was unremarkable on the initial exam. Due to poor images on a transthoracic echocardiography (TTE), a transesophageal echocardiography (TEE) and soft tissue chest CT scan was also performed which revealed a severely stenotic bicuspid aortic valve with fusion of the left and noncoronary cusps as well as an ascending aorta dilatation of 4.8 cm and aortic root dilatation of 4.5 cm with concern for an aortic root abscess (Figures 1(a), 1(b), and 2). The patient's hospital course was complicated by an embolic stroke and embolic phenomenon of his right thumb, requiring stabilization prior to surgical intervention. The patient underwent an uncomplicated bioprosthetic aortic valve replacement with a 23 mm Magna Ease Tissue valve, a patch exclusion of the left coronary sinus abscess, and aortoplasty. A coronary artery bypass grafting with a saphenous vein graft to the left anterior descending (LAD) artery was also performed, as the abscess had involved the LAD artery as well. The final pathological report demonstrated thrombotic vegetations on the valve leaflets consistent with acute endocarditis. Once stabilized, the patient was discharged to acute rehabilitation on a 6-week course of IV nafcillin based on culture sensitivities.

About four months after discharge, the patient presented to an outpatient cardiology clinic for a routine postoperative follow-up. At that time, he was asymptomatic and reported having completed the antibiotic course. Physical exam, however, was notable for a left lower sternal harsh holosystolic murmur. He underwent stat TTE, which revealed an abnormal aortic valve with a possible leak near the patch. Upon arrival back to the hospital, TEE revealed a normally seated bioprosthetic aortic valve with no abnormal valvular motion or apparent dysfunction but had a large ventral septal defect (VSD) involving the lower border of the valve which entered the right ventricle adjacent to the septal leaflet of the tricuspid valve (Figure 3). It also showed an aortopulmonary artery fistula connecting the sinus of Valsalva to the pulmonary artery and moderate dilatation of the aortic root with an aneurysmal appearance (Figure 4). Given the level of complexity of the case, he was transferred to a tertiary care

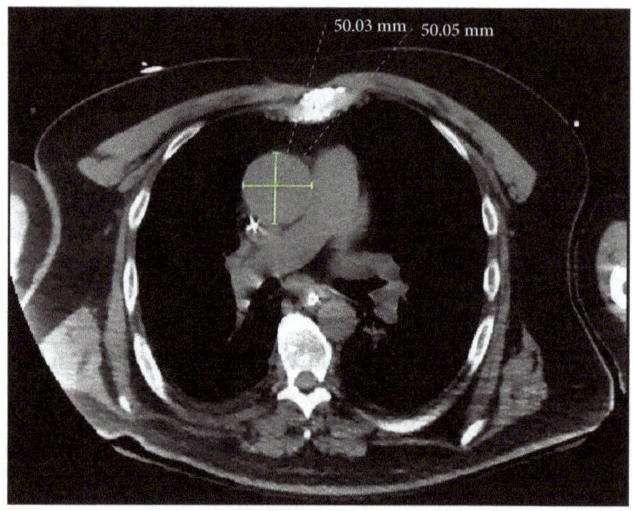

Figure 2: Soft-tissue axial view of CT chest demonstrating dilated aortic root.

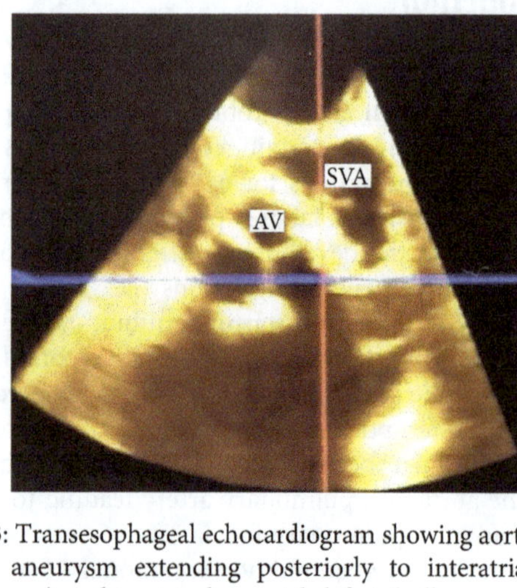

Figure 3: Transesophageal echocardiogram showing aortic sinus of Valsalva aneurysm extending posteriorly to interatrial septum (white arrow) and ventricular septal defect (yellow arrow). View: color Doppler, apical four chamber.

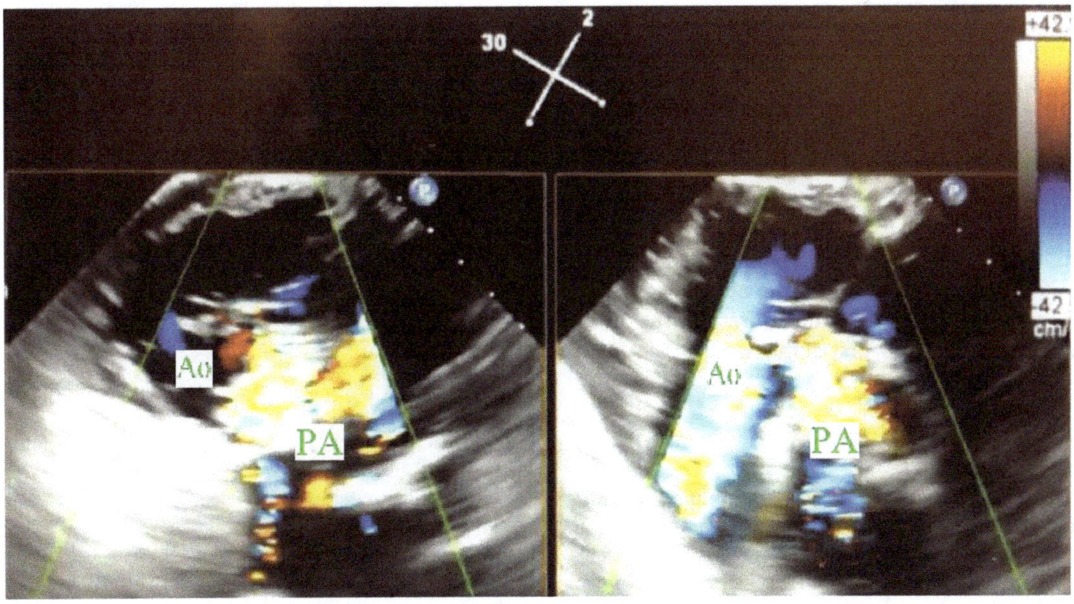

FIGURE 4: Transesophageal echocardiogram showing aortopulmonary fistula. View: color Doppler, long axis view—upper esophageal. AO: ascending aorta; PA: pulmonary artery.

facility, at which he successfully underwent freestyle aortic root (23 mm) and ascending aortic replacement (24 mm), reimplantation of SVG to LAD bypass graft, and VSD closure.

3. Discussion

For surgical management of infective endocarditis, bioprosthetic SAVR is a successful technique with normally minimal complications as compared to other modalities [6, 7]. Aortopulmonary artery fistula formation following bioprosthetic SAVR is an extremely rare but potentially lethal complication of the procedure. Aortopulmonary fistulas can form secondary to infective endocarditis fistulation, thoracic aortic aneurysm rupture, a ruptured sinus of Valsalva aneurysm, or as a complication of procedures performed on the aorta or pulmonic valve. In the present case, the patient had an extensive paravalvular infective endocarditis that formed from an aortic root aneurysm which required aortic valve replacement surgery as a result. Additionally, the patient's blood cultures identified *Staphylococcus* as the causative organism of the infective endocarditis, which has been shown to be the most common organism associated with any type of fistula formation [5]. Though it is hard to differentiate the main cause that led to the development of the fistula, the negative blood cultures and absence of systemic symptoms helped us rule out a recurrent infection. Therefore, the fistula formation was determined to likely be a complication of the valve replacement surgery.

Additionally, a ruptured sinus of Valsalva aneurysm can result in an aortopulmonary fistula formation [7]. A sinus of Valsalva aneurysm is an enlargement of the aortic root area between the aortic valve annulus and the sinotubular ridge. It is found in roughly 0.09% of the general population, and it has been associated with endocarditis [8]. An aortic root aneurysm was identified in the present case, and we believe that the surgical intervention on the right sinus of Valsalva aneurysm led to the development of the aortopulmonary fistula and possibly also to the ventricular septal defect. However, of note, postoperative echocardiography was not completed. Thus, the VSD could have been iatrogenic, as it is a rarely known complication following surgical repair of cardiac valves. A postoperative echocardiography is of utmost importance as it would have elucidated the VSD.

Furthermore, although there were no clinical signs or symptoms of right heart failure, right ventricular overload was evident on echocardiogram. Given the large size of the ventricular septal defect and the aortopulmonary fistula, the patient would be expected to show symptoms of right heart failure, such as dyspnea, hemoptysis, chest pain, orthopnea, or syncope. Interestingly, the patient had no symptoms when the structural defects were identified at routine follow-up. This demonstrates how imperative follow-up visits are for this patient population given that an aortopulmonary fistula can present without symptoms and an early and accurate diagnosis can be life-saving. It also highlights the importance of obtaining postoperative echocardiography. [2].

4. Conclusions

Iatrogenic ventricular septal defect and aortopulmonary artery fistula are extremely rare and lethal complications of bioprosthetic SAVR and reconstruction in the setting of acute infective endocarditis. These fistulas can lead to rapid deterioration of the patient and so early and accurate identification is crucial to the survival of the patient. However, these fistulas can initially present asymptomatically, and so, close follow-up after discharge must be emphasized and encouraged for all patients. Future studies could reevaluate follow-up guidelines in this patient population to better prevent such devastating results.

Disclosure

Khalid Y and Dasu N are co-first authors.

Authors' Contributions

YK, ND, MD, KD, PJ, and AP were responsible for the study concept and design, data collection, and drafting of the manuscript. ND and YK edited the contents and grammar of the manuscript. AS supervised the entirety of the study. Y. Khalid and N. Dasu are co-first authors.

References

[1] AATS Surgical Treatment of Infective Endocarditis Consensus Guidelines Writing Committee Chairs, G. B. Pettersson, J. S. Coselli et al., "2016 The American Association for Thoracic Surgery (AATS) consensus guidelines: surgical treatment of infective endocarditis: executive summary," *The Journal of Thoracic and Cardiovascular Surgery*, vol. 153, no. 6, pp. 1241–1258.e29, 2017.

[2] R. K. Premchand, B. B. Rao, and K. Partani, "A rare case of acquired aortopulmonary fistula with bicuspid aortic valve: report of successful surgical repair," *Case Reports*, vol. 2014, no. - nov181, article bcr2014207374, 2014.

[3] D. Izzo, K. Savino, C. Castellani et al., "Post-traumatic aortopulmonary fistula after Bentall procedure," *Journal of Cardiovascular Echography*, vol. 30, no. 1, pp. 29–32, 2020.

[4] K. Damien, H. Noa, T. David, and M. Hijazi Ziyad, "Aortopulmonary fistula after transcatheter pulmonary valve replacement," *Circulation. Cardiovascular Interventions*, vol. 6, no. 6, article e67, 2013.

[5] S. Klassen, C. G. Mihos, M. J. Birmingham, K. Gadoua, and E. Yucel, "Infective endocarditis of the aortic valve complicated by aorta-to-pulmonary artery fistula," *CASE*, vol. 3, no. 3, pp. 110–114, 2019.

[6] S. Rouzé, E. Flécher, M. Revest et al., "Infective endocarditis with paravalvular extension: 35-year experience," *The Annals of Thoracic Surgery*, vol. 102, no. 2, pp. 549–555, 2016.

[7] M. R. Moon, D. C. Miller, K. A. Moore et al., "Treatment of endocarditis with valve replacement: the question of tissue versus mechanical prosthesis," *The Annals of Thoracic Surgery*, vol. 71, no. 4, pp. 1164–1171, 2001.

[8] M. Weinreich, P.-J. Yu, and B. Trost, "Sinus of Valsalva aneurysms: review of the literature and an update on management," *Clinical Cardiology*, vol. 38, no. 3, pp. 185–189, 2015.

37

Giant Pericardial Lipoma Inducing Cardiac Tamponade and New Onset Atrial Flutter

Connor Charles Kerndt[1] **Alexander Michael Balinski**[2] **and Hayk Vahe Papukhyan**[3]

[1]*Michigan State University College of Osteopathic Medicine, East Lansing, MI 48824, USA*
[2]*Oakland University William Beaumont School of Medicine, Rochester, MI 48309, USA*
[3]*Department of Internal Medicine, Henry Ford Macomb Hospital, Clinton Township, MI 48038, USA*

Correspondence should be addressed to Connor Charles Kerndt; kerndtconnor@gmail.com

Academic Editor: Hajime Kataoka

Although pericardial lipomas are both rare and benign, rapid or excessive growth can induce potentially fatal conditions such as pericarditis, arrhythmia, and cardiac tamponade. This case illustrates an example where a 65-year-old with atypical chest tightness unveiled a 10 × 15 cm anterior pericardial mass with circumferential effusion and progressive deterioration to cardiac tamponade. Initial transthoracic echocardiogram imaging was technically difficult in this patient due to habitus and body mass, which failed to illustrate underlying effusion. Recurrent bouts of refractory supraventricular tachycardia prompted further investigation of this patient's presentation with transesophageal echocardiogram, which showed evidence of an echogenic mass with cardiac tamponade. An urgent pericardial window and pericardial lipectomy immediately relieved this hemodynamically compromising condition. Subsequent atrial flutter resulted with the removal of the anterior fat pad during surgery, complicating recovery.

1. Introduction

Pericardial tumors are exceptionally rare, composing only 6.7-12.8% of all primary cardiac neoplasms [1, 2]. Cardiac tumors can present asymptomatically with incidental findings on imaging or arise with a myriad of symptoms dependent on location, size, and subtype. Pericardial lipomas are benign pericardial neoplasms with a predominance of adipose cells which generally grow insidiously but can expand to compress and irritate adjacent structures via mass effect [3]. Rarely, they can induce fluid infiltration into the pericardial sac due to inflammatory mechanisms, resulting in pericarditis [4].

2. Case Presentation

A 65-year-old female presented to the emergency department with pleuritic chest pain, tachycardia, and eructation. The chest pain was characterized as a "band-like" chest tightness that radiated to the left axilla accompanied with associated shortness of breath, racing heart, and belching. The patient denied nausea, emesis, diaphoresis, and loss of motor/sensory function. The past medical history was significant for type II diabetes, tobacco use, obesity, and hyperlipidemia. The patient's body mass index (BMI) was calculated to be 35.4 upon admission. Family history revealed heart disease in the mother and a noncontributory surgical history. The patient was normotensive, afebrile, and tachycardic with a pulse of 128 bpm and SpO2 of 94%. Physical exam initially presented without pathologic findings.

In light of tachycardia, multiple risk factors, and pleuritic chest pain, a pulmonary embolism workup ensued. Electrocardiogram (EKG) showed sinus tachycardia of 139 bpm (Figure 1(a)), and chest X-ray indicated cardiomegaly (Figure 2(a)). Subsequent blood work demonstrated a negative D-dimer of 0.3 ug/mL with unremarkable thyroid-stimulating hormone (TSH) and serial troponins. Additional tests showed an elevated white blood cell (WBC) count of 23.8 K/uL and lactic acid of 2.3 mmol/L (Table 1). A computerized tomography scan for pulmonary embolism (CT/PE)

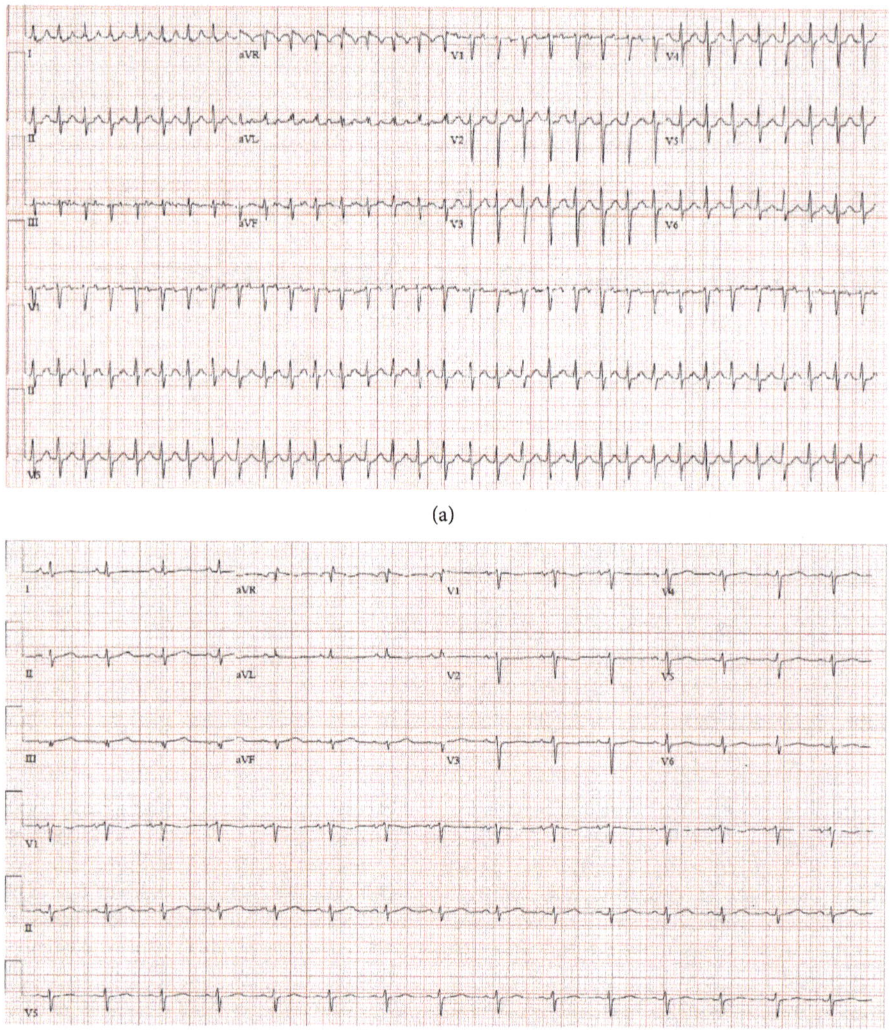

(a)

(b)

Figure 1: EKG before (a) and after (b) pericardial lipoma resection. (a) Findings: supraventricular tachycardia (197 bpm) with low voltage QRS. (b) Findings: normal sinus rhythm (91 bpm).

was then performed which displayed pericardial effusion, patchy bilateral pulmonary infiltrate, and pleural effusions (Figure 3). The setting of tachycardia, leukocytosis, and pulmonary infiltrate initiated sepsis protocol. Based on abnormal EKG findings and clinical presentation, the patient was given ketorolac with colchicine for concern of potential pericarditis, as well as azithromycin and ceftriaxone for concern of potential bilateral atypical pneumonia. The patient was then transferred to the intensive care unit (ICU), cardiology was consulted, and a STAT transthoracic echocardiogram (TTE) was ordered.

Transthoracic echocardiogram findings were limited and failed to show cardiac tamponade or visualization of the pulmonic valve (Figure 2(c)). Given the patient habitus and unknown underlying tumor, the TTE was suboptimal. Later that night, the patient's tachycardia increased to over 200 bpm, prompting cardioversion. An initial dose of 10 mg intravenous (IV) diltiazem returned the patient to sinus tachycardia temporarily but rebounded to supraventricular tachycardia (SVT). A dose of metoprolol 5 mg IV successfully cardioverted her to sinus tachycardia. The patient was then further stabilized with oxygen and pantoprazole. Given the inconclusive TTE, the patient proceeded to transesophageal echocardiogram (TEE) after stabilization to reevaluate a potential mass and evidence of tamponade. The TEE displayed right ventricular collapse, right atrial collapse, large pericardial effusion, evidence of tamponade, and an echogenic mass in the pericardial effusion (Figure 4). Cardiothoracic surgery deemed the patient a candidate for a pericardial window procedure to treat the effusion and tamponade. While a cardiac MRI was briefly considered, the evidence of tamponade and recurrent SVT prompted immediate surgical intervention rather than additional imaging studies.

The surgical procedure unsheathed a large 10×15 cm lipoma in the retrosternal space. This mass was excised and sent to pathology for analysis. Underneath the prepericardial pad, a bulging pericardium was exposed. A small incision in the pericardium expressed 400 mL of dark serosanguinous fluid from around the heart which was sent for cytology, culture, and cell count (Table 2). During surgery, the

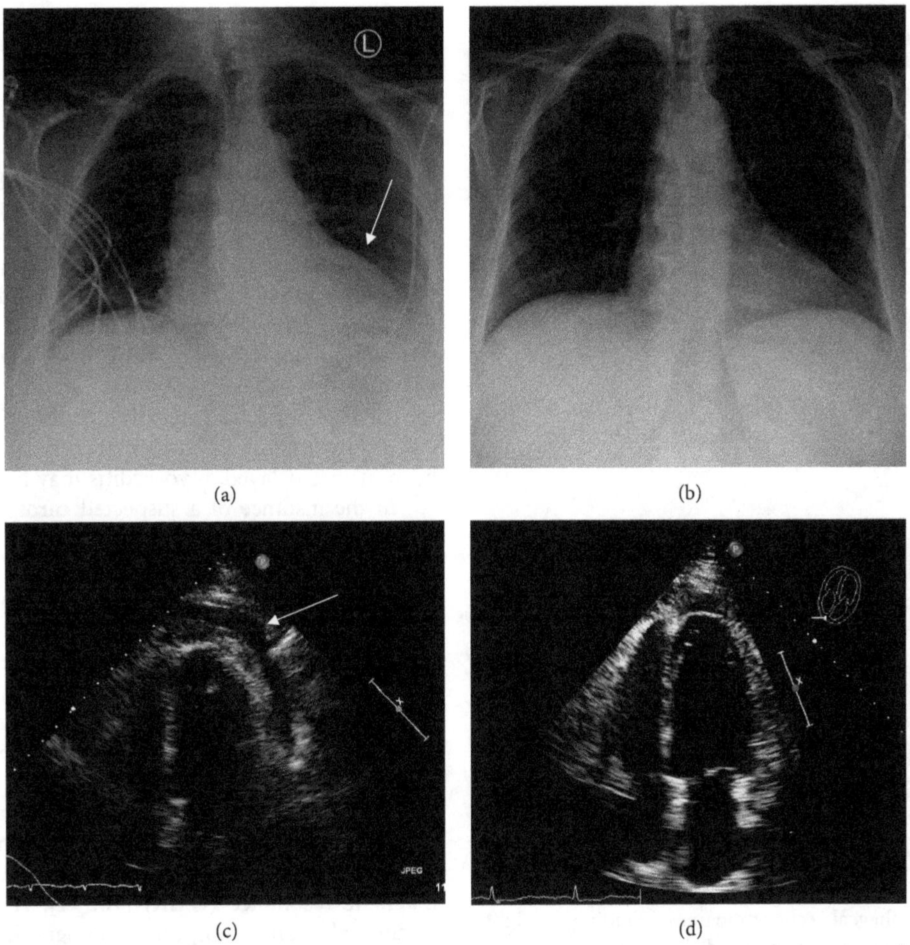

Figure 2: CXR/TTE before (left) and after (right) pericardial lipoma resection. (a) Findings: enlarged cardiac silhouette with epicardial fat pad sign. Impression: cardiomegaly with mild left basilar atelectasis. (b) Findings: the cardiomediastinal silhouette appears WNL. No evidence of pulmonary vascular congestion. Impression: no acute process. (c) Findings: moderately sized pericardial effusion presents circumferentially around the entire heart. (d) Findings: no evidence of cardiac tamponade and minimal remnant pericardial effusion.

Table 1: Preliminary laboratory values.

CBC labs	Patient's value	Reference range	Additional tests	Patient's value	Reference range
WBC	23.8	3.8–10.6 K/uL	BUN	14	10–25 mg/dL
RBC	4.93	4.15-5.55 M/uL	Cr	.77	<1.03 mg/dL
Hg	14.2	12.0–15.0 g/dL	D-dimer	.3	0–0.50 ug/mL
Hct	37.2	36–46%	Lactic acid	2.1	0–2.1 mmol/L
Plt	390	150–450 K/uL	Troponin	<40, <40	0–50 ng/L

pericardium was noted to be thickened and inflamed; thus, a 3 × 3 cm biopsy was sent for histologic analysis. The epicardium was also noted to have chronic and acute inflammatory changes. A chest tube was then inserted, and the patient was taken to recovery after extubation.

Pericardial biopsy demonstrated fibroadipose tissue consistent with an inflammatory pericarditis (Figure 5) and benign adipocytes consistent with pericardial lipoma (Figure 6). The pericardial fluid cytology was negative for malignancy and failed to culture acid-fast organisms. Fluid amylase, glucose, protein, triglycerides, and cholesterol were all within normal limits (Table 2). Effusion lactate dehydrogenase (LDH) was greatly elevated at 1,324 IU/L. Given the lab values, etiology was deemed to be an inflammatory pericarditis.

Postoperatively, the patient was initially unremarkable and transferred to the surgical ICU. Later that night, the patient developed new onset atrial flutter status post pericardial window and was placed on diltiazem for rate control. After insufficient rate control, sotalol was added to the treatment regimen along with apixaban for anticoagulation due to the patient's CHADSVASC score of 3. The patient was stabilized in the ICU, and SVT was managed until stabilization for 6 days. Colchicine and ibuprofen were

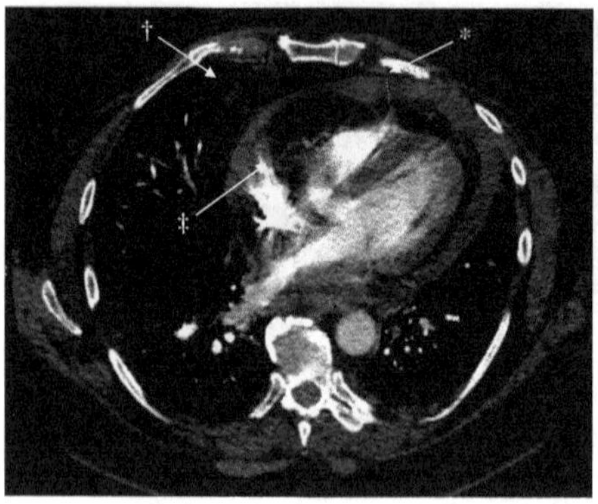

FIGURE 3: CT pulmonary angiography. Findings: *pericardial effusion: 15.4 mm (shown). †pericardial mass; ‡epicardial fat.

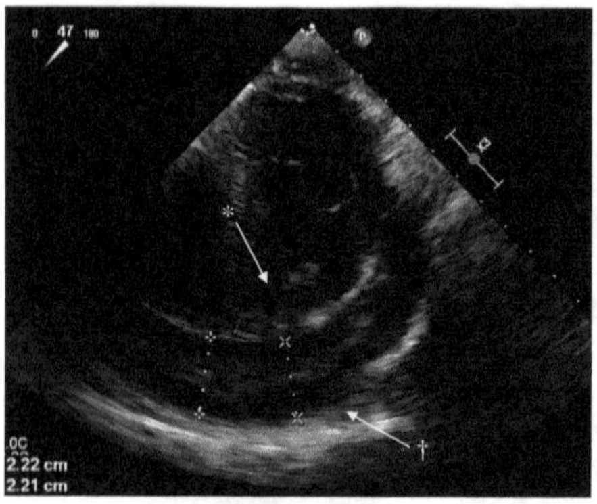

FIGURE 4: Transesophageal echocardiogram. Findings: *right ventricular diastolic collapse with †pericardial effusion.

prescribed as initial treatment for the patient's inflammatory pericarditis. Repeat echocardiogram showed no evidence of tamponade and minimal remnant pericardial effusion (Figure 2(d)). The patient's chest tube was removed, and she was discharged postoperatively on day 6 with apixaban 5 mg, colchicine 0.6 mg, diltiazem 30 mg, and sotalol 80 mg. The patient was instructed to follow up with outpatient cardiology to monitor recovery and manage her new postoperative arrhythmia.

3. Discussion

Cardiac lipomas are typically asymptomatic, benign heart tumors composed of mature adipocytes void of cellular atypia originating from the subendocardium [5]. However, these lipomas can turn symptomatic in rare circumstances when allowed to grow sufficiently substantial in size. Large cardiac lipomas can cause a wide spectrum of symptoms such as chest pain, exertional dyspnea, arrhythmia, syncope, and lower extremity edema depending on their size and location [3]. Reports have also implicated these neoplasms as causes of sudden death [6]. Pericardial lipomas are an especially rare subset of cardiac lipomas and can present with unique complications due to their location.

Typically, pericardial lipomas are asymptomatic, with incidental findings found on computerized tomography (CT) or magnetic resonance imaging (MRI) [3]. It is in rare circumstances that these lipomas present symptomatically and even more unusual to be substantial enough to induce cardiac tamponade. In this case, there were two leading theories regarding causalities of cardiac tamponade: cardiac compression by pericardial lipoma leading to hemodynamic compromise or inflammation resulting in fibrosis and pericardial fluid accumulation due to extracellular matrix destruction and increased vascular filtration [7]. For this patient, biopsies of the cardiac muscle and pericardium confirmed that cardiac tamponade was induced by activation of proinflammatory markers from the patient's giant 10×15 cm anterior pericardial lipoma. Lymphocytic infiltration of the cardiac muscle was negative for fibrosis, suggesting acute phase presentation of disease (Figure 7). Had intervention been further delayed, myocarditis may have ensued.

In the instance of a suspected cardiac tumor, transthoracic echocardiogram is most commonly the initial method of imaging investigation due to its ease of access and noninvasive application [8]. With 90% sensitivity and 95% specificity, echocardiography provides dynamic evaluation when detecting cardiac tumors with capacity for physiologic characterization of consequences [9]. However, transesophageal echocardiography may provide a better, unobstructed view of the heart as it is not limited by an acoustic window and is uninterrupted by the chest wall or lungs [10]. In nonemergent situations, enhanced evaluation and confirmatory testing for a suspected cardiac lipoma can be achieved with cardiac computerized tomography (CCT) and cardiac magnetic resonance (CMR) [10, 11]. A positron emission tomography and computed tomography (PET-CT) scan should also be obtained when attempting to accurately identify the presence or absence of metabolic activity within a suspected mass and reveal possible sites of lesion metastasis. Ultimately, diagnosis of a nonspecific cardiac mass requires specimen biopsy to understand its composition and origin.

Upon diagnosis of a pericardial lipoma, surgical excision by median sternotomy is indicated as both the therapeutic and diagnostic course of treatment [8]. With the incidence of postoperative atrial fibrillation after major thoracic surgery being not uncommon at >30% [12, 13], monitoring for postoperative arrhythmias (usually atrial fibrillation or flutter) has become common practice for these procedures [14]. However, this elevated awareness does not mean arrhythmias are of little consequence, as resultant hemodynamic compromise and thromboembolism are serious contributors to morbidity and mortality in these patients [15]. Prophylactic drug therapy is currently the best method for avoiding postoperative arrhythmic complications and should be considered when managing a patient after the excision of a pericardial lipoma [16]. Sotalol has demonstrated efficacy as a prophylactic agent for postoperative arrhythmias when compared to placebo, with amiodarone being useful as an additional agent in high-risk patients [17]. Alternatively, recent evidence suggests that preservation of the anterior cardiac fat pad during lipoma resection may also reduce the risk of postoperative arrhythmias [18]. While this modified technique does have the potential to reduce the incidence of postoperative arrhythmia, it is uncertain as to whether it would

TABLE 2: Fluid analysis consistent with inflammatory pericarditis.

Test	Patient's value	Reference range	Tests/culture	Patient's value	Reference range
Albumin	2.6	0–4.6 g/dL	TAG	67	0–200 mg/dL
Amylase	16	0–100 IU/L	RBC	67,481	Cu/mm (N/A)
Cholesterol	125	0–200 mg/dL	WBC	4,228	Cu/mm (N/A)
Glucose	86	0–100 mg/dL	Bacteria culture	Negative	N/A
LDH	1,342	0–220 IU/L	Fungal culture	Negative	N/A
Protein	67	<8.2 g/dL	AFB culture	Negative	N/A

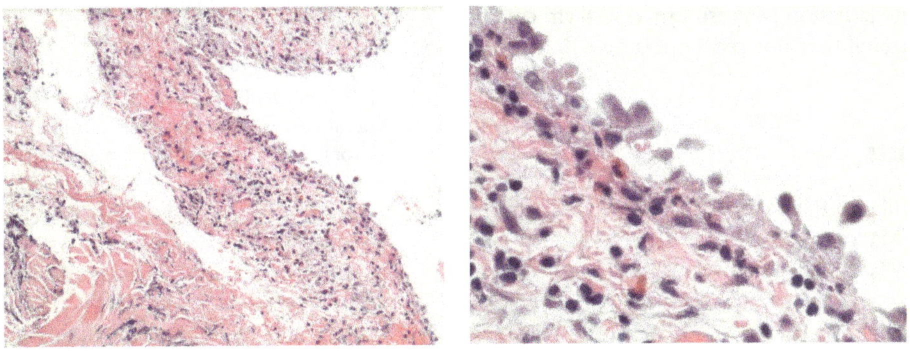

(a) (b)

FIGURE 5: Pericardial biopsy on low power (a) and high power 40x (b). Findings: inflamed hemorrhagic pericardium with lymphocytic involvement.

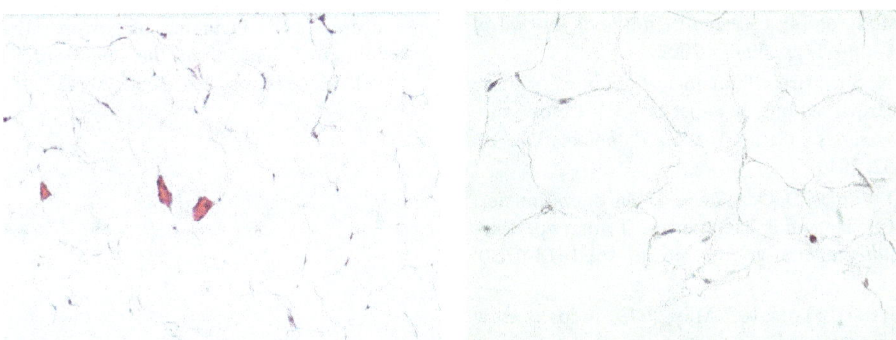

(a) (b)

FIGURE 6: Pericardial lipoma biopsy on low power (a) and high power 40x (b). Findings: benign adipocytes consistent with lipoma. Negative for malignancy.

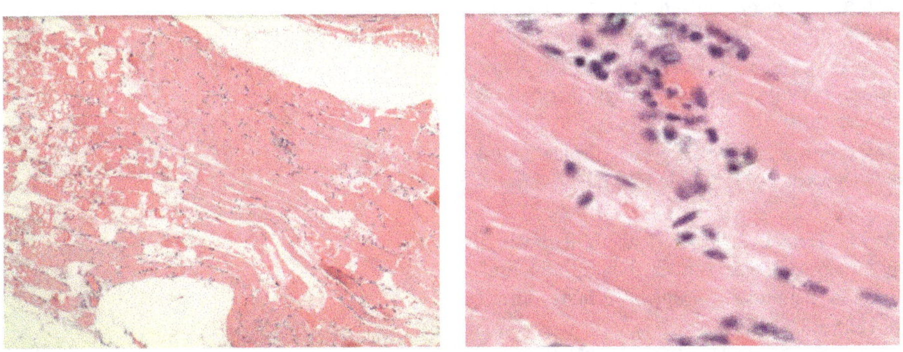

(a) (b)

FIGURE 7: Cardiac biopsy on low power (a) and high power 40x (b). Findings: Lymphocytic infiltration into cardiac muscle, suggestive of myocarditis.

have significantly decreased the likelihood of postoperative arrhythmia and concomitant life-long medical therapy in this case.

4. Summary

Chest pain, while a common presentation, can be benign or potentially fatal. Casting a wide differential while working up chest pain, rather than defaulting judgment to solely common presentations, can have a significant impact on patient care. While patients with benign pericardial tumors carry a good prognosis, acute irritation can result in long-term complications and even fatality if not recognized and managed correctly.

Acknowledgments

The authors would like to thank the Department of Pathology at Henry Ford Macomb Hospital for their assistance in evaluating the biopsy specimens that were critical to the completion of this case report.

References

[1] Q. Meng, H. Lai, J. Lima, W. Tong, Y. Qian, and S. Lai, "Echocardiographic and pathologic characteristics of primary cardiac tumors: a study of 149 cases," *International Journal of Cardiology*, vol. 84, no. 1, pp. 69–75, 2002.

[2] J. Patel and M. N. Sheppard, "Pathological study of primary cardiac and pericardial tumours in a specialist UK Centre: surgical and autopsy series," *Cardiovascular Pathology*, vol. 19, no. 6, pp. 343–352, 2010.

[3] C. S. Restrepo, D. Vargas, D. Ocazionez, S. Martínez-Jiménez, S. L. Betancourt Cuellar, and F. R. Gutierrez, "Primary pericardial tumors," *Radiographics*, vol. 33, no. 6, pp. 1613–1630, 2013.

[4] "Cardiac tumors - UpToDate," May 2019, https://www.uptodate.com/contents/cardiac-tumors.

[5] S. Wu, P. Teng, Y. Zhou, and Y. Ni, "A rare case report of giant epicardial lipoma compressing the right atrium with septal enhancement," *Journal of Cardiothoracic Surgery*, vol. 10, no. 1, p. 150, 2015.

[6] I. N. Bagwan and M. N. Sheppard, "Cardiac lipoma causing sudden cardiac death," *European Journal of Cardio-Thoracic Surgery*, vol. 35, no. 4, pp. 727–727, 2009.

[7] J. Scallan, V. H. Huxley, and R. J. Korthuis, *Capillary fluid exchange: regulation, functions, and pathology*, Morgan & Claypool Life Sciences, 2010.

[8] C. M. Steger, "Intrapericardial giant lipoma displacing the heart," *ISRN Cardiology*, vol. 2011, Article ID 243637, 4 pages, 2011.

[9] R. Engberding, W. G. Daniel, R. Erbel et al., "Diagnosis of heart tumours by transoesophageal echocardiography: a multicentre study in 154 patients," *European Heart Journal*, vol. 14, no. 9, pp. 1223–1228, 1993.

[10] L. Barbuto, A. Ponsiglione, W. del Vecchio et al., "Humongous right atrial lipoma: a correlative CT and MR case report," *Quantitative Imaging in Medicine and Surgery*, vol. 5, no. 5, pp. 774–777, 2015.

[11] S. Singh, M. Singh, D. Kovacs, D. Benatar, S. Khosla, and H. Singh, "A rare case of a intracardiac lipoma," *International Journal of Surgery Case Reports*, vol. 9, pp. 105–108, 2015.

[12] P. D. Bhave, L. E. Goldman, E. Vittinghoff, J. Maselli, and A. Auerbach, "Incidence, predictors, and outcomes associated with postoperative atrial fibrillation after major noncardiac surgery," *American Heart Journal*, vol. 164, no. 6, pp. 918–924, 2012.

[13] L. L. Creswell, R. B. Schuessler, M. Rosenbloom, and J. L. Cox, "Hazards of postoperative atrial arrhythmias," *The Annals of Thoracic Surgery*, vol. 56, no. 3, pp. 539–549, 1993.

[14] S. Jayaprakash, "Clinical presentations, diagnosis, and management of arrhythmias associated with cardiac tumors," *Journal of Arrhythmia*, vol. 34, no. 4, pp. 384–393, 2018.

[15] G. Peretto, A. Durante, L. R. Limite, and D. Cianflone, "Postoperative arrhythmias after cardiac surgery: incidence, risk factors, and therapeutic management," *Cardiology Research and Practice*, vol. 2014, Article ID 615987, 15 pages, 2014.

[16] D. C. Burgess, M. J. Kilborn, and A. C. Keech, "Interventions for prevention of post-operative atrial fibrillation and its complications after cardiac surgery: a meta-analysis," *European Heart Journal*, vol. 27, no. 23, pp. 2846–2857, 2006.

[17] I. Koniari, E. Apostolakis, C. Rogkakou, N. G. Baikoussis, and D. Dougenis, "Pharmacologic prophylaxis for atrial fibrillation following cardiac surgery: a systematic review," *Journal of Cardiothoracic Surgery*, vol. 5, no. 1, p. 121, 2010.

[18] J. E. Cummings, I. Gill, R. Akhrass, M. A. Dery, L. A. Biblo, and K. J. Quan, "Preservation of the anterior fat pad paradoxically decreases the incidence of postoperative atrial fibrillation in humans," *Journal of the American College of Cardiology*, vol. 43, no. 6, pp. 994–1000, 2004.

38

Therapeutic Potential of a Vasopressin V2 Receptor Antagonist for Calcium Channel Blocker-Associated Edema with Vasospastic Angina

Kojiro Toda, Masashi Fujino, Kota Murai, and Teruo Noguchi

Department of Cardiovascular Medicine, National Cerebral and Cardiovascular Centre, Suita, Japan

Correspondence should be addressed to Masashi Fujino; fujinom@ncvc.go.jp

Academic Editor: Manabu Shirotani

Calcium channel blocker- (CCB-) associated peripheral edema does not resolve without CCB discontinuation or dose reduction. However, renin–angiotensin system (RAS) inhibitors have been reported to be effective for CCB-associated edema. We report a case of vasospastic angina with refractory CCB-associated edema. A 78-year-old man had refractory edema induced by a CCB. It was successfully treated with tolvaptan, an active vasopressin V2 receptor antagonist. The aim of this case report is to understand the mechanism and treatment of CCB-associated peripheral edema and how tolvaptan affects peripheral edema.

1. Introduction

Calcium channel blockers (CCBs) are commonly used antihypertensive drugs. Peripheral edema is a common dose-dependent adverse effect. CCB-associated peripheral edema is thought to result from preferential arteriolar dilatation. Renin–angiotensin system (RAS) inhibitors can reduce CCB-associated peripheral edema by decreasing postcapillary resistance, which normalizes intracapillary pressure and reduces fluid extravasation. No other medications for CCB-associated peripheral edema have been reported. We describe successful treatment of CCB-associated peripheral edema using tolvaptan, an active vasopressin V2 receptor antagonist, in a patient with vasospastic angina who had been resistant to conventional diuretic and RAS inhibitor therapy.

2. Case Presentation

A 78-year-old man was admitted to our hospital with bilateral lower extremity swelling. He could not put on shoes of his usual size due to severe edema. His blood pressure was 126/62 mmHg, and pulse was 83 beats/min. Compared to his usual body weight, there was a 10 kg increase, up to 71 kg. Physical examination was notable for pitting edema on both lower extremities (Figures 1(a) and 1(b)). Furthermore, he had edema on his face and upper extremities. His jugular veins were not dilated.

His medical history included vasospastic angina, chronic kidney disease, and paroxysmal atrial fibrillation. Two months prior, he was diagnosed with vasospastic angina because of transient ST-segment elevation on an electrocardiogram during a heart attack, which was relieved by sublingual nitroglycerin (Figures 2(a) and 2(b)). Coronary angiography showed stenosis of the left anterior descending artery, which improved with nitroglycerin injection into the left coronary artery via a catheter (Figures 3(a) and 3(b)). He was prescribed nifedipine 40 mg daily because he had experienced angina with amlodipine 5 mg per day, but angina with ST-segment elevation recurred several times. Finally, he was discharged after being gradually titrated to nifedipine 80 mg per day, diltiazem 200 mg per day, and nitroglycerin patch 27 mg per 24 hours.

The differential diagnosis included CCB-associated peripheral edema, congestive heart failure, kidney failure, cirrhosis, hypothyroidism, and deep venous thrombosis. Laboratory tests revealed elevated creatinine (1.25 mg/dL)

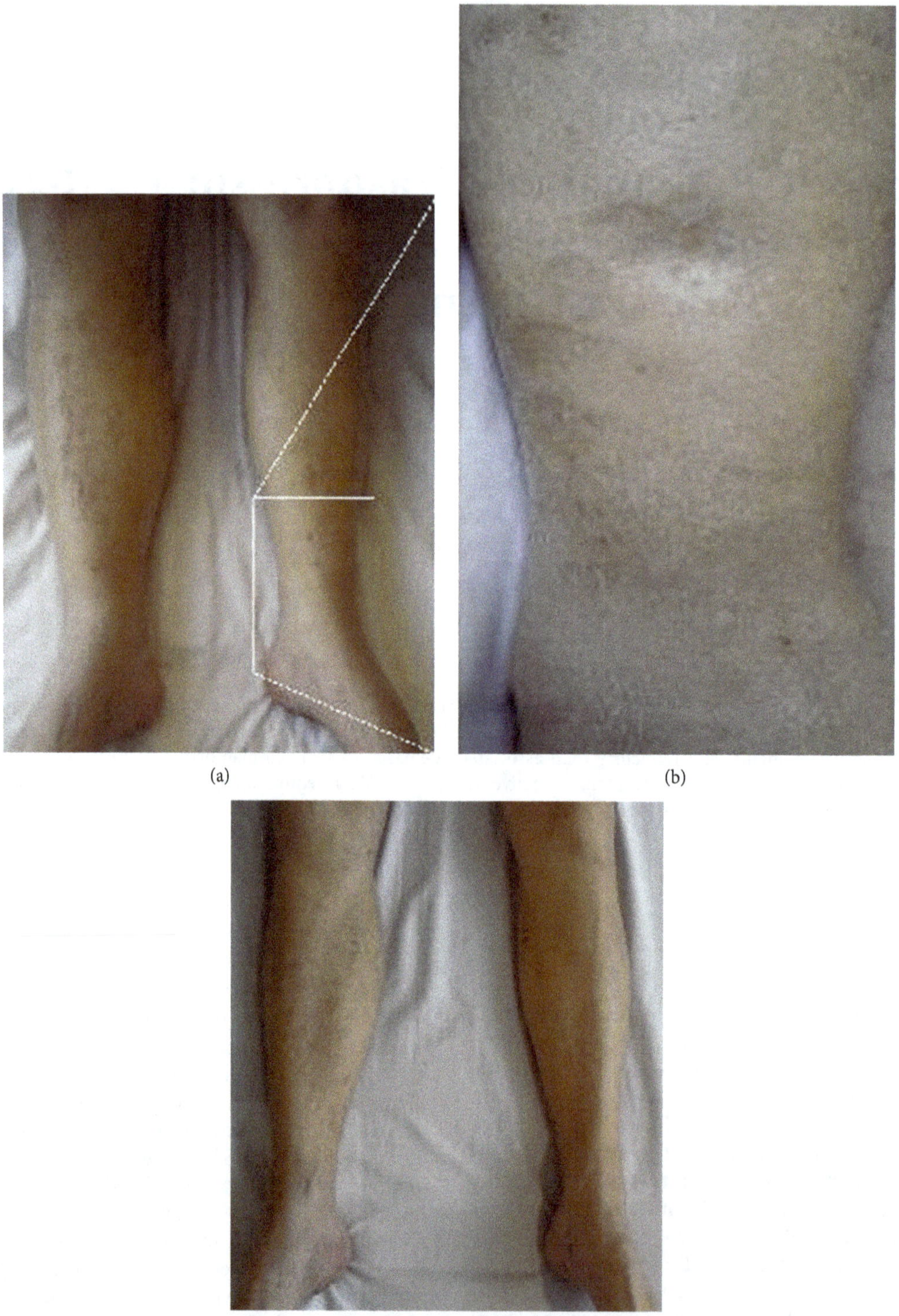

(a) (b) (c)

FIGURE 1: Photographs of the lower extremities. (a) Severe edema of the lower extremities. (b) Pitting edema in a magnified area of (a). (c) Tolvaptan reduced edema without side effects, leading to a body weight decrease of 12 kg.

and B-type natriuretic peptide (128 pg/mL; normal range < 18 pg/mL), but no significant changes from baseline. Albumin, liver function, and thyroid hormone levels were within normal limits. The electrocardiogram showed atrial fibrillation with no remarkable ST-segment changes. Chest radiography revealed a cardiothoracic ratio of 48%, but both costophrenic angles were dull. Echocardiography revealed a normal left ventricular ejection fraction of 60%, left ventricular diastolic/systolic diameter of 51/33 mm, interventricular septum/posterior wall thickness of 10/9 mm, mild

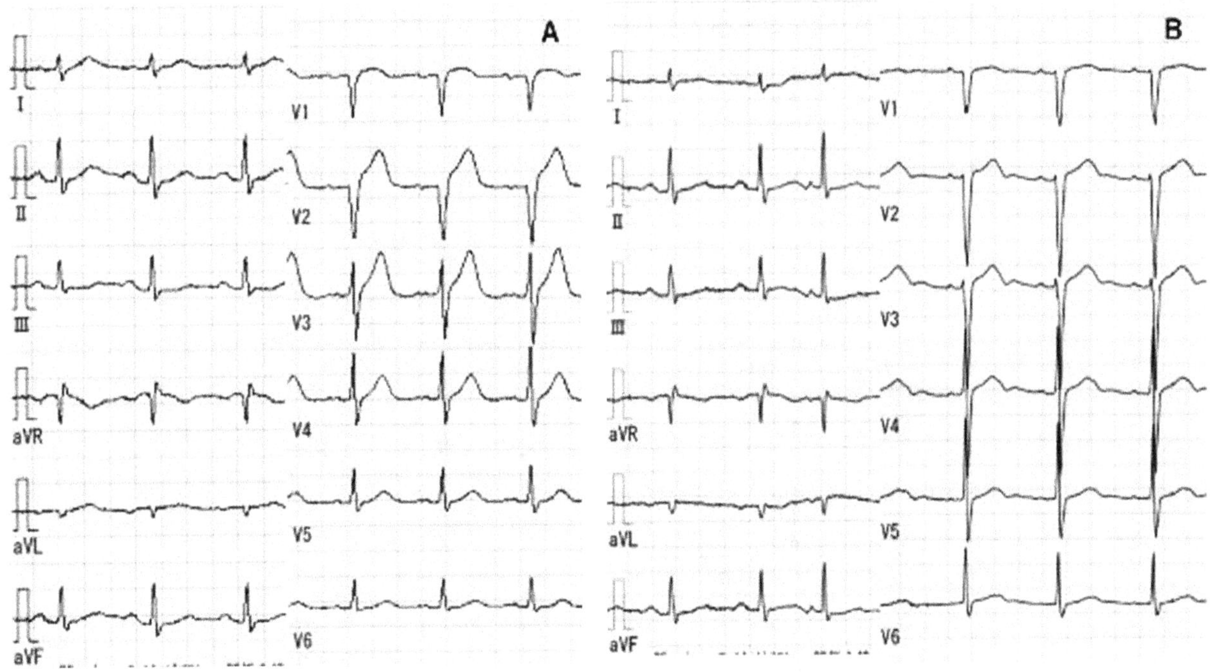

(a) (b)

Figure 2: Electrocardiography findings. (a) ST-segment elevation in leads V2–4 during a heart attack. (b) After lingual nitroglycerin therapy, ST-segment elevations resolved.

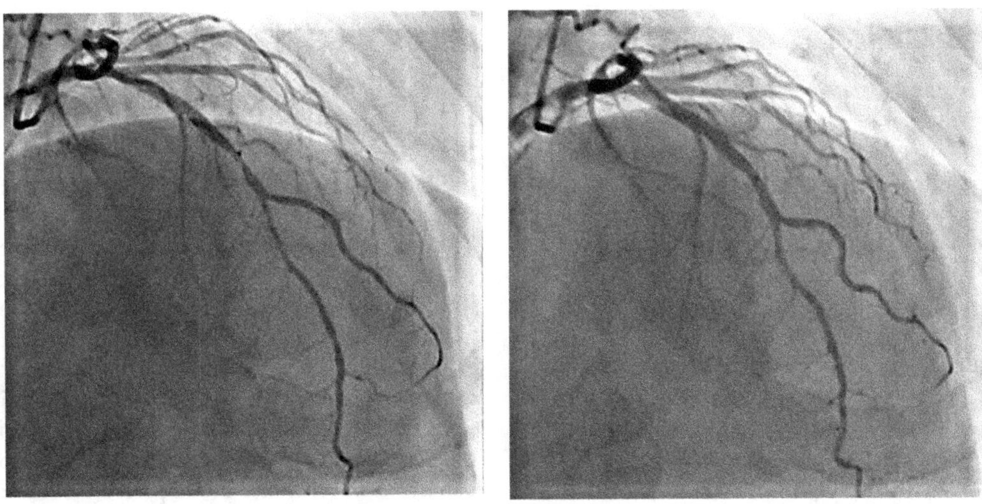

(a) (b)

Figure 3: Coronary angiography findings. Left coronary angiography before (a) and after (b) nitroglycerin injection via a catheter, which dilated the stenosis in the middle of the left anterior descending coronary artery.

tricuspid regurgitation, and preserved function of the other cardiac valves. Based on these results, we made a diagnosis of CCB-associated peripheral edema.

As initial treatment, enalapril 2.5 mg per day and furosemide 20 mg per day were administered. The patient could not tolerate a higher dose of enalapril because of dizziness due to hypotension. Furosemide was discontinued because it decreased renal function. After adding spironolactone 25 mg per day, he lost 4 kg of body weight, but edema and pleural effusion remained. Concerned about the recurrence of angina, the patient disagreed with CCB discontinuation or dose reduction. When we tried the active vasopressin V2 receptor antagonist tolvaptan at 7.5 mg per day, his urine output increased and his edema gradually resolved (Figure 1(c)). He lost 12 kg of body weight; his weight decreased to 59 kg. He had no adverse side effects while taking tolvaptan, such as hypernatremia. Renal function remained stable. After taking tolvaptan, laboratory tests revealed serum sodium of

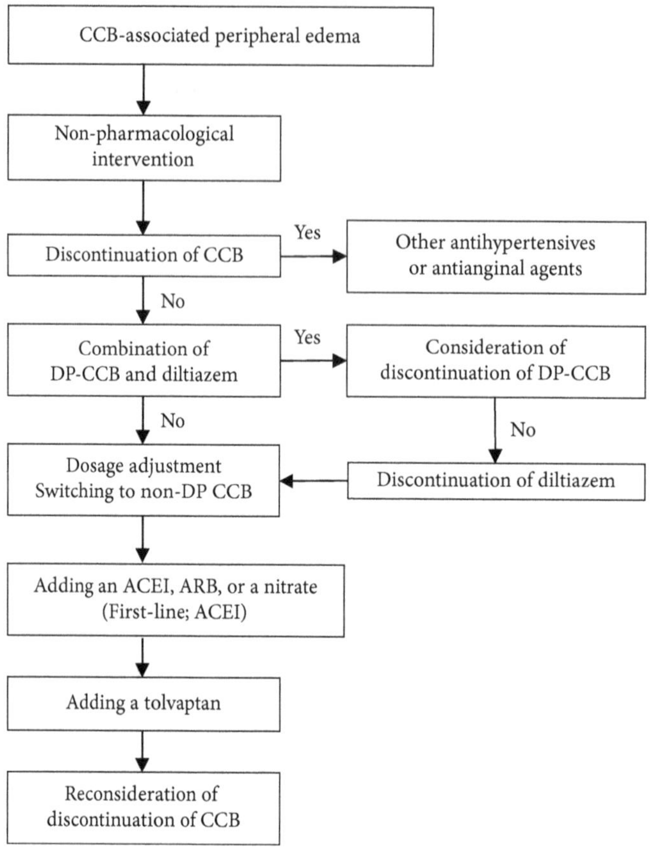

FIGURE 4: Treatment strategies for patients with CCB-associated peripheral edema. Abbreviations: ACE: angiotensin-converting enzyme; ARB: angiotensin II receptor blocker; CCB: calcium channel blocker; DP: dihydropyridine.

140 mEq/L, creatinine of 1.21 mg/dL, and B-type natriuretic peptide of 81.0 pg/mL. After discharge, the frequency of tolvaptan was decreased to every other day, with no recurrences of peripheral edema and no side effects from tolvaptan.

3. Discussion

This case indicated that tolvaptan has favorable effects on CCB-associated peripheral edema. Peripheral edema is a common adverse effect of CCBs. The incidence of peripheral edema is both dose- and duration-dependent. The incidence might exceed 80% with very high doses of dihydropyridine CCBs [1]. Furthermore, conventional racemic amlodipine causes edema more commonly than the S-isomer of amlodipine [2]. Treatment of CCB-associated peripheral edema consists of CCB dose reduction or discontinuation. A previous meta-analysis reported that combining angiotensin-converting enzyme (ACE) inhibitors or angiotensin II receptor blockers (ARBs) with CCBs reduces the incidence of CCB-associated edema by 38%. The CCB discontinuation rate due to peripheral edema with RAS inhibitors was 62% lower than with CCB monotherapy [3]. In addition, ACE inhibitors seem to be more effective than ARBs in reducing CCB-associated peripheral edema [3]. However, edema is sometimes refractory. Peripheral edema is considered to be the result of peripheral arteriolar dilatation, which increases the pressure gradient between arteriolar and venule capillaries and leads to extravasation of intravascular fluid. RAS inhibitors decrease postcapillary resistance, which normalizes intracapillary pressure and reduces fluid extravasation. This patient required high doses of nifedipine and diltiazem to control angina. The combination of these two drugs increases the blood concentration of nifedipine and potentiates its antihypertensive effects. Thus, he could not tolerate ACE inhibitors at a sufficiently high dose. Dihydropyridine-associated edema occasionally occurs despite the use of RAS inhibitors in addition to a diuretic. Exchanging nifedipine for extended-release diltiazem or felodipine led to patient tolerability and blood pressure control [4]. Although there has been a case report showing that the combination of dihydropyridine and diltiazem lowers blood pressure through their interaction [5], there have been no reports of refractory edema due to that interaction.

This patient was concerned about the recurrence of angina. Thus, he disagreed with CCB discontinuation or dose reduction. Furthermore, since he had mild chronic kidney disease, the edema was extremely severe and his response to conventional diuretics was poor. Refractory peripheral edema developed; low-dose RAS inhibitor therapy did not reduce the edema.

Tolvaptan has a diuretic effect with a mechanism that is different from that of conventional diuretics. Tolvaptan is an orally active vasopressin V2 receptor antagonist that blocks arginine vasopressin from binding to V2 receptors in the distal nephron, which induces the excretion of electrolyte-free water without changing the total level of electrolyte excretion [6]. Although loop diuretics predominantly decrease extracellular water (ECW) rather than intracellular water (ICW), a previous study that involved bioimpedance analysis showed that tolvaptan ameliorates body fluid retention and induces equivalent reductions in ICW and ECW without worsening renal function [7]. Another study showed that tolvaptan restores body fluids by the efficient reduction of intracellular fluid than hemodialysis, by reducing the volume of intracellular fluid by a greater amount and maintaining more fluid in the extracellular space [8]. Tolvaptan induces diuresis of free water and an increase in serum sodium. Because the serum sodium concentration and the interstitial sodium concentration is identical, tolvaptan then induces an increase in the osmolarity of both the intravessel compartment and the interstitial compartment which would accelerate the oncotic forces leading to fluid movement from the intracellular compartment to the interstitial compartment. Tolvaptan helps maintain a lower intravessel volume and promote efficient diuresis, which ultimately decreases the fluid in the interstitium (i.e., edema). To treat CCB-associated peripheral edema, tolvaptan might work by helping fluid move from the intracellular compartment to the interstitial compartment. Furthermore, tolvaptan is reported to be effective for patients with chronic kidney disease [9]. In addition, dihydropyridine CCBs have a sodium diuretic effect; peripheral edema is not due to salt retention [10]. Therefore, classical diuretic treatment is not expected to be effective. However, tolvaptan was effective for this patient with CCB-associated peripheral edema. Figure 4 shows the strategy for patients with CCB-associated peripheral edema [11].

This case demonstrated that tolvaptan had a favorable effect on CCB-associated peripheral edema. It also suggested that an oral vasopressin V2 receptor antagonist could reduce CCB-associated peripheral edema in a patient with refractory edema even after CCB dose reduction or RAS inhibitor therapy.

Abbreviations

ACE: Angiotensin-converting enzyme
ARB: Angiotensin II receptor blocker
CCB: Calcium channel blocker
ECW: Extracellular water
ICW: Intracellular water
RAS: Renin-angiotensin system.

Acknowledgments

Masashi Fujino is supported by a Grant-in-Aid for Young Scientists from the Japan Society for the Promotion of Science (20K17138).

References

[1] F. H. Messerli, "Vasodilatory edema: a common side effect of antihypertensive therapy," *Current Cardiology Reports*, vol. 4, no. 6, pp. 479–482, 2002.

[2] J. Dalal, J. C. Mohan, S. S. Iyengar et al., "S-Amlodipine: an isomer with difference—time to shift from racemic amlodipine," *International Journal of Hypertension*, vol. 2018, Article ID 8681792, 14 pages, 2018.

[3] H. Makani, S. Bangalore, J. Romero, O. Wever-Pinzon, and F. H. Messerli, "Effect of renin-angiotensin system blockade on calcium channel blocker- associated peripheral edema," *The American Journal of Medicine*, vol. 124, no. 2, pp. 128–135, 2011.

[4] J. Handler, "Managing calcium channel blocker-related peripheral edema," *Journal of Clinical Hypertension*, vol. 6, no. 7, pp. 400–402, 2004.

[5] J. C. Busse, R. E. de Velasco, and E. L. Pellegrini, "Combined use of nifedipine and diltiazem for the treatment of severe hypertension," *Southern Medical Journal*, vol. 84, no. 4, pp. 502–504, 1991.

[6] R. W. Schrier, P. Gross, M. Gheorghiade et al., "Tolvaptan, a selective oral vasopressin V2-receptor antagonist, for hyponatremia," *The New England Journal of Medicine*, vol. 355, no. 20, p. 2099, 2006.

[7] T. Masuda, T. Murakami, Y. Igarashi et al., "Dual impact of tolvaptan on intracellular and extracellular water in chronic kidney disease patients with fluid retention," *Internal Medicine*, vol. 55, no. 19, p. 2759, 2016.

[8] H. Kawabata, H. Iwatani, Y. Yamamichi, K. Shirahase, N. Nagai, and Y. Isaka, "Tolvaptan efficiently reduces intracellular fluid: working toward a potential treatment option for cellular edema," *Internal Medicine*, vol. 58, no. 5, pp. 639–642, 2019.

[9] J. Sen, E. Chung, and D. McGill, "Tolvaptan for heart failure in chronic kidney disease patients: a systematic review and meta-analysis," *Heart, Lung & Circulation*, vol. 27, no. 8, pp. 928–939, 2018.

[10] M. Epstein, G. D. M. Anna, and F. Hayley, "Natriuretic effects of calcium antagonists in humans: a review of experimental evidence and clinical data," *Cardiovascular Drug Reviews*, vol. 9, no. 4, pp. 398–412, 1991.

[11] J. J. Saseen, "Pharmacologic treatment of hypertension," in *Cardiovascular Therapeutics (Fourth Edition) a Companion to Braunwald's Heart Disease*, pp. 474–489, Saunders, 2013.

39

Cold at the Core: Osborn Waves in Neurosarcoidosis-Induced Central Hypothermia

Gregory Scott Troutman,[1] Jason Salamon,[2] Matthew Scharf,[3] and Jeremy A. Mazurek[4]

[1]*Sidney Kimmel Medical College at Thomas Jefferson University, Philadelphia, PA, USA*
[2]*Department of Medicine, Division of Cardiology, Morristown Medical Center, Atlantic Medical Group, Morristown, NJ, USA*
[3]*Department of Medicine, Division of Sleep Medicine, Robert Wood Johnson University Hospital, New Brunswick, NJ, USA*
[4]*Department of Medicine, Division of Advanced Heart Failure and Transplant Cardiology, Hospital of the University of Pennsylvania, Philadelphia, PA, USA*

Correspondence should be addressed to Gregory Scott Troutman; gst002@jefferson.edu

Academic Editor: Hajime Kataoka

Osborn waves, or J waves, initially described by John Osborn in 1953 in hypothermic dog experiments, are highly sensitive and specific for hypothermia. Initially thought to be secondary to a hypothermia-induced "injury current," they have more recently been attributed to a voltage differential between epicardial and endocardial potassium (I_{to}) currents. While the exact conditions required to induce such waves have been debated, numerous clinical scenarios of environmental and iatrogenic hypothermia have been described. Below, we report a novel case of hypothermia—that of neurosarcoidosis-induced central hypothermia with resultant Osborn waves and other associated findings found on electrocardiogram (ECG).

1. Introduction

Osborn waves, or J waves, initially attributed to a hypothermia-induced "injury current," have more recently been attributed to a differential between epicardial and endocardial potassium (I_{to}) currents creating a voltage gradient and the observed J wave [1, 2]. While not pathognomonic for hypothermia, the presence of J waves, most commonly seen in the anterior and lateral precordial leads, is highly sensitive and specific for hypothermia [3, 4].

Neurosarcoidosis is a relatively uncommon, often debilitating condition affecting approximately 5% of patients with sarcoidosis. Pituitary disease can cause thyroid, gonadal, and adrenal abnormalities or panhypopituitarism. Hypothalamic involvement can further result in central diabetes insipidus and dysthermia (either hypothermia or hyperthermia). Management often involves systemic corticosteroids and the replacement of all deficient hormones to correct the endocrine dysfunction [5].

Below, we describe the case of a patient with neurosarcoidosis who presented with hypothermia and prominent Osborn waves on electrocardiogram (ECG) in the setting of significant pituitary and hypothalamic dysfunction.

2. Case Report

A 40-year-old African-American male with neurosarcoidosis involving the hypothalamus and pituitary (Figure 1) presented to an urban academic medical center with altered mental status. On arrival, the patient was lethargic but responsive to verbal stimuli and the physical examination was otherwise unremarkable. The patient was noted to be hypothermic (32°C) and hypernatremic (176 mEq/L). Admission ECG revealed sinus bradycardia at 41 beats per minute, first-degree AV block (PR interval 280 ms), premature atrial contractions, prolonged QRS (160 ms) and QT (QTc 584 ms) intervals, and Osborn waves most prominent in the precordial lateral leads (Figure 2(a)).

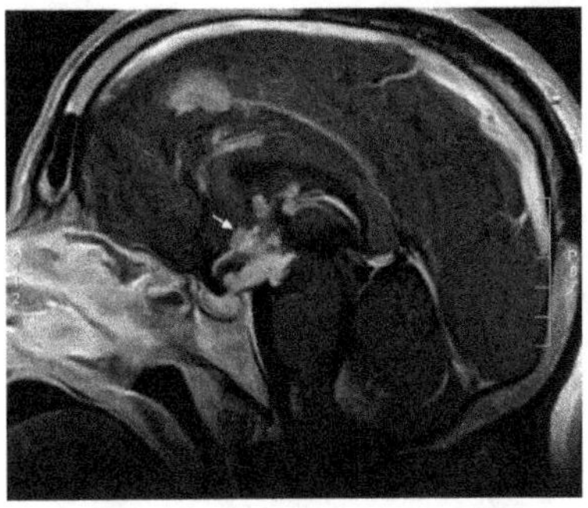

FIGURE 1: Brain magnetic resonance image showing neurosarcoidosis involving the hypothalamus and pituitary.

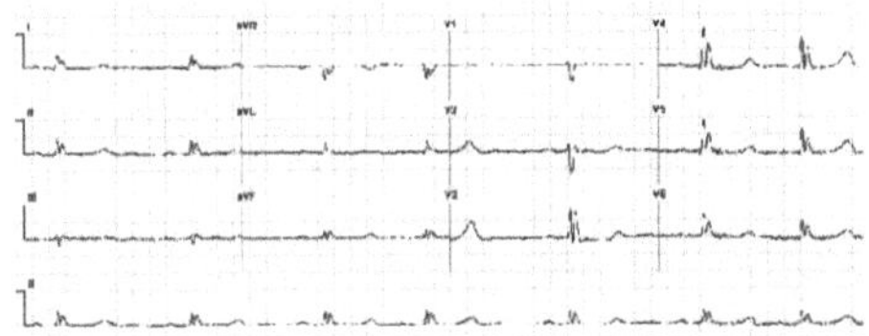

(a)

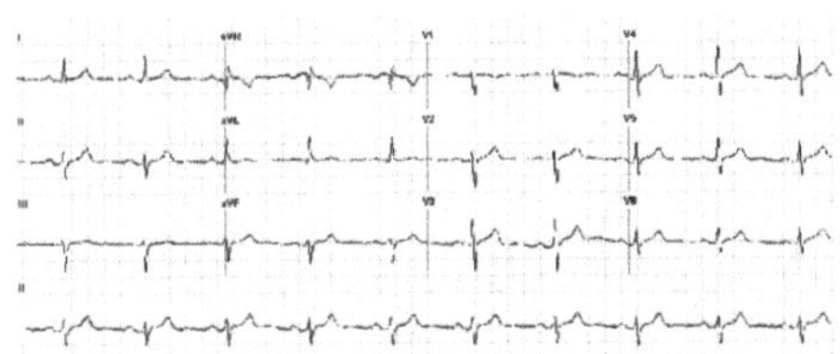

(b)

FIGURE 2: (a) Electrocardiogram at 32°C revealing sinus bradycardia with premature atrial contractions, Osborn waves most prominent in the precordial lateral leads, prolonged PR and QT intervals. (b) Electrocardiogram after initiation of treatment reveals an increase in heart rate to 60 beats per minute and an improvement of the PR (210 ms), QRS (98 ms), and QT (QTc 432 ms) intervals.

The patient was admitted to the intensive care unit where careful intravenous fluid management and administration of intranasal desmopressin were initiated. After 24 hours, with the improvement of his serum sodium, the patient's mental status improved. The patient was warmed via external warming blankets, with resolution of the above electrocardiographic findings (Figure 2(b)). The remainder of the patient's treatment included corticosteroids, testosterone, levothyroxine, and desmopressin, and he was discharged home ten days after presentation.

3. Discussion

Neurosarcoidosis is a debilitating condition that affects a minority of patients (~5%) with sarcoidosis. As a systemic granulomatous disease, sarcoidosis can affect both the central and peripheral nervous systems with the neurological manifestations varying depending on the areas of disease involvement [6, 7]. Pituitary disease and hypothalamic involvement can result in severe endocrine dysfunction including panhypopituitarism and central diabetes insipidus and dysthermia (either hypothermia or hyperthermia), respectively, as were seen in this patient [4–7].

Osborn waves, or J waves, initially described as a hypothermia-induced "injury current," have more recently been attributed to a differential between epicardial and endocardial potassium (I_{to}) currents creating a voltage gradient and the observed J wave [1, 2]. Though not necessarily pathognomonic for hypothermia, the presence of J waves is highly sensitive and specific for hypothermia. Most commonly seen in the anterior and lateral precordial leads is the amplitude of the J wave which is inversely proportional to the degree of hypothermia and is present in 80% of individuals with a temperature below 35°C. Other electrocardiographic findings include PR, QRS, and QT prolongation, as in this patient, as well as supraventricular and ventricular arrhythmias in more severe hypothermia [3].

Since its original description, it has been suggested that hypothermia must be accompanied by some other disturbance (i.e., acidosis) to result in the development of the Osborn wave [1, 3]. Subsequent reports, however, have suggested a hypothalamic or neurogenic cause for the J waves as seen in patients with subarachnoid hemorrhage [3, 8]. Experimental animal experiments inducing subarachnoid hemorrhage have confirmed similar ECG findings to that of hypothermia suggesting a possible relationship between hypothalamic dysfunction and autonomic catecholamine imbalance with a resultant disorder of myocardial rhythm and function [9, 10].

Thus, our patient represents an unusual cause of hypothermia with classic findings on ECG. These findings, unlike prior reports, may represent effects of both systemic hypothermia and hypothalamic dysfunction. To our knowledge, this is the first report of neurosarcoidosis-induced hypothermia with associated Osborn waves along with other associated ECG changes, all of which resolved with warming, steroid and hormone replacement, and supportive care.

References

[1] J. J. Osborn, "Experimental hypothermia: respiratory and blood pH changes in relation to cardiac function," *American Journal of Physiology-Legacy Content*, vol. 175, no. 3, pp. 389–398, 1953.

[2] G. X. Yan and C. Antzelevitch, "Cellular basis for the electrocardiographic J wave," *Circulation*, vol. 93, no. 2, pp. 372–379, 1996.

[3] A. Mattu, W. J. Brady, and A. D. Perron, "Electrocardiographic manifestations of hypothermia," *The American Journal of Emergency Medicine*, vol. 20, no. 4, pp. 314–326, 2002.

[4] O. Eroglu, S. Serbest, T. Kufeciler, and A. Kalkan, "Osborn wave in hypothermia and relation to mortality," *The American Journal of Emergency Medicine*, 2018.

[5] T. M. Burns, "Neurosarcoidosis," *Archives of Neurology*, vol. 60, no. 8, pp. 1166–1168, 2003.

[6] D. L. Vargas and B. J. Stern, "Neurosarcoidosis: diagnosis and management," *Seminars in Respiratory and Critical Care Medicine*, vol. 31, no. 4, pp. 419 427, 2010.

[7] B. J. Stern, W. Royal III, J. M. Gelfand et al., "Definition and consensus diagnostic criteria for neurosarcoidosis: from the neurosarcoidosis consortium–consensus group," *JAMA Neurology*, 2018.

[8] J. De Sweit, "Changes simulating hypothermia in the electrocardiogram in subarachnoid hemorrhage," *Journal of Electrocardiology*, vol. 5, no. 2, pp. 193–195, 1972.

[9] L. Offerhaus and J. van Gool, "Electrocardiographic changes and tissue catecholamines in experimental subarachnoid haemorrhage," *Cardiovascular Research*, vol. 3, no. 4, pp. 433–440, 1969.

[10] L. A. Coghlan, B. J. Hindman, E. O. Bayman et al., "Independent associations between electrocardiographic abnormalities and outcomes in patients with aneurysmal subarachnoid hemorrhage," *Stroke*, vol. 40, no. 2, pp. 412–418, 2009.

40

Diagnostic Management and Surgical Treatment of Isolated Tricuspid Regurgitation

Arthur Cicupira Rodrigues de Assis,[1] Gustavo Andre Boeing Boros,[1] Lea Maria Macruz Ferreira Demarchi,[2] Thiago Luis Scudeler,[1] and Paulo Cury Rezende[1]

[1]*MASS Research Unit, Instituto do Coração (InCor), Hospital das Clínicas da Faculdade de Medicina da Universidade de São Paulo, São Paulo, Brazil*

[2]*Pathology Department, Instituto do Coração (InCor), Hospital das Clínicas da Faculdade de Medicina da Universidade de São Paulo, São Paulo, Brazil*

Correspondence should be addressed to Paulo Cury Rezende; rezendepaulo@hotmail.com

Academic Editor: Dietmar Kivelitz

Severe tricuspid regurgitation is especially caused by pulmonary hypertension. Primary tricuspid regurgitation in the absence of pulmonary hypertension and of unknown etiology is a very rare condition with scarce data about its diagnosis, treatment, and follow-up. The particularities of surgery indication and outcomes are still not clearly known. A 72-year-old woman with a medical history of coronary artery bypass grafting three years ago presented with shortness of breath and low limb edema. Physical examination revealed a prominent bilateral jugular turgescence, hepatomegaly, peripheral edema, and a left midsternal border holosystolic murmur, suggestive of tricuspid regurgitation. The echocardiogram confirmed the diagnosis and showed preserved right and left ventricular dimensions and function. Coronary angiography showed no new obstructive lesions and patent surgical grafts. Right cardiac catheterization revealed mild pulmonary hypertension and increased right atrium pressure. Cardiac magnetic resonance showed mild right ventricular dilation with normal systolic function and normal left chambers. No late gadolinium enhancement was detected. Because of persistent symptoms, even after optimization of medical therapy, the patient was submitted to tricuspid valve replacement surgery. Immediately after the surgery, the patient developed significant right ventricular dysfunction, with the need of continuous hemodynamic support. She had progressive clinical recovery that was confirmed by serial echocardiograms that showed improvement in right ventricular volume and function. The patient was discharged with no signs or symptoms of right heart failure. The histopathological examination showed significant and diffuse myxomatous degeneration of the leaflets. No signs of infection or vegetation nor disruption of strands were observed. This report illustrates a very rare case of symptomatic primary isolated severe tricuspid regurgitation caused by myxomatous degeneration of the leaflets. The thoroughly diagnostic workup is presented, and only the histopathological analysis of the leaflets revealed the etiologic process. Surgical treatment indicated before the onset of right ventricular failure was essential to patient's full recovery.

1. Introduction

The major etiology of tricuspid regurgitation (TR) is secondary to pulmonary hypertension, but primary disease occurs in about 10% of the cases [1]. In this setting, congenital and acquired diseases should be considered, such as Ebstein's anomaly, atrioventricular septal defects, myxomatous prolapse, endocarditis, rheumatic disease, carcinoid syndromes, and blunt trauma. Secondary TR is most related to right ventricular remodeling in pulmonary hypertension. Interestingly, atrial fibrillation (AF) may be considered the cause of tricuspid insufficiency rather than the consequence, especially when it is long lasting. In the acute setting, right ventricular infarction can result in papillary muscle damage and subsequent acute atrioventricular valvar regurgitation, although mitral valve is the most common.

Recently, some authors have identified that the incidence of isolated TR is increasing [1, 2]. This is mainly explained because of the use of implantable right cardiac devices and increased AF prevalence. Rarer are the cases when no causes are identified. The diagnostic management in such cases and the appropriate treatment are also challenging. Although the surgical treatment with the substitution of the impaired native valve by a prosthesis is a definitive therapeutic option, there are few data about the diagnostic workup and outcomes in such patients. Challenges are both in the acute phase after surgery and in the long-term follow-up. In this case report, the authors present one patient with stable multivessel coronary artery disease who developed symptoms of right heart failure and was diagnosed with severe isolated tricuspid regurgitation. The diagnostic workup and the surgical substitution of the tricuspid valve by a bioprosthesis are reported and discussed.

2. Case Presentation

A 72-year-old woman was evaluated for newly diagnosed symptomatic right heart failure, with preserved left ventricular ejection fraction and no history of precipitating factors. She complained of progressive dyspnea, orthopnea, and paroxysmal nocturnal dyspnea in the last 5 months. Prominent bilateral jugular turgescence, moderate hepatomegaly and ascites, and peripheral edema were present. Cardiac auscultation revealed an irregular rhythm and a left midsternal border holosystolic murmur, suggestive of TR.

The patient's medical history included coronary artery bypass grafting (CABG), diabetes mellitus, and dyslipidemia. CABG was performed on May 20, 2014, elective, with cardiopulmonary bypass (CPB). CPB duration was 117 minutes, and anoxia time was 70 minutes. Revascularization was anatomically complete and included the following grafts: left internal mammary artery to the anterior descending coronary artery, saphenous vein to the ramus diagonalis of the left main coronary artery, saphenous vein to the inferior interventricular artery, and saphenous vein to the second obtuse marginal of the circumflex coronary artery. There were no complications in the entire perioperative period. She remained asymptomatic during all outpatient visits every 6 months, with no clinical signs of heart failure, valvular insufficiency, or atrial fibrillation. Five months before this outpatient visit, she started with symptoms and signs of right heart failure, three years after CABG, on May 22, 2017. There was no history of previous arrhythmias. No history of fever, diaphoresis, weight loss, or trauma was reported.

The electrocardiogram showed newly diagnosed AF. Transthoracic echocardiography revealed significant enlargement of the right atrium, preserved right and left ventricular dimensions and function, and severe TR (an additional movie file shows this in more detail (see Additional file 1 at https://drive.google.com/file/d/1dI5rywG2qCX7lSrrmFuC1_IPkNvy6p1H/view)). No signs of tricuspid or mitral prolapse were observed. Coronary angiography showed no new obstructive lesions compared to previous exams and patent surgical grafts. Right cardiac catheterization revealed mild pulmonary hypertension (mean artery pulmonary pressure 33 mmHg), along with increased right atrium pressure (21 mmHg). Cardiac magnetic resonance showed the right atrium diameter and volume severely increased (antero-posterior diameter was 63 mm, and area was 27cm^2) and mild right ventricular dilation along with normal systolic function; the tricuspid valve annulus diameter was not enlarged (30 mm in diastole); left chambers were unremarkable (Additional file 1). Subjective analysis was compatible with severe TR; no late gadolinium enhancement was detected. Additional investigation of rheumatological and oncological diseases revealed no etiological diagnosis.

The patient developed limiting symptoms of dyspnea, even after optimization of diuretic therapy, and was admitted at our hospital for surgery eleven months after symptom onset and six months after starting the optimization of medical therapy. A tricuspid valve replacement surgery was performed with a bovine pericardial prosthesis (Braile Biomedical®), with the use of cardioplegia and CPB. CPB duration was 60 minutes, and anoxia time was 34 minutes. No surgical intervention for atrial fibrillation (such as Maze procedure) was performed in order to do not prolong the intervention. Immediately after CPB, the patient developed significant right ventricular dysfunction. Hemodynamic support with aggressive preload management with high doses of intravenous diuretics, vasoactive drugs, and nitric oxide was introduced to control right ventricular failure. Serial transthoracic echocardiograms showed progressive improvement in the right ventricular volume and function, achieving normal parameters 1 week after the procedure. Analysis of the bioprosthetic valve showed no signs of dysfunction. The patient was weaned from mechanical ventilation after 48 hours and remained in the intensive care unit (ICU) for 10 days. In the ICU, she developed acute kidney injury in the first 72 hours after surgery that progressively recovered with the improvement in right cardiac function.

Despite a long hospital stay due to deep wound infection, treated with large-spectrum antibiotics and daily care by wound-infection specialized nurses, the patient showed progressive clinical recovery. The paroxysmal atrial fibrillation was treated with antiarrhythmics and anticoagulation.

In the follow-up visits, she presented well and had no signs or symptoms of right heart failure. Antiarrhythmics were progressively withdrawn, as well as anticoagulation because the patient sustained sinus rhythm after many months of follow-up.

The anatomical study of the native tricuspid valve showed glistening and dome-shaped cusps (Figure 1(a)) and irregularly thickened and branched chordae (Figure 1(b)). The histopathological examination of the tricuspid valve showed no signs of infection or vegetation nor disruption of strands (Figure 2(a)). A significant and diffuse mixomatous degeneration was observed in the leaflets (Figure 2(b)). A very small healed infarct in papillary muscle of unspecified origin was observed (Figure 2(c)).

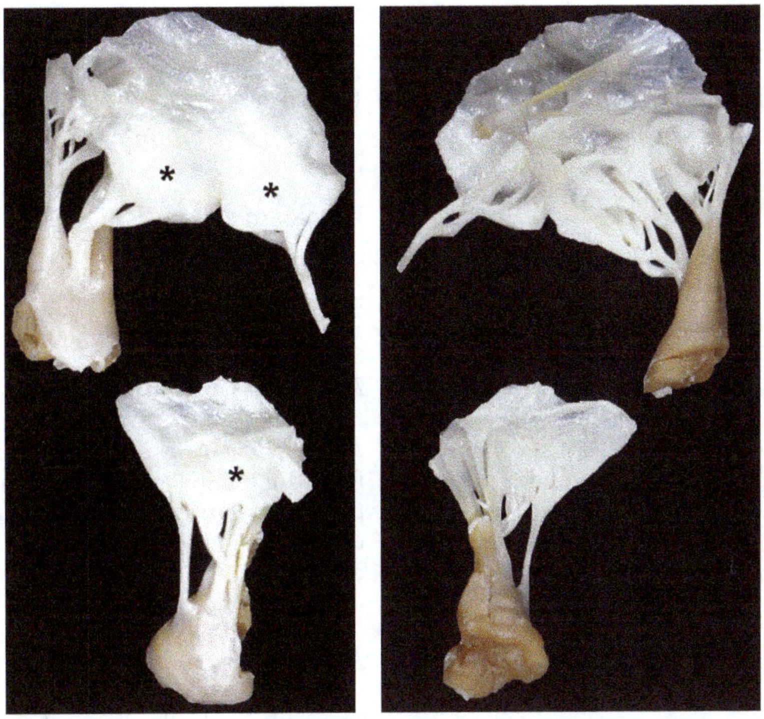

FIGURE 1: Surgical specimen from tricuspid valve repair. (a) Atrial aspect: cusps are glistening and dome-shaped (*). (b) Ventricular aspect: chordae are irregularly thickened and branched.

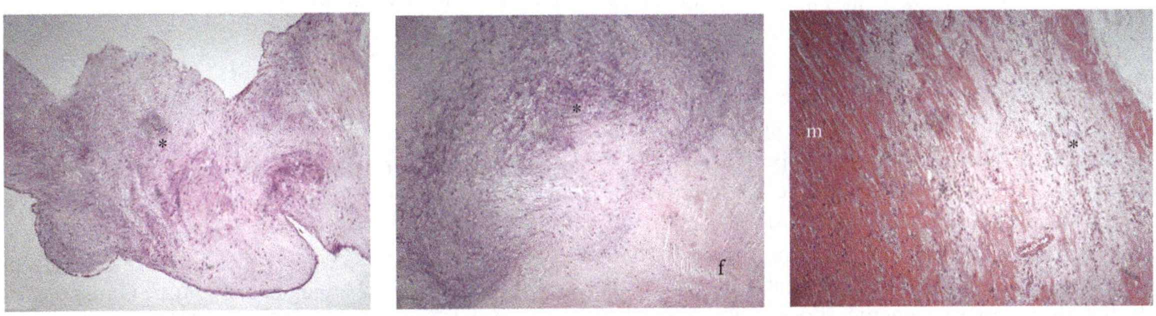

FIGURE 2: Photomicrographs from tricuspid valve. (a, b) Myxomatous degeneration (*) and fibrosis (f) of the spongiosa layer. (c) Healed infarct (*) in papillary muscle (m).

3. Discussion and Conclusions

The incidence of isolated severe TR is increasing, because of the higher prevalence of AF and the growing indication of cardiac devices [1, 2]. However, there are still no specific guidelines about diagnostic approach and management. The patient showed severe symptoms and signs of right heart failure, but no other organ impairment, such as renal or hepatic dysfunction, and this contributed to the good evolution. After confirmation of TR, an extensive investigational approach was performed. We ruled out moderate to severe pulmonary hypertension, long-term arrhythmias, and ischemic, rheumatologic, and storage diseases. The presence of AF was considered a result of severe regurgitation with subsequent right atrial enlargement and remodeling, since there was no history or documentation of arrhythmias in the regular follow-up started in 2013. Moreover, CMR showed the tricuspid valve annulus not to be enlarged. This finding strongly suggests that AF was not the cause of severe TR in this case, because echocardiographic studies of severe TR of unknown etiology in patients with AF have identified extreme annular dilation as the driving mechanism [3], suggesting, thus, that AF may be a cause rather than the consequence in such cases. Finally, the histopathological examination of the valve excluded the diagnosis of endocarditis and confirmed the myxomatous degeneration of the leaflets as the etiology of the severe TR.

Myxomatous degeneration especially affects the mitral valve apparatus, causing the prolapse of mitral valve cusps. About 30 to 40% of these patients may also have a prolapse of the tricuspid valve [4]. However, in this patient, no involvement of the mitral valve was detected, and no prolapse of tricuspid or mitral valves were observed by echocardiograms or cardiac magnetic resonance.

The main contemporary guidelines supported the approach of this case with good recommendation classes, but low levels of evidence (class I, level of evidence C, according to the European Society of Cardiology [5]; class IIa, level of evidence C, according to American Heart Association/American College of Cardiology [6]). Surgical treatment for severe TR is mainly signaled if simultaneous left valve treatment is indicated. Low levels of evidence are justified by the paucity of surgeries in this setting [7]. Studies evaluating mortality are retrospective and describe mortality of 2 to 20% in 30 days after surgery [1]. Our review of literature found one retrospective study comparing surgical and drug treatments that demonstrated a non-statistical mortality benefit in the surgical group in 10-year survival analysis [8].

The option for the replacement instead of the repair of the valve apparatus was discussed with the surgical team before the procedure. Because of anatomical characteristics that were not favorable to repair, and in order to do not prolong CPB and surgery times, replacement was the option for this patient.

Although our patient had only preoperative mild dilation of the right ventricle with normal ejection fraction and no evidence of severe pulmonary hypertension, acute right ventricular failure occurred after cardiopulmonary bypass. The acute increase in the right ventricular afterload with the surgical resolution of tricuspid regurgitation is often poorly tolerated by the right ventricle that can evolve to severe dysfunction and cardiogenic shock right after the surgery. In this setting, aggressive diuretic therapy, inotropes, and nitric oxide were essential to the progressive improvement of right ventricular function.

In conclusion, the authors report a very rare case of severe isolated tricuspid regurgitation, from the clinical presentation, investigative process, surgical treatment, and outcomes. A thoroughly diagnostic workup associated with an early indication for surgery before the development of severe right ventricular dysfunction contributed to the good clinical evolution of the patient.

Abbreviations

AF: Atrial fibrillation
CMR: Cardiac magnetic resonance
CPB: Cardiopulmonary bypass
TR: Tricuspid regurgitation.

Consent

A written informed consent to publish was obtained from the patient.

Disclosure

The funder had no influence during the preparation of this manuscript.

Authors' Contributions

ACRA and GABB drafted the manuscript. LAMFD performed the histological examination of the valve and contributed in writing the manuscript. TLS and PCR made critical revision of the manuscript for important intellectual content.

Acknowledgments

The authors thank all members of the MASS Research group for the hard work in this manuscript. Medical writing support was provided by Ann Conti Morcos, from MorcosMedia. Funding was provided by a research grant from the Zerbini Foundation, São Paulo, Brazil, to the payment of medical writing support.

References

[1] E. A. Fender, C. J. Zack, and R. A. Nishimura, "Isolated tricuspid regurgitation: outcomes and therapeutic interventions," *Heart*, vol. 104, no. 10, pp. 798–806, 2018.

[2] Y. Topilsky, V. T. Nkomo, O. Vatury et al., "Clinical outcome of isolated tricuspid regurgitation," *JACC: Cardiovascular Imaging*, vol. 7, no. 12, pp. 1185–1194, 2014.

[3] H. Utsunomiya, Y. Itabashi, H. Mihara et al., "Functional tricuspid regurgitation caused by chronic atrial fibrillation: a real-time 3-dimensional transesophageal echocardiography study," *Circulation. Cardiovascular Imaging*, vol. 10, no. 1, article e004897, 2017.

[4] P. M. Shah and A. A. Raney, "Tricuspid valve disease," *Current Problems in Cardiology*, vol. 33, no. 2, pp. 47–84, 2008.

[5] Joint Task Force on the Management of Valvular Heart Disease of the European Society of Cardiology (ESC), European Association for Cardio-Thoracic Surgery (EACTS), A. Vahanian et al., "Guidelines on the management of valvular heart disease (version 2012)," *European Heart Journal*, vol. 33, no. 19, pp. 2451–2496, 2012.

[6] R. A. Nishimura, C. M. Otto, R. O. Bonow et al., "2014 AHA/ACC guideline for the management of patients with valvular heart disease: a report of the American College of Cardiology/American Heart Association Task Force on Practice Guidelines," *Journal of the American College of Cardiology*, vol. 63, no. 22, pp. e57–185, 2014.

[7] C. M. Vassileva, J. Shabosky, T. Boley, S. Markwell, and S. Hazelrigg, "Tricuspid valve surgery: the past 10 years from the Nationwide Inpatient Sample (NIS) database," *The Journal of Thoracic and Cardiovascular Surgery*, vol. 143, no. 5, pp. 1043–1049, 2012.

[8] J. W. Lee, J. M. Song, J. P. Park, J. W. Lee, D. H. Kang, and J. K. Song, "Long-term prognosis of isolated significant tricuspid regurgitation," *Circulation Journal*, vol. 74, no. 2, pp. 375–380, 2010.

41

Incidental Finding of Giant Coronary Artery Aneurysms Successfully Treated with Medical Therapy

Rony Shammas, Prasanna Sengodan, and Assad Movahed

Division of Cardiology, Vidant Medical Center-East Carolina University at Brody School of Medicine, Greenville, NC, USA

Correspondence should be addressed to Assad Movahed; movaheda@ecu.edu

Academic Editor: Ertugrul Ercan

We report a case of a 30-year-old male who presented with signs and symptoms of respiratory infection with left lower lobe consolidation and cardiomegaly on a chest radiography. The presence of cardiomegaly lead to further cardiac evaluation revealing giant coronary aneurysms. The patient was treated conservatively with Coumadin and aspirin and has done well at four years of follow-up.

1. Background

Coronary artery aneurysms (CAAs) are defined as a focal dilation of coronary segments of at least 1.5 times the adjacent normal segment, whereas the term coronary artery ectasia is used to define similar, but more diffuse, lesions. The overall incidence ranges from 0.3 to nearly 5%. With more widespread use of coronary angiography, CAAs have been increasingly identified as an incidental finding. Giant CAAs defined as dilation of the artery greater than 4 times the reference diameter are rare.

2. Case Description

A 30-year-old male with a history of cerebral palsy, autism, and scoliosis presented to the emergency department with complaints of left-sided pleuritic chest pain, shortness of breath, and fever.

Initial work-up revealed a white blood cell count of 19,300 and a chest radiography (Figure 1) showed left lower lobe consolidation, cardiomegaly, and a calcified mass in the left lung base. Electrocardiogram (EKG) showed sinus tachycardia with a rate of 114 with right axis deviation and non-specific ST-T changes (Figure 2). He was initially treated for pneumonia and subsequently underwent an echocardiogram (Figure 3) due to findings of cardiomegaly on the chest radiograph. This revealed a large extra cardiac mass alongside the left ventricle with normal left and right ventricular size and function.

Computed tomographic scan of the chest (Figure 4) showed large mostly thrombosed proximal and mid left anterior descending artery (LAD) aneurysm measuring 7.7 cm in addition to a smaller calcified distal aneurysm which corresponds to the mass seen on the chest radiography. The LAD lumen appeared to be patent (asterisk). Coronary angiography (Figure 5) confirmed the presence of multiple aneurysms within the left main coronary artery and LAD with slow flow. The large mid LAD aneurysm was not well delineated on the angiogram due to the absence of calcification. No aneurysmal changes were noted in the right coronary or left circumflex arteries.

Due to the extensive and diffuse nature of the aneurysmal changes which involved the whole length of the LAD in addition to the substantial amount of organized thrombus, surgical intervention was not felt to be feasible. The patient was placed on Coumadin, atorvastatin, and aspirin and has not had a cardiac event over a 4-year follow-up period.

3. Discussion

Coronary artery aneurysms are defined as a focal dilation of coronary segments of at least 1.5 times the adjacent normal segment, whereas the term coronary artery ectasia is used to define similar, but more diffuse, lesions [1]. The right

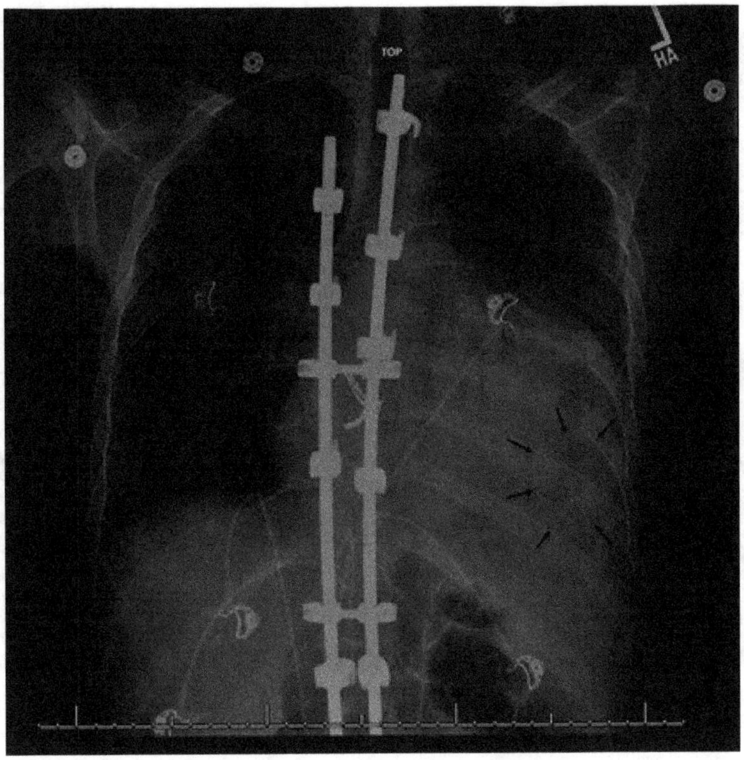

FIGURE 1: Chest radiography showing left lower lobe consolidation, cardiomegaly, and a calcified mass in the left lung base.

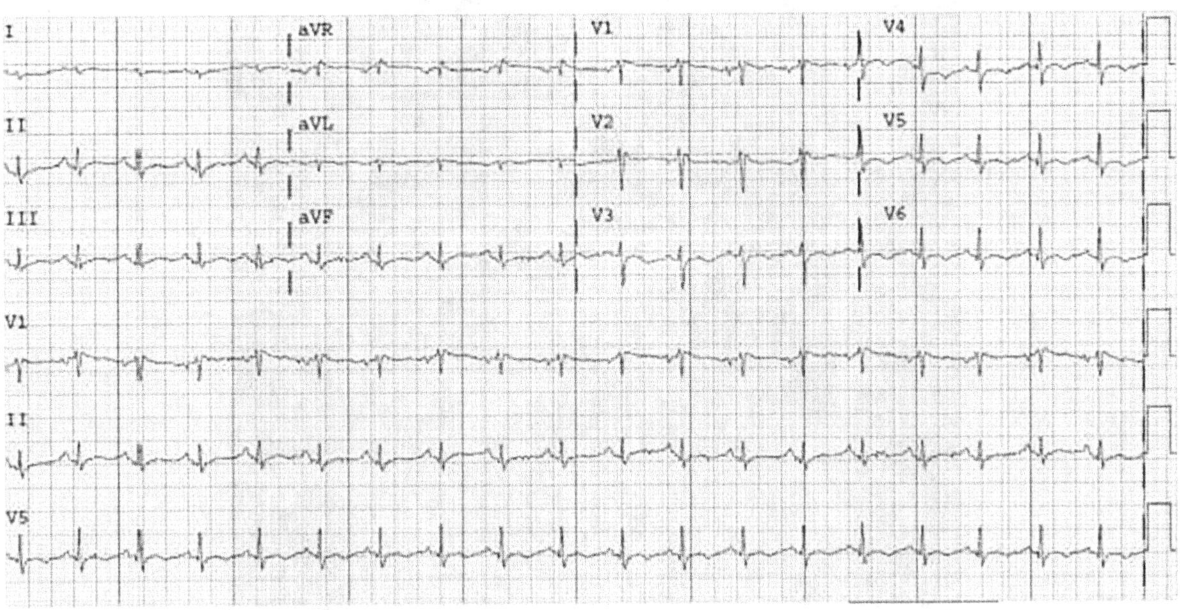

FIGURE 2: Electrocardiogram (EKG) showed sinus tachycardia with a rate of 114 with right axis deviation and nonspecific ST-T changes.

coronary artery is usually the most affected artery (40%) followed by the left anterior descending (32%), and the left main being the least affected artery (3.5%) [2]. Mechanisms underlying their formation including a molecular basis (a possible role of matrix metalloproteinases (MMPs)) are being investigated as suggested by Lamblin et al. [3]. They report that the 5A/5A genotype of MMP-3 was significantly more frequent in patients with coronary aneurysms than in controls. The pathogenesis of the formation of CAAs is not clear; however, a few mechanisms have been proposed including individual genetic susceptibility, atherosclerosis, and iatrogenic injury following percutaneous interventions, in addition to congenital etiology, vasculitis, and connective tissue disorders such as Kawasaki disease and Marfan syndrome. Fibromuscular dysplasia, a nonatherosclerotic and non-inflammatory vascular disease, commonly associated

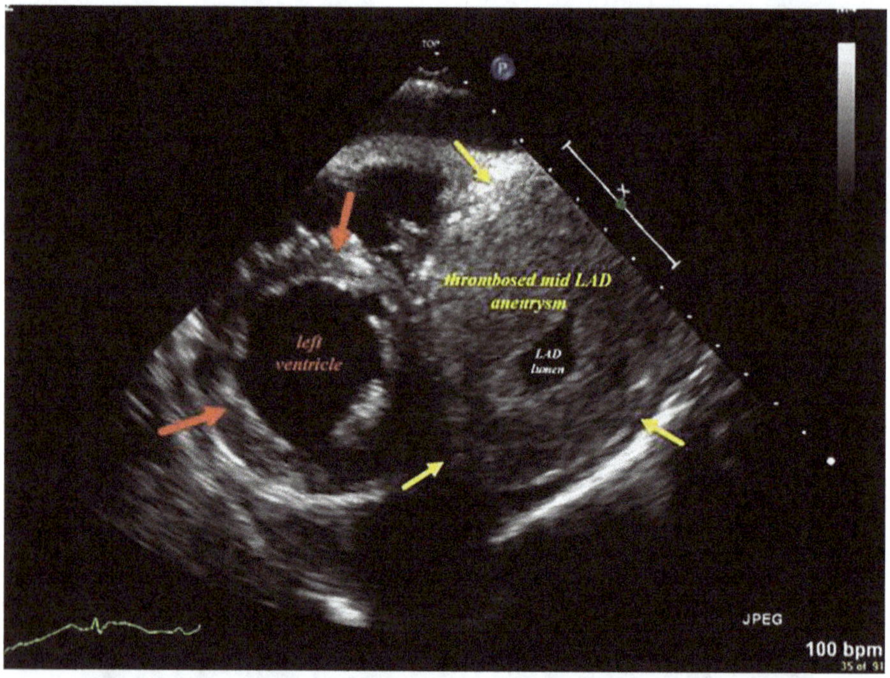

Figure 3: Two-dimensional transthoracic echocardiogram short axis view showing a large extracardiac mass (yellow arrows) alongside the left ventricle (red arrows).

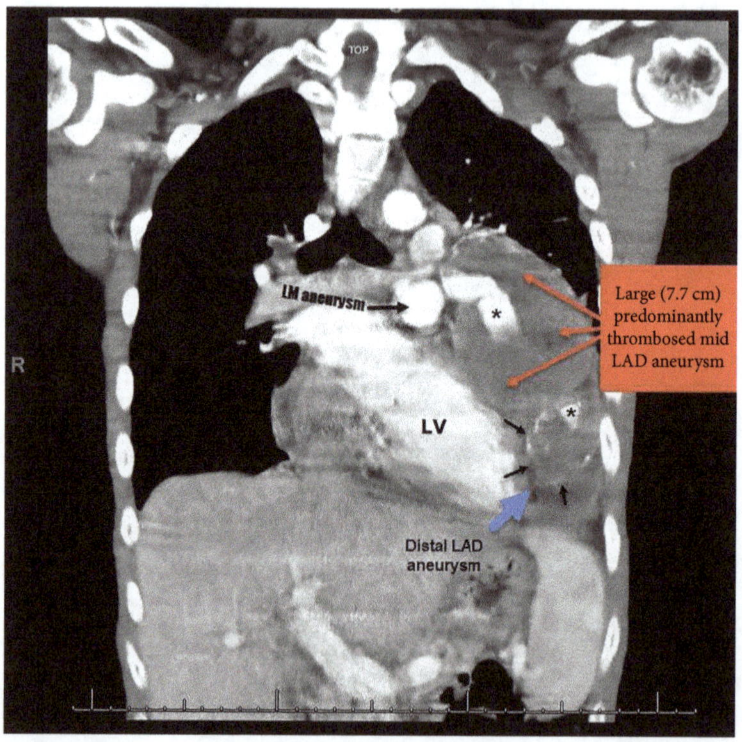

Figure 4: Computed tomographic scan shows a large mostly thrombosed proximal and mid left anterior descending artery (LAD) aneurysm (red arrows) measuring 7.7 cm in addition to a smaller calcified distal aneurysm (blue arrow). The opacified left main (LM) aneurysm is also seen.

with lesions of the internal carotid and renal arteries, has also been linked to CAA [4].

The two common classifications of CAAs are either saccular or fusiform. Saccular aneurysms are found to be more common in the left anterior descending artery than in other coronary arteries [5, 6]. The clinical presentation of CAAs can vary widely and mostly depends on the underlying etiology. The slow flow of blood on the irregular internal surface

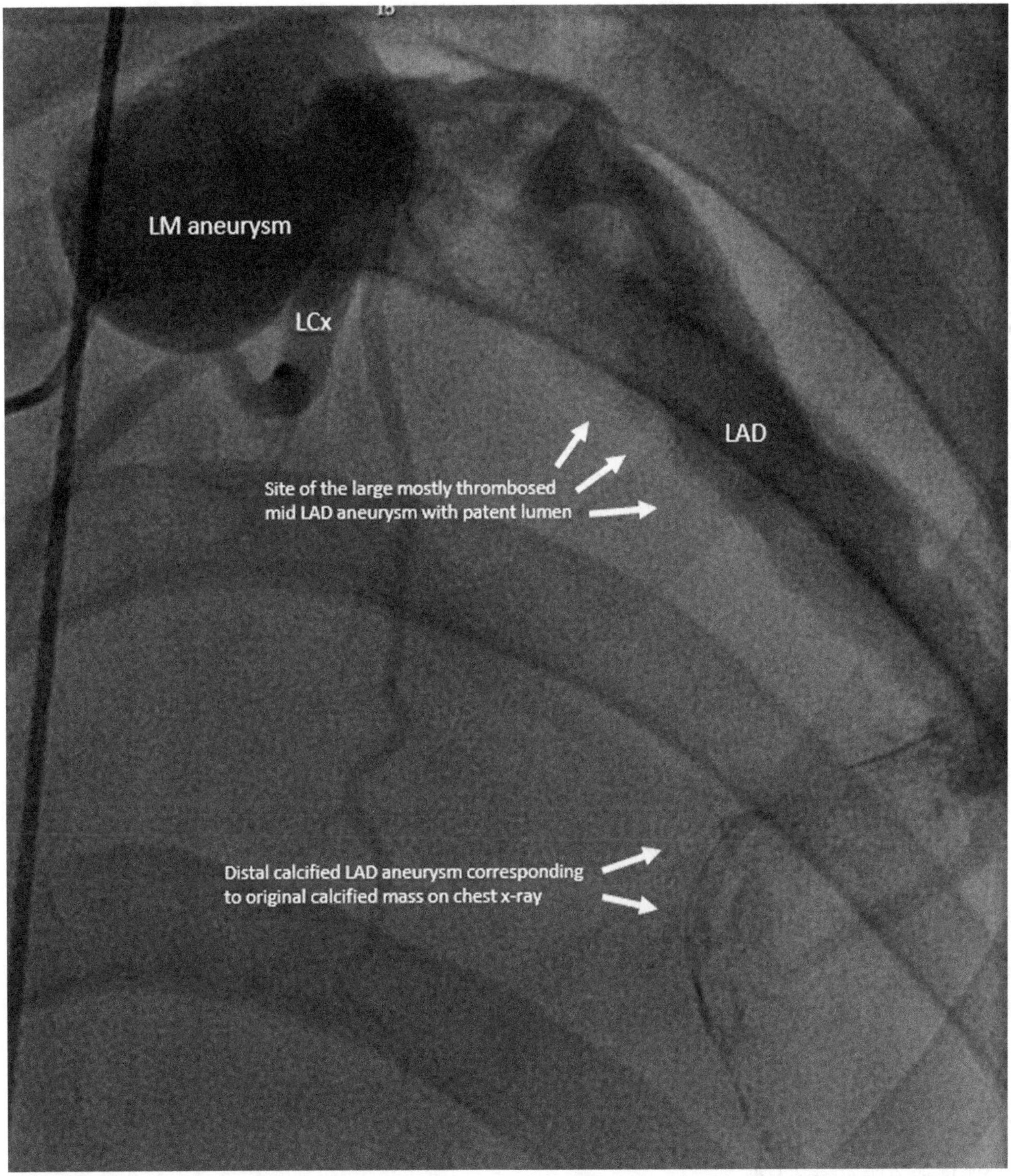

FIGURE 5: Coronary angiography showing multiple aneurysms within the left main (LM) coronary artery and left anterior descending artery (LAD) with slow flow. The top arrows point to the large mostly thrombosed aneurysm and the lower arrows show the location of the smaller calcified distal aneurysm.

of the aneurysm wall predisposes to the formation of thrombi with potential for subsequent embolization, resulting in ischemic symptoms [6–9].

Although CAAs are mostly detected incidentally during angiography, they are much less likely to show up on a chest radiograph or echocardiogram as in our case. Other useful modalities for diagnosis are computed tomography and cardiac magnetic resonance angiography. During angiography, delayed antegrade contrast filling, segmental back flow, and contrast stasis in the dilated coronary segment often hamper optimal imaging [10]. Intravascular ultrasound can be extremely helpful to supplement angiography and may be considered to help distinguish between true aneurysm, pseudoaneurysm, and segments with aneurysmal appearance which may be due to stenosis.

Since the natural history and prognosis are related to multiple factors, the decisions around treatment should be tailored to each patient and should consider many aspects such as the clinical presentation, etiology, aneurysm size, location, association with infections, and the presence and extent of any coexisting atherosclerosis [2, 11, 12]. In general, the smaller the size of the aneurysm and earlier the treatment is initiated, the lower the chance of major adverse cardiac outcomes [13–15]. Doi et al. suggested a possible advantage of anticoagulation in patients with CAA and acute coronary syndrome [16]. Percutaneous intervention may be performed in certain cases, using covered stents; however, substantial thrombus burden, sizing, and landing zone assessment may be problematic. Surgical options include resection of the aneurysm, proximal and/or distal ligation, and aneurysmal thrombectomy, with or without bypass grafting. The role of newer anticoagulants in the management of CAAs remains to be studied.

References

[1] Y. Luo, J. Tang, X. Liu et al., "Coronary artery aneurysm differs from coronary artery ectasia: angiographic characteristics and cardiovascular risk factor analysis in patients referred for coronary angiography," *Angiology*, vol. 68, no. 9, pp. 823–830, 2017.

[2] M. Syed and M. Lesch, "Coronary artery aneurysm: a review," *Progress in Cardiovascular Diseases*, vol. 40, no. 1, pp. 77–84, 1997.

[3] N. Lamblin, C. Bauters, X. Hermant, J. M. Lablanche, N. Helbecque, and P. Amouyel, "Polymorphisms in the promoter regions of MMP-2, MMP-3, MMP-9 and MMP-12 genes as determinants of aneurysmal coronary artery disease," *Journal of the American College of Cardiology*, vol. 40, no. 1, pp. 43–48, 2002.

[4] F. Zack, H. Terpe, U. Hammer, and R. Wegener, "Fibromuscular dysplasia of coronary arteries as a rare cause of death," *International Journal of Legal Medicine*, vol. 108, no. 4, pp. 215–218, 1996.

[5] S. Harikrishnan, K. R. Sunder, J. M. Tharakan et al., "Saccular coronary aneurysms: angiographic and clinical profile and follow-up of 22 cases," *Indian Heart Journal*, vol. 52, no. 2, pp. 178–182, 2000.

[6] P. A. Tunick, J. Slater, I. Kronzon, and E. Glassman, "Discrete atherosclerotic coronary artery aneurysms: a study of 20 patients," *Journal of the American College of Cardiology*, vol. 15, no. 2, pp. 279–282, 1990.

[7] W. C. Alford Jr., W. S. Stoney, G. R. Burrus, R. A. Frist, and C. S. Thomas Jr., "Recognition and operative management of patients with arteriosclerotic coronary artery aneurysms," *The Annals of Thoracic Surgery*, vol. 22, no. 4, pp. 317–321, 1976.

[8] R. Bhindi, L. Testa, O. J. Ormerod, and A. P. Banning, "Rapidly evolving giant coronary aneurysm," *Journal of the American College of Cardiology*, vol. 53, no. 4, p. 372, 2009.

[9] H. M. Y. Chia, K. H. Tan, and G. Jackson, "Non-atherosclerotic coronary artery aneurysms: two case reports," *Heart*, vol. 78, no. 6, pp. 613–616, 1997.

[10] A. Manginas and D. V. Cokkinos, "Coronary artery ectasias: imaging, functional assessment and clinical implications," *European Heart Journal*, vol. 27, no. 9, pp. 1026–1031, 2006.

[11] P. S. Swaye, L. D. Fisher, P. Litwin et al., "Aneurysmal coronary artery disease," *Circulation*, vol. 67, no. 1, pp. 134–138, 1983.

[12] P. S. Pahlavan and F. Niroomand, "Coronary artery aneurysm: a review," *Clinical Cardiology*, vol. 29, no. 10, pp. 439–443, 2006.

[13] K. G. Friedman, K. Gauvreau, A. Hamaoka-Okamoto et al., "Coronary artery aneurysms in Kawasaki disease: risk factors for progressive disease and adverse cardiac events in the US population," *Journal of the American Heart Association*, vol. 5, no. 9, 2016.

[14] E. Bonacina, A. Brucato, and M. Vertemati, "Kawasaki's disease: morphology of coronary artery aneurysms," *Pathology*, vol. 39, no. 1, pp. 187-188, 2007.

[15] Y. Sasaguri and H. Kato, "Regression of aneurysms in Kawasaki disease: a pathological study," *The Journal of Pediatrics*, vol. 100, no. 2, pp. 225–231, 1982.

[16] T. Doi, Y. Kataoka, T. Noguchi et al., "Coronary artery ectasia predicts future cardiac events in patients with acute myocardial infarctionhighlights," *Arteriosclerosis, Thrombosis, and Vascular Biology*, vol. 37, no. 12, pp. 2350–2355, 2017.

42

Torsades De Pointes Electrical Storm Induced by H1N1 in a Patient with KCNH2 Variant of Unknown Significance

Bashar Khiatah[1] **Jonathan Dukes,**[2] **Christina Desai**[3] **and Amanda Frugoli**[4]

[1]*Department of Internal Medicine, Community Memorial Hospital, 147 N Brent St, Ventura, CA 93003, USA*
[2]*Electrophysiology, Cardiology Associate Medical Group, USA*
[3]*Internal Medicine, Community Memorial Hospital, USA*
[4]*GME Department, Community Memorial Hospital, USA*

Correspondence should be addressed to Bashar Khiatah; bkhiatah@cmhshealth.org

Academic Editor: Ertugrul Ercan

This report describes a case of an electrical storm of Torsades De Pointes in a structurally normal heart, following an H1N1 infection in the presence of a genetic variant of unknown significance. The patient was successfully treated with isoproterenol. This case highlights the dilemma of evaluating novel genetic testing results in a clinical setting.

1. Clinical Case

A 60-year-old male with an implantable cardioverter-defibrillator (ICD) presented to the emergency room (ER) for being shocked multiple times. He was hemodynamically stable with a blood pressure of 115/72 and a heart rate of 93. He reported fever, muscle aches, runny nose, and a productive cough with white sputum for the last 2 days. The physical exam was unremarkable except for mild erythema in the oropharynx with no exudate.

His past medical history was significant for recurrent Torsades De Pointes (TdP) in association with aspiration pneumonia in 2014 status post-ICD placement; heart catheterization at that time showed completely normal coronary arteries. He denies any family history of cardiac disease in his parents or grandparents.

Differential diagnoses at this point included emergent interrogation of the ICD device which confirmed the diagnosis of TdP. Thus, the differential was for the eliciting factor which was broadly similar to the data found in Table 1.

Upon further investigations and after interrogating his pacemaker, eleven shocks for ventricular tachycardia (V-Tach) and TdP were confirmed. Electrocardiogram (ECG) showed sinus rhythm (Figure 1), first-degree AV block, left bundle branch block (LBBB) pattern, a wide QRS complex as a result of the left bundle branch block, and a delayed QRS transition zone; QTc interval was not prolonged according to when corrected to the LBBB. (LBBB;QTcH = $458 + 1.75 \times (100 - 60) = 528$ ms, final QTc = QTcH $- 120 \times 0.5 = 364$ ms, QTc = 468). Mildly elevated troponin is at 0.71 ng/mL with normal electrolyte, complete blood count (CBC), thyroid-stimulating hormone (TSH), arterial blood gas (ABG), and urine drug screen. Influenza screen positive for type A was confirmed later using polymerase chain reaction (PCR) H1N1. Transthoracic echo (TTE), chest X-ray, and myocardial perfusion scan were normal.

In ER, an amiodarone drip and a bolus were started by the ER physician. Oseltamivir was started, 2 grams of magnesium was given, and he was admitted to the intensive care unit. Overnight, the patient was shocked for multiple runs of TdP and V-Tach as shown in Figure 2(a). Isoproterenol drip was started and titrated to a heart rate of 100-110, which controlled his electrical storm. ICD was set at 100 beats per minute on DDD mode (Figure 2(b)). Over the next 24 hours, he did not have any episodes and was transitioned to quinidine 300 mg every 8 hours. His ICD was at the end of device life, and the patient was scheduled for device replacement. After his device was replaced, he experienced 3 runs of TdP which he was shocked for (Figure 2(c)). Thus, quinidine dose was increased to 648 every 12 hours.

Table 1: Causes of polymorphic ventricular arrhythmia [1].

Structural heart diseases	Structurally normal heart	
	Primary causes	Secondary causes
(i) Ischemic heart diseases (ii) Acute or recent myocardial infarction, prior myocardial infarction (iii) Nonischemic cardiomyopathy (iv) Dilated cardiomyopathy (v) Hypertrophic cardiomyopathy (vi) Arrhythmogenic right ventricular dysplasia/cardiomyopathy (vii) Valvular heart diseases (viii) Corrected congenital heart diseases (ix) Myocarditis (x) Cardiac sarcoidosis (xi) Chagas disease (xii) Metastatic cardiac tumor	(i) Idiopathic (ii) Brugada syndrome (iii) Early repolarization syndrome (iv) Long QT syndrome (v) Short QT syndrome (vi) Catecholaminergic polymorphic ventricular tachycardia	(i) Electrolyte abnormalities (ii) Toxic/drug-related (iii) Endocrinologic (iv) Perioperative (v) Iatrogenic (T-wave pacing)

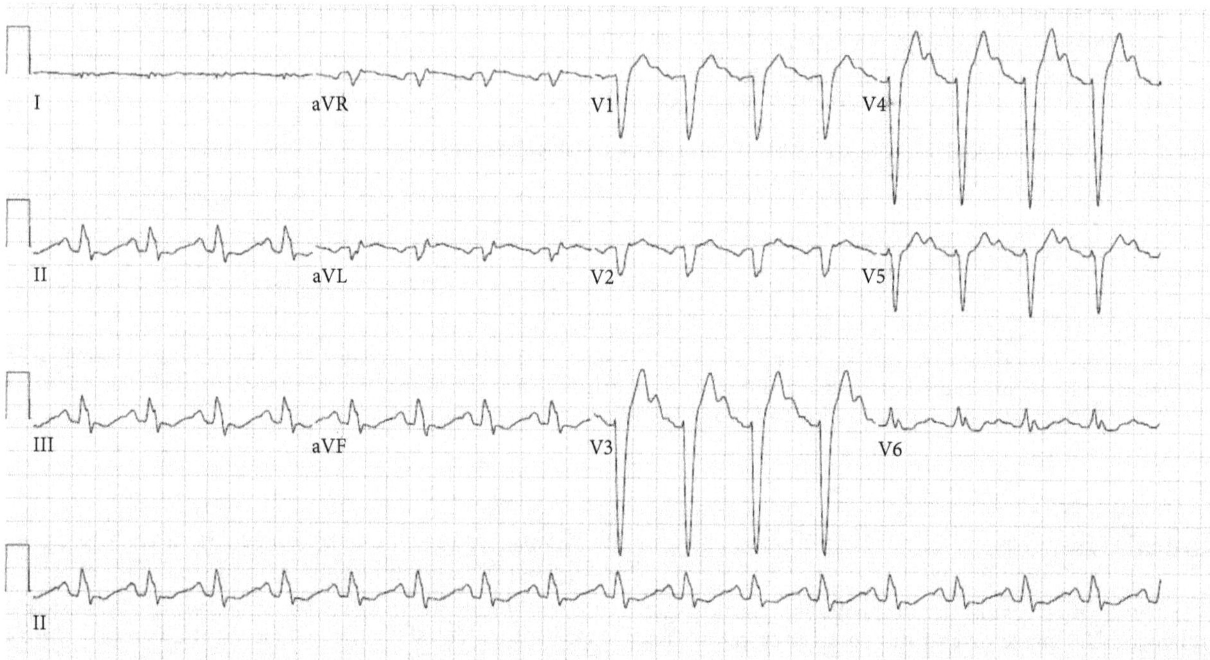

Figure 1: Sinus rhythm with first-degree AV block, left bundle branch block pattern, and delayed QRS transition zone. QTc interval was not prolonged when corrected to the left bundle branch block (LBBB).

After 7 days of initial presentation and 48 hours of episodes free, the patient was discharged home (Figure 2(d)) ($QTcH = 420 + 1.75(100 - 60) = 490$ ms, final $QTc = QTcH - 180 \times 0.5 = 400$ ms). An outpatient exercise treadmill stress test was scheduled to look for abnormal QT prolongation with exercise and was found negative. Later on (12 weeks after presentation), the genetic cardiac arrhythmia panel revealed; five variants of uncertain significance were detected, one variant of KCNH2 and LDB3 genes, and three of the TTN gene. The patient was called in for a follow-up and switched to nadolol 80 mg qday gradually, since LQTS was a concern despite negative ECG and stress test.

2. Discussion

The definition of cardiac electrical storm (ES) is electrical instability of the heart manifesting as recurrent ventricular arrhythmia in a short period of time (>3 in 24 hr). Despite the significant improvement of survival with ICD placement in these patients, ES remains to hold high mortality and morbidity and has a negative impact on long-term outcomes [1]. It is imperative to improve the treatment strategy for ES since the incidence rate of ES is not low (10–28% in patients with an ICD implanted for secondary prevention and 4% for primary prevention) [1]. Given the wide etiologies of Torsades De Pointes (Table 1), it is vital to identify the cause to guide the treatment [1]. Thus, the workup should include ECG, cardiac structural studies with a TTE, myocardial perfusion scan or heart cath, a cardiac enzyme with full electrolyte and basic metabolic panel, thyroid study, blood gas, CBC, blood cultures, chest X-ray, drug screen, home medication review, and finally a cardiac arrhythmia gene panel.

Recognizing the genetic substrate underlying the inherited arrhythmia syndromes has remarkably improved the

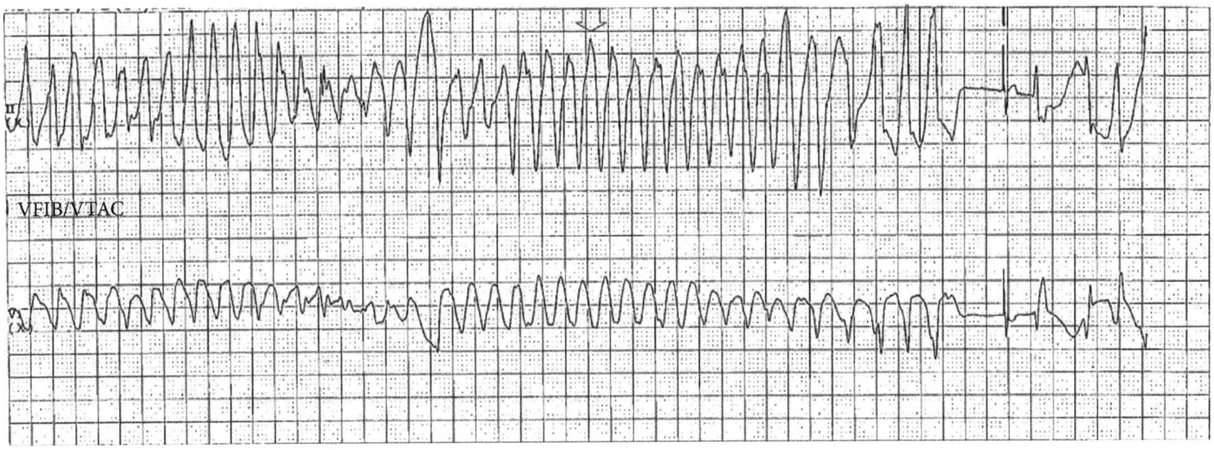

(a)

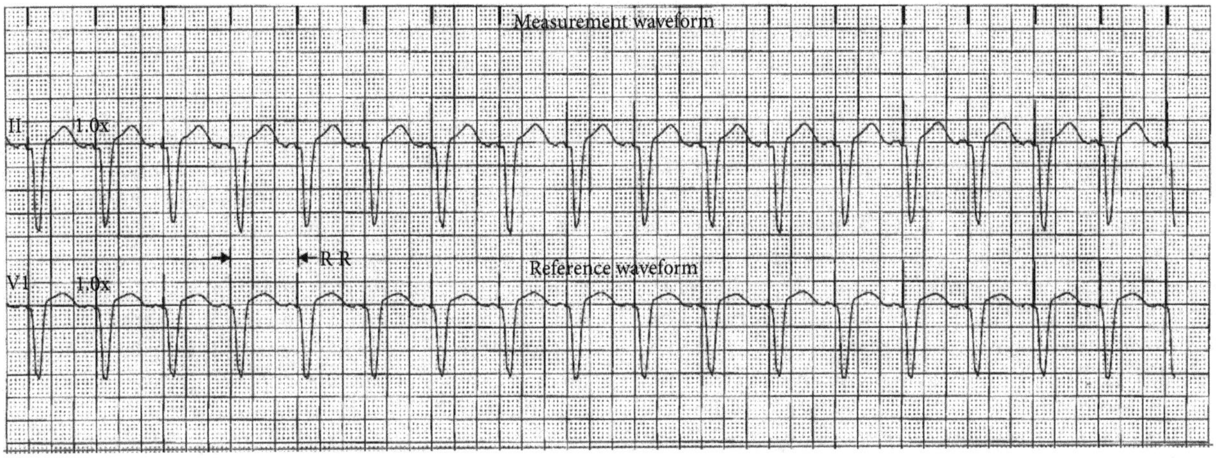

(b)

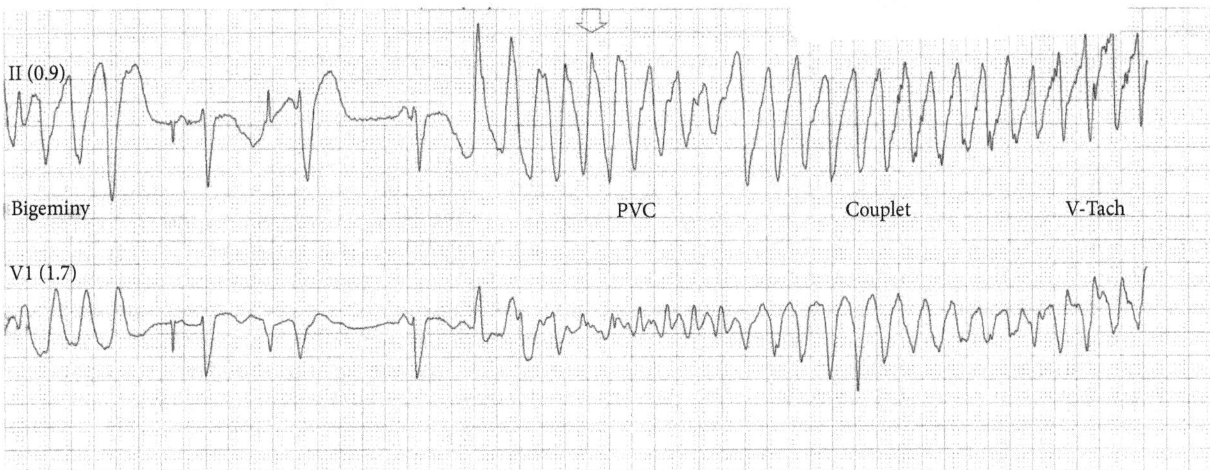

(c)

FIGURE 2: Continued.

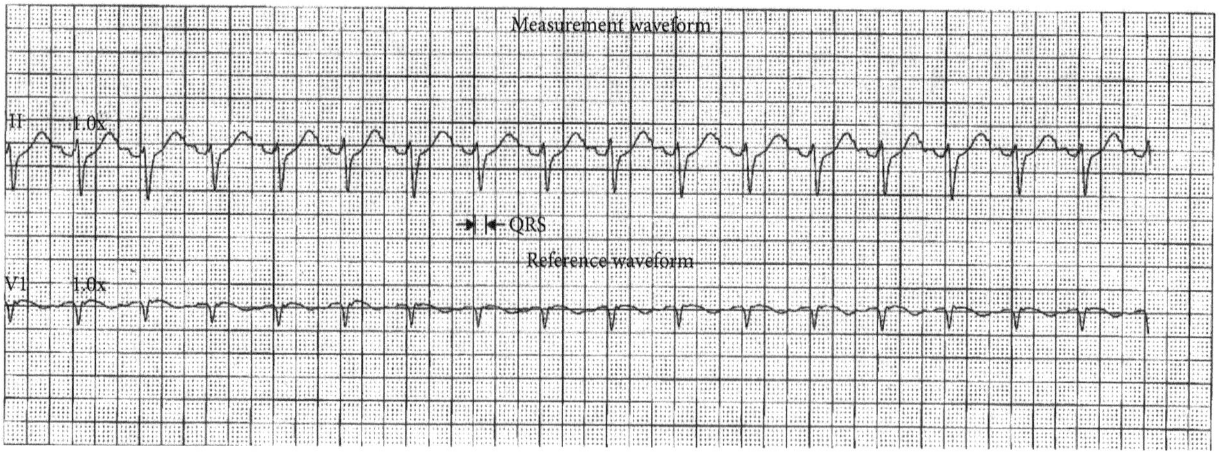

(d)

Figure 2: (a) Torsades De Pointes, first episode in the hospital. (b) Setting the ICD at 100 beats per minute. (c) Torsade De Pointes after the replacement of ICD. (d) Dual AV-paced normal ECG by discharge time.

field of the molecular basis of cardiac electrophysiology, including arrhythmia mechanism and the role of the different ion channels [2, 3]. Genotype-phenotype study relationships, performed mainly for the LQTS, have uncovered the importance of genetic aspects of disease and proved that the patient's management should consider the nature of the gene affected. Any abnormality in ion channel function can result in a disastrous complication that presents as an ECG abnormality and arrhythmias and is usually referred to as cardiac channelopathy. Gene testing for genes coding the cardiac ion channels demonstrated a specific type of inheritable arrhythmogenic disorders that occur in a structurally normal heart and also brought the genetic cardiac channelopathy into focus. These genetic disorders include the LQTS, SQTS, catecholaminergic polymorphic ventricular tachycardia, idiopathic atrial fibrillation, and Brugada syndrome. One of these channels is the potassium channels that are the primary contributors to the repolarization process, which appeared to underlie LQTS in case of dysfunction especially when mutations in genes encoding for pore-forming α-subunits (KCNQ1, KCNH2) of these channels are detected [2, 3]. KCNH2 (potassium voltage-gated channel subfamily H member 2), one of many genes, reported having a refractory fever-induced TdP and VF in two related LQT2 patients with the A558P mutation in KCNH2. ECG in these patients showed increased QTc with fever [4]. Currently, more than 1300 KCNH2 variants are recognized in the public genetic archive ClinVar, 5, with almost a third designated as variants of unknown significance [5]. Despite the numerous variants detected for KCNH2, the specific one found in our patient was never reported. Our patient's genetic report showed, a variant of uncertain significant of KCNH2 gene with heterozygous nucleic acid change C.1756 C<G and p.Leu586Val amino acid alteration that has an autosomal dominant inheretance pattern. This have raised many view points; firstly, although the variants in question have not been described previously, a more detailed analysis is warranted as they may be novel disease-causing mutations. Secondly, although the patient has a suspected hereditary LQTS and coding variants in KCNH2, the variants previously have not been described as mutations. Reliably determining whether the variants are causative is therefore not possible. Finally, the patient has a suspected hereditary LQTS consistent with KCNH2 variant, which result in changes to the protein in charge of potassium channel structure; therefore, the variants are likely causative.

Since the ES is an emergency, it is initially managed with the advanced cardiac life support (ACLS) protocol [6], regardless of the etiology of the electrical storm. In advanced settings, the treatment is more etiology specific with pharmacologic choices of amiodarone, quinidine, propranolol, metoprolol, and isoproterenol or interventional therapies with ICD or ablations [7–11]. Neumar et al. compared the combination of IV amiodarone and oral propranolol to the combination of IV amiodarone and oral metoprolol in the management of ES in ICD patients and found amiodarone and propranolol to be superior, safe, and effective in ES management [6]. Isoproterenol showed high efficacy in idiopathic ventricular fibrillation (IVF) patients due to its effectiveness in controlling ventricular fibrillation (VF) and attenuation of the J waves, which showed augmentation prior to the VF onset and was diminished to below the diagnostic level with isoproterenol treatment [9]. In patients with idiopathic VF and Brugada syndrome, the long-term reproducibility of the EP efficacy of quinidine is excellent [10]. In another specific patient population, radiofrequency catheter ablation (RFCA) of refractory V-Tach in patients with myocarditis and RFCA of drug-refractory V-Tach were found to be feasible, safe, and effective [12].

But what if the inducing factor is H1N1 infection without the genetic predisposition or myocarditis? Or the upper respiratory infection with H1N1 in the setting of KCNH2, p.Leu586Val variant is the combination inducing this TdP ES?

In our case, the patient had TdP in 2014 that was believed to be induced by his aspiration pneumonia, and since then, the patient was symptoms free until the recent H1N1 that caused his ES. Oseltamivir was given, which has a safety profile far outweighs the side effects that includes 5-10% nausea, vomiting, and no known arrhythmic side effects that might complicate the patient's situation [13]. While myocarditis has been reported in association with influenza pandemics and interpandemic periods [12], in this case, the lack of different degrees of heart failure (ranging from cardiogenic shock to subtly progressive chronic heart failure), chest pain, bradyarrhythmias, tachyarrhythmias (including sudden cardiac death), negative biochemical markers of myocardial necrosis, normal echocardiographic features, and responding to quinidine is arguing against myocarditis. On the other hand, prodromal symptoms were present and no biopsy was performed.

Also, it has been reported that H1N1 could induce ES in a patient with LQTS which was treated with perfusing magnesium sulfate, increasing the resting pacing rate from 40 to 85 bpm, and increasing propranolol dosage [14]. In contrast, in our patient case with confirmed H1N1 infection in the setting of a negative genetic panel, a successful treatment was achieved with isoproterenol drip and increase pacing rate to 100 bpm with subsequent transition to high dose quinidine. In a follow-up appointment, he was symptom-free for a month with no arrhythmic attacks or pacemaker malfunction. The exercise stress test did not show any abnormal QT prolongation while also acknowledging the sensitivity of this test in unmasking LQTS.

3. Conclusion

While more studies are required to understand the effect of H1N1 in patients with genetic variants of uncertain significance, it is worthwhile to consider the potential effect of H1N1 influenza infection in triggering an electrical storm in this population. This may have a great impact as ventricular arrhythmias are a cause of sudden death.

References

[1] M. Maruyama and T. Yamamoto, "Electrical storms: recent advances," in *Cardiac Arrhythmias: From Basic Mechanism to State-of-the-Art Management*, A. S. Kibos and B. P. Knight, Eds., pp. 285–292, Springer-Verlag, London, 2014.

[2] A. A. Wilde and C. R. Bezzina, "Genetics of cardiac arrhythmias," *Heart*, vol. 91, no. 10, pp. 1352–1358, 2005.

[3] R. De Zio, A. Gerbino, C. Forleo et al., "Functional study of a KCNH2 mutant: novel insights on the pathogenesis of the LQT2 syndrome," *Journal of Cellular and Molecular Medicine*, vol. 23, no. 9, pp. 6331–6342, 2019.

[4] A. S. Amin, L. J. Herfst, B. P. Delisle et al., "Fever-induced QTc prolongation and ventricular arrhythmias in individuals with type 2 congenital long QT syndrome," *The Journal of Clinical Investigation*, vol. 118, no. 7, pp. 2552–2561, 2008.

[5] C. G. Vanoye and A. L. George Jr., "Decoding KCNH2 variants of unknown significance," *Heart Rhythm*, vol. 17, no. 3, pp. 501-502, 2020.

[6] R. W. Neumar, C. W. Otto, M. S. Link et al., "Part 8: adult advanced cardiovascular life support: 2010 American Heart Association Guidelines for Cardiopulmonary Resuscitation and Emergency Cardiovascular Care," *Circulation*, vol. 122, 18_suppl_3, pp. S729–S767, 2010.

[7] S. Chatzidou, C. Kontogiannis, D. I. Tsilimigras et al., "Propranolol versus metoprolol for treatment of electrical storm in patients with implantable cardioverter-defibrillator," *Journal of the American College of Cardiology*, vol. 71, no. 17, pp. 1897–1906, 2018.

[8] European Heart Rhythm Association, Heart Rhythm Society, D. P. Zipes et al., "ACC/AHA/ESC 2006 guidelines for management of patients with ventricular arrhythmias and the prevention of sudden cardiac death: a report of the American College of Cardiology/American Heart Association Task Force and the European Society of Cardiology Committee for Practice Guidelines (writing committee to develop guidelines for management of patients with ventricular arrhythmias and the prevention of sudden cardiac death)," *Journal of the American College of Cardiology*, vol. 48, no. 5, pp. e247–e346, 2006.

[9] Y. Aizawa, M. Chinushi, K. Hasegawa et al., "Electrical storm in idiopathic ventricular fibrillation is associated with early repolarization," *Journal of the American College of Cardiology*, vol. 62, no. 11, pp. 1015–1019, 2013.

[10] B. Belhassen, A. Glick, and S. Viskin, "Excellent long-term reproducibility of the electrophysiologic efficacy of quinidine in patients with idiopathic ventricular fibrillation and Brugada syndrome," *Pacing and Clinical Electrophysiology*, vol. 32, no. 3, pp. 294–301, 2009.

[11] L. Di Biase, P. Santangeli, D. J. Burkhardt et al., "Endo-epicardial homogenization of the scar versus limited substrate ablation for the treatment of electrical storms in patients with ischemic cardiomyopathy," *Journal of the American College of Cardiology*, vol. 60, no. 2, pp. 132–141, 2012.

[12] A. Dello Russo, M. Casella, M. Pieroni et al., "Drug-refractory ventricular tachycardias after myocarditis," *Circulation. Arrhythmia and Electrophysiology*, vol. 5, no. 3, pp. 492–498, 2012.

[13] F. Y. Aoki, U. D. Allen, H. G. Stiver, and G. A. Evans, "The use of antiviral drugs for influenza: guidance for practitioners 2012/2013," *The Canadian Journal of Infectious Diseases & Medical Microbiology*, vol. 23, no. 4, pp. e79–e92, 2012.

[14] J. S. Marques, A. Veiga, J. Nóbrega, M. J. Correia, and J. de Sousa, "Electrical storm induced by H1N1 A influenza infection," *EP Europace*, vol. 12, no. 2, pp. 294-295, 2010.

43

Multiple Coronary Fistulas as a Rare Cause of Stable Angina Pectoris

Jasna Čerkez Habek,[1] Tea Friščić,[1] Jozica Šikić,[1] Marko Perčić,[1] Dean Strinić,[1] and Daria Ljubas Perčić[2]

[1]*Department of Cardiology, Clinic of Internal Medicine, "Sveti Duh" University Hospital, School of Medicine, University of Zagreb, Zagreb, Croatia*
[2]*Department of Neonatology, Clinic of Gynecology and Obstetrition, "Sveti Duh" University Hospital, School of Medicine, University of Zagreb, Zagreb, Croatia*

Correspondence should be addressed to Marko Perčić; markopercicmef@gmail.com

Academic Editor: Antonio de Padua Mansur

Congenital coronary artery-left ventricular multiple microfistulas (CA-LVMMFs) are rare anomalies in adults. They are more often found in female patients, and they usually originate from the distal segments of the coronary arteries, but they can originate from a proximal segments of a coronary arteries, and these patients are likely to be identified and treated in the pediatric age group. They are mostly asymptomatic. When symptoms and complications occur, they include angina, myocardial infarction, atrial heart failure, arrhythmias, and endocarditis. The management of CA-LVMMFs is controversial, but it is generally agreed that conservative medical management is the primary treatment of choice. Our case describes a rare form of CA-LVMMFs draining into the left ventricle in a female patient presenting with fatigue, atypical anginal symptoms, atrial fibrillation, and premature ventricular complexes, without concomitant obstructive coronary artery disease.

1. Introduction

Coronary artery fistulas (CAFs), congenital or acquired due to trauma and iatrogenic causes, are defined as a direct communication of a coronary artery with a cardiac chamber, great vessel, or other vascular structure, bypassing the myocardial capillary bed [1]. Incidence of CAFs is speculative since many are never detected or detected while imaging for another indication. Angiographic series have revealed that the frequency of CAFs in adults is approximately 0.1-0.8% [2, 3]. CAFs have two distinctive angiographic appearances, which could be solitary or multiple and drain into different vascular bed/cardiac chambers [4]. Most CAFs are small, and the patient is usually asymptomatic, but when symptoms and complications occur, they include angina, myocardial infarction, heart failure, arrhythmias, and endocarditis [5]. The management of CAFs is controversial, and recommendations are based on cases or small retrospective series [2]. We report a rare case of CA-LVMMF without concomitant coronary artery disease (CAD).

2. Case Presentation

A 70-year-old female patient with a medical history of chronic myeloid leukemia that was diagnosed five years ago, chronic obstructive pulmonary disease, peripheral artery disease (PAD) with a recently implanted stent in the left superficial femoral artery, permanent atrial fibrillation (AF), and ventricular extrasystole was admitted to the emergency department because of complaints of fatigue, dyspnea and constant, and retrosternal chest pain not related to exertion, described as heaviness which started a week ago. Her chronic therapy already included apixaban and clopidogrel because of PAD and AF. ECG showed AF with single premature ventricular contraction (PVC) and no significant changes in the ST segment. Physical examination was

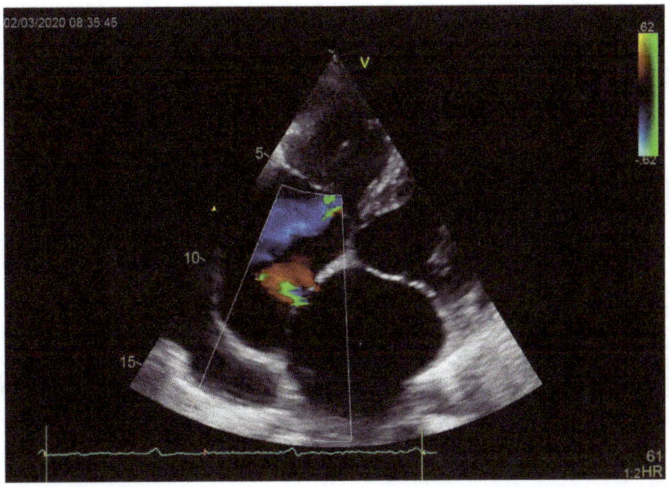

FIGURE 1: Atrial septal defect with left to right shunt. Both atria are enlarged. Tricuspid regurgitation jet is also visible.

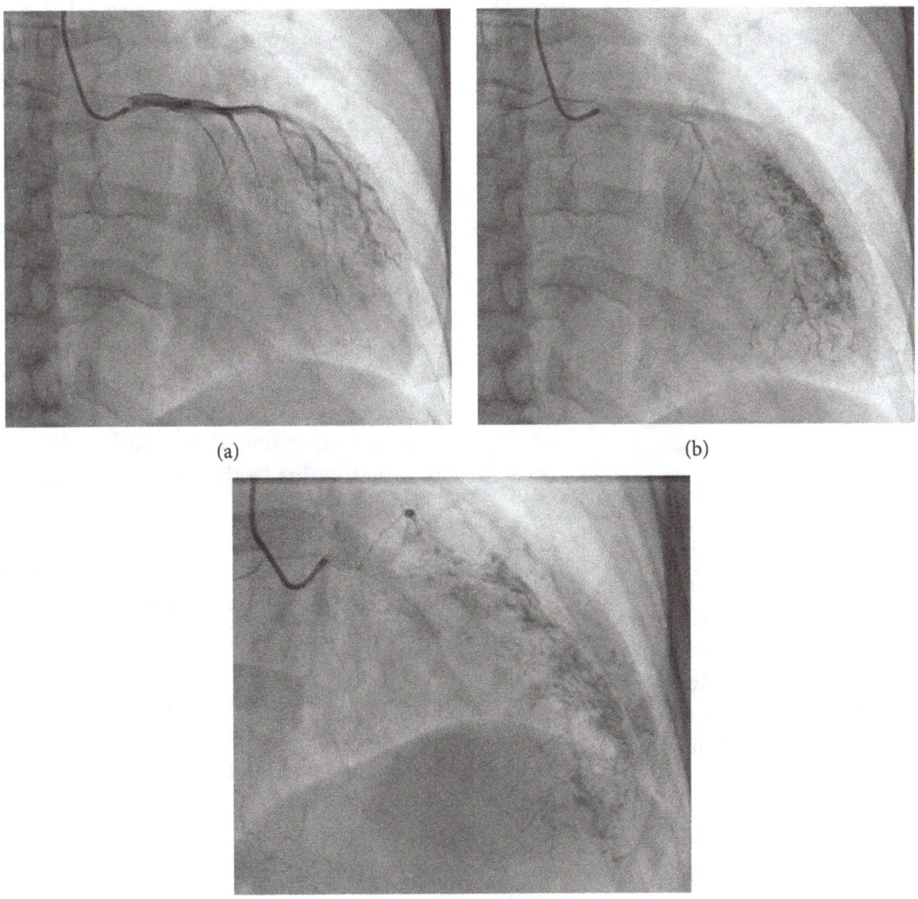

(a) (b)

(c)

FIGURE 2: (a) Left coronary artery. (b and c) Multiple microfistulas draining in the left ventricle.

normal. Her blood pressure was 150/100 mmHg, and her heart rate was 85/minute. The laboratory test results were with in normal range, including the troponin level. Coronary angiography has been indicated, and she was admitted to cardiology department. Echocardiography showed normal global and segmental systolic function of the left and right ventricle (Simpson method ejection fraction was 55% and TAPSE 22 mm), moderate diastolic dysfunction of the left ventricle, enlarged left and right atria (LAA 28 cm2 and RAA 30 cm2), mild dilatation of the right ventricle, moderate mitral regurgitation (RV 40 mL and ERO 0.3) due to degenerative alterations of posterior mitral leaflet, and moderate/severe tricuspid regurgitation with RVSP of 50 mmHg. In the area of fossa ovalis, an atrial septal defect (ASD) with

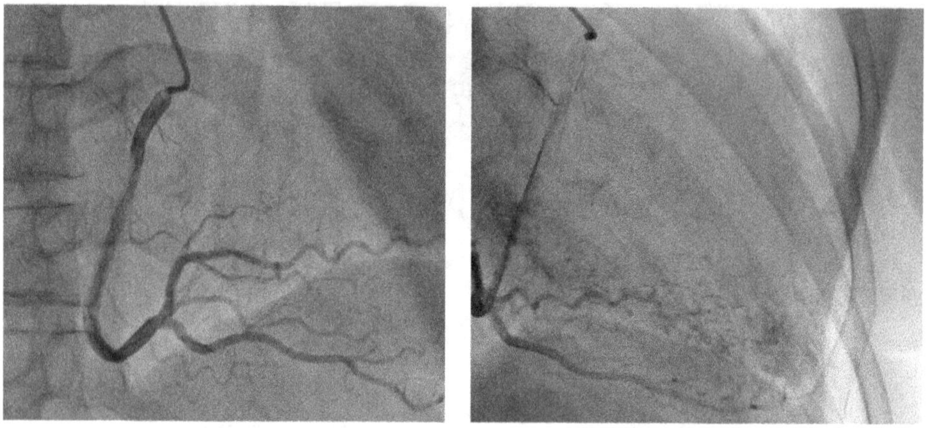

(a) (b)

FIGURE 3: (a) Right coronary artery. (b) Multiple microfistulas draining in the left ventricle.

left to right shunt was detected with a Qp : Qs 1.3 (Figure 1). Coronary angiography excluded significant obstructive CAD (Figures 2(a) and 3(a)) but showed left ventricle opacification through extensive multiple CA-LVMMF in the late phase of contrast injection to the left coronary arteries (Figures 2(b) and 2(c)) and the right coronary artery (Figure 3(b)). Patient had no chest pain during the hospitalization and was discharged with apixaban, clopidogrel, metoprolol, ramipril, and amlodipine. Two months after the discharge, she had an embolectomy of the right superficial femoral artery, despite apixaban and clopidogrel. On the follow-up in the cardiology clinic, she had no chest pain or palpitation, with occasional dyspnea and 736 PVC in Holter monitor; clopidogrel was excluded from the therapy.

3. Discussion

Congenital coronary artery-left ventricular multiple microfistulas (CA-LVMMFs) have infrequent anomalies in adults. CAFs develop early in the embryogenesis, between the sixth and eighth week of gestation, when enlargement of the capillary network from which coronary arteries develop occurs [6]. Approximately 10-30% of patients with CAF also have another congenital cardiovascular anomaly such as tetralogy of Fallot, patent ductus arteriosus, and atrial septal defect [7]. They are more often found in female patients originating from the distal segment of the coronary arteries, but they can originate from a proximal segment of a coronary artery, they are usually larger, and these patients are likely to be identified and treated in the pediatric age group [8]. CA-LVMMFs can lead to angina pectoris and coronary insufficiency even without CAD. Younger patients are generally asymptomatic, but CAF-related symptoms are secondary to fistula size and the volume shunted through, rather than age alone. Typical symptoms are dyspnea, fatigue, palpitation, and angina [9]. According to a Dutch survey of coronary artery fistulas in adult cardiology, the population main-presenting symptoms were angina pectoris and dyspnea in 70% of the patients, ECG showed pathologic changes in 75%, chest X-ray revealed cardiomegaly in 38% of the patients, and congestive heart failure was documented in 10% of the patients. The origin of the fistulas was the left coronary artery in 71% and the right coronary artery in 29% with majority (97%) originating from the mid or distal segments of the coronary vessels [8]. According to Levin et al. 3% of solitary CAFs terminate into the left ventricle [10]. Angina in the absence of CAD is thought to be a consequence of the "steal" phenomenon, which induces ischemia by diverting blood from the high-resistance myocardial capillary bed into the low-resistance fistula [10]. Patients with multiple fistulas in the left ventricle usually present with typical or atypical anginal symptoms [5]. The hemodynamic consequences of CAF vary depending on shunt size, shunt site, and other underlying cardiac diseases. A coronary fistula that drains to the left atrium results in no left to right shunt but causes a volume load similar to mitral regurgitation. Similarly, a coronary artery fistula that drains to the left ventricle produces hemodynamic changes similar to aortic insufficiency [3]. Heart failure is more likely to be seen in adults with concomitant CAD and AF [8]. Surgical strategy for CA-LVMMFs has sporadically been reported in the literature, but patients with multiple fistulae draining into LV without any significant volume overload are generally treated conservatively. Medical management is the primary treatment of choice [8].

4. Conclusion

Our case describes a rare form of CA-LVMMFs draining into the left ventricle and ASD in a female patient presenting with fatigue, atypical anginal symptoms, AF, and PVCs, without concomitant CAD or myocardial infarction who has been treated without any specific therapy.

Disclosure

This study was performed as part of the employment of the authors with the employer University Hospital Sveti Duh.

References

[1] M. Vavuranakis, C. A. Bush, and H. Boudoulas, "Coronary artery fistulas in adults: incidence, angiographic characteristics, natural history," *Catheterization and cardiovascular diagnosis*, vol. 35, no. 2, pp. 116–120, 1995.

[2] C. Tuncer, B. Eryonucu, T. Batyraliev et al., "Angiographic characteristics of coronary artery fistulas," *Turk Kardiyoloji Dernegi Arsivi*, vol. 42, no. 5, pp. 456–460, 2014.

[3] L. A. Latson, "Coronary artery fistulas: how to manage them," *Catheterization and Cardiovascular Interventions*, vol. 70, no. 1, pp. 111–118, 2007.

[4] S. A. Said, "Current characteristics of congenital coronary artery fistulas in adults: a decade of global experience," *World Journal of Cardiology*, vol. 3, no. 8, pp. 267–277, 2011.

[5] P. Iyer and R. Yelisetti, "Multiple left anterior descending coronary artery to left ventricular fistula - a case series and literature review," *Journal of Community Hospital Internal Medicine Perspectives*, vol. 7, no. 4, pp. 258–261, 2017.

[6] W. N. O'Connor, J. B. Cash, C. M. Cottrill, G. L. Johnson, and J. A. Noonan, "Ventriculocoronary connections in hypoplastic left hearts: an autopsy microscopic study," *Circulation*, vol. 66, no. 5, pp. 1078–1086, 1982.

[7] R. Holzer, R. Johnson, G. Ciotti, M. Pozzi, and D. Kitchiner, "Review of an institutional experience of coronary arterial fistulas in childhood set in context of review of the literature," *Cardiology in the Young*, vol. 14, no. 4, pp. 380–385, 2004.

[8] S. A. Said and T. van der Werf, "Dutch survey of congenital coronary artery fistulas in adults: coronary artery-left ventricular multiple micro-fistulas: multi-center observational survey in the Netherlands," *International Journal of Cardiology*, vol. 110, no. 1, pp. 33–39, 2006.

[9] T. Tirilomis, I. Aleksic, T. Busch, D. Zenker, W. Ruschewski, and H. Dalichau, "Congenital coronary artery fistulas in adults: surgical treatment and outcome," *International Journal of Cardiology*, vol. 98, no. 1, pp. 57–59, 2005.

[10] D. C. Levin, K. E. Fellows, and H. L. Abrams, "Hemodynamically significant primary anomalies of the coronary arteries. Angiographic aspects," *Circulation*, vol. 58, no. 1, pp. 25–34, 1978.

Cardiac Arrest and Successful Extracorporeal Cardiopulmonary Resuscitation as a Result of a Refeeding Syndrome in a Young Female with Anorexia Nervosa

Daniela Waddell,[1] Felix Meincke,[1] Samer Hakmi,[1] Hendrick van der Schalk,[1] Niklas Schenker,[1] Jonas Hahn,[1] Anna Moschner,[1] Mintje Bohné,[1] Da-Un Chung,[1] Stephan Willems,[1] Dietmar Kivelitz,[2] and Edda Bahlmann[1]

[1]*Department of Cardiology, Asklepios Clinic St. Georg, Hamburg, Germany*
[2]*Department of Radiology, Asklepios Clinic St. Georg, Hamburg, Germany*

Correspondence should be addressed to Daniela Waddell; d.waddell@asklepios.com

Academic Editor: Hajime Kataoka

Anorexia nervosa is a potentially life-threatening eating disorder, characterized by an abnormally low body weight. This case report illustrates a 22-year old female with cardiac arrest due to a refeeding syndrome in a patient with anorexia nervosa. It features the successful use of extracorporeal cardiopulmonary resuscitation in a case of severe left ventricular dysfunction resulting in a favorable outcome. *Conclusion.* We present the first case of a cardiac arrest due to a refeeding syndrome in anorexia nervosa featuring the successful use of an extracorporeal cardiopulmonary resuscitation approach as a bridge to full recovery.

1. Introduction

In female patients hospitalized due to eating disorders, nearly half of the patients were categorized as having AN [1]. AN is a psychiatric disease with a high mortality rate, 85% occurring in young women [2]. Reported mortality rates for AN range from 1.36% to 20% [3]. Death is commonly resulting from sudden cardiac death in one-third of all deaths associated with AN or suicide [4, 5]. However, sudden cardiac death in refeeding syndrome is not that frequent in AN [6–9]. In a case review, 3 of 48 adolescent females admitted with AN developed life-threatening complications associated with refeeding in AN [7]. Of these, one presented with a severe cardiac complication, an asystolic cardiac arrest [7]. Typically, but not in all cases of sudden death in AN with refeeding [9], these clinical findings are associated with hypophosphatemia [6]. This is the first report documenting cardiac arrest and successful extracorporeal cardiopulmonary resuscitation as a result of a refeeding syndrome in a young female with AN.

2. Case Presentation

A 22-year-old female (height 1.72 cm, weight 40 kg, and body mass index 13.5 kg/m^2) was admitted to our emergency room while receiving cardiopulmonary resuscitation for 45 minutes. Rhythm upon arrival was ventricular fibrillation. Since return of spontaneous circulation could not be achieved by all medical measures provided, the patient was immediately transferred to the catheter laboratory. Extracorporeal cardiopulmonary resuscitation via venoarterial extracorporeal membrane oxygenation (va-ECMO) was established. Due to severe left ventricular (LV) dysfunction, an Impella® pump was added to ensure sufficient LV output. Subsequently, percutaneous coronary angiogram was performed and showed no coronary disease (Figure 1(a)). The patient's history was noticeable for anorexia nervosa (AN) with several hospitalizations for renutrition, at the last several months prior to emergency admission. During the last few days prior to sudden cardiac death and after excessive caloric restriction, our patient began to increase her caloric intake to

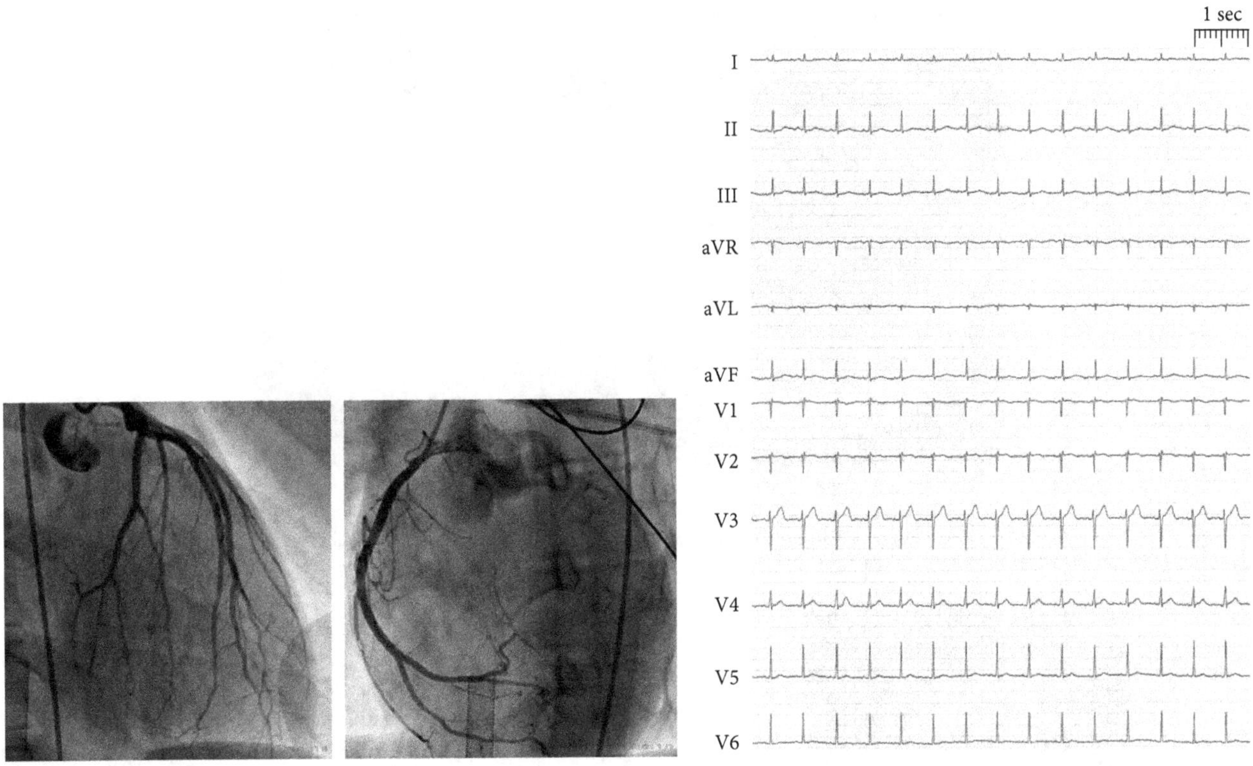

(a) (b)

Figure 1: 12-lead electrocardiogram shows sinus tachycardia (heart rate 98 beats/min), and prolongation of the corrected QT interval was detected (660 ms).

improve her nutritional state to avoid complications at an upcoming doctor's appointment. Prior to admission, our patient was an outpatient; did not receive medical refeeding or preventive treatment with supplementation of vitamins, phosphorus, or micronutrients; and did not had a history of binge episodes.

Initial blood analysis showed a severe electrolyte disorder with potassium depletion (1.38 mmol), hypocalcemia (ionized calcium 1.75 mmol/l), hyponatremia (117 mmol/l), hypochloremia (54 mmol/l), hypophosphatemia (0.28 mmol/l), and hypoproteinemia (total protein 30.2 g/l; albumin 28.9 g/l). In addition, laboratory data indicated a high level of lactate (18 mmol/l) combined with a normal pH of 7.38. Initial sugar levels were elevated (blood glucose 430 mmol/l). The first performed echocardiogram confirmed severe LV dysfunction. In the electrocardiogram, a sinus tachycardia and prolongation of the corrected QT interval were detected (660 ms) (Figure 1(b)). Electrolytes were substituted. Transient anisocoria and simultaneous severe coagulopathy under va-ECMO therapy led to a cranial computed tomography (CT), showing small bilateral subdural hematoma (Figure 2(a)). Most likely, the patient had aspirated during resuscitation; therefore, calculated antibiotic therapy with ampicillin/sulbactam was given. After initiating inodilatative support with levosimendan, cardiac output significantly improved within the next 24 hours. The Impella® pump and va-ECMO were subsequently removed on day 3. After the patient's respiratory situation had stabilized, extubation took place on day 5. Neurological assessment 10 days after admittance showed a mild difference in reflexes such as vertical saccade. Cranial magnetic resonance imaging (MRI), performed on day 16, revealed unchanged small bilateral subdural hematoma (Figure 2(b)). Subsequent cardiac MRI performed after 2 weeks showed a recovered LV ejection fraction and no signs of myocarditis (Figure 3). The patient was dismissed after 3 weeks of hospitalization without neurological deficit to a psychiatric care station for further treatment of AN.

3. Discussion

Silent LV dysfunction in patients with AN in the starvation phase is common [10], and its identification is of importance to prevent heart failure, a complication that often develops during clinical refeeding [6]. Causes of heart failure in AN patients with severe malnutrition often include deficiencies of magnesium, phosphorus, thiamine, and selenium [11–13]. It is suggested by de Simone et al. in 1994 that an abrupt increase in preload developing during refeeding might precipitate heart failure [10]. There were not enough elements for a chronic LV dysfunction preceding cardiac arrest in our patient. Rather, a massive LV dysfunction without an associated chronic LV dysfunction decompensated by a refeeding syndrome is likely. This hypothesis is supported by the imagery data and the rapid return "ad integrum" of the LV function after resuscitation. LV dysfunction together with the electrolyte abnormalities that can occur as a result of starvation and malnutrition caused by AN [14, 15] or during refeeding [6] (that is, hypomagnesaemia, hypokalemia,

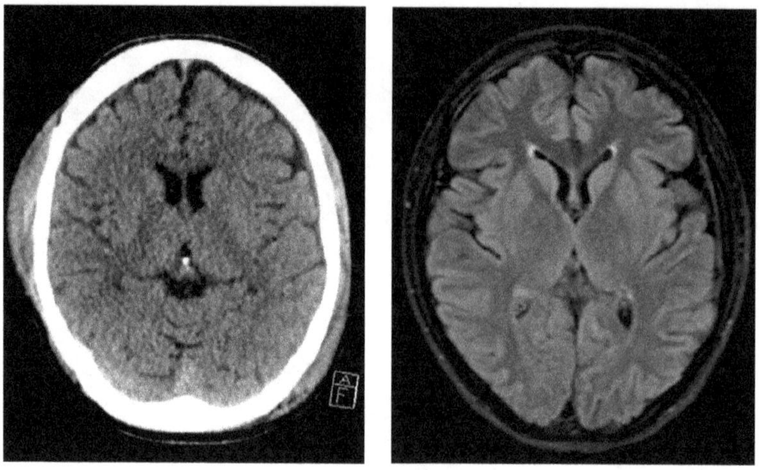

(a) (b)

FIGURE 2: Cranial CT scan (a) and cranial MRI scan (b) revealed evidence of a small right-sided subdural and intracerebral hematoma.

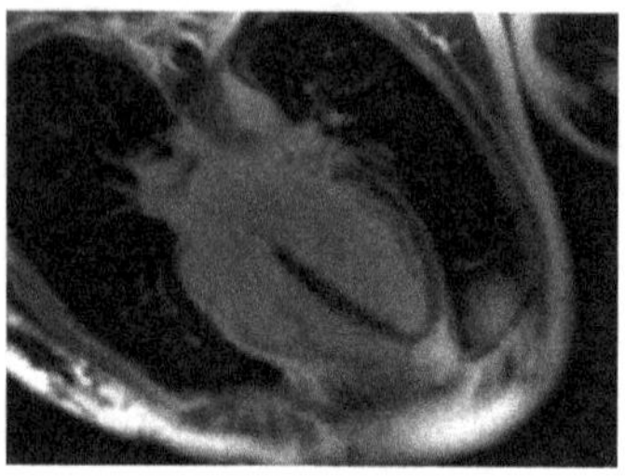

FIGURE 3: Cardiac MRI demonstrates a 4-chamber late enhancement view without pathological findings.

and hypophosphatemia, and hypocalcemia), severely present in our patient, can lead to sudden cardiac death in these patients [7, 10]. However, a more recent study with a more aggressive approach to nutritional rehabilitation to avoid ineffective refeeding in AN showed no evidence for developing moderate or severe hypophosphatemia [16]. Thus, a multivisceral failure associated with an increasing undernutrition, besides a refeeding syndrome hypothesis, might also be considered as a cause of cardiac failure in our patient.

Prolongation of the corrected QT interval due to the severe electrolyte disorder, present in our patient, is a known predictor of serious cardiac arrhythmias in AN [17]. Cardiotoxicity and arrhythmogenesis in these patients might also be related to elevated sympathetic activity [18]. Sudden cardiac death due to catecholamine cardiomyopathy is described in one case of a 22-year-old female [19]. Similar to the potentially lethal phenomenon of Takotsubo cardiomyopathy [20, 21], cardiac abnormalities in patients with AN are in fact reversible conditions after weight recovery [4, 22].

As usually described, refeeding syndrome in our patient also occurred within four days of starting to refeed [6–8]. Gradually increasing the caloric intake while carefully monitoring patients is therefore recommended for treating AN patients [23].

During fasting, the body switches its main fuel source from carbohydrates to fat tissue fatty acids and amino acids as the main energy sources. As result of a disturbed glucose metabolism and insulin secretion in refeeding, electrolyte disturbance typically takes the form of a hypokalemic, hypochloremic, and metabolic alkalosis [24]. The initial presentation with a pH-neutral severe lactatemia thereby likely is interpreted as a result of the prolonged hunger metabolism and also severe thiamin depletion. Dependent edema, often complicating refeeding and associated with lowered plasma proteins, could not be distinguished from treatment-dependent volume overload due to a severe cardiogenic shock in this case. Prolonged advanced life support including mechanical circulatory and temporary LV support devices in the setting of cardiac arrest unresponsive to resuscitation efforts and severely depressed LV function, as recommended in current guidelines [25], resulted in a favorable neurologic outcome in our patient.

In the presence of a reversible condition, an implantable cardioverter defibrillator therapy as secondary prevention of sudden cardiac death was not indicated in our patient [26]. However, the fact that only 51% had achieved a full recovery in a prospective long-term follow-up study including 84 AN patients [27] requires careful further surveillance of our patient.

Takeaway lessons of this case report:

(1) Severe electrolyte disturbance due to refeeding or as a result of severe starvation in patients with AN can result in sudden cardiac death even without a preceding cardiac dysfunction

(2) Careful monitoring in early phase of refeeding is of major importance

(3) Extracorporeal resuscitation is recommended as bridge to recovery treatment strategy in cardiac arrest and acute heart failure in AN

Authors' Contributions

The authors DW, FM, SH, HS, NS, JH, AM, MB, DC, SW, DK, and EB were all involved in the clinical management of the patient and conduction of the case report, FM in addition established the va-ECMO and performed the coronary angiogram, and DK was responsible for the interpretation of CT and MRI images.

References

[1] R. Patel, M. R. Sardar, A. Greway et al., "Cardiovascular impact of eating disorders in adults: a single center experience and literature review," *Heart Views*, vol. 16, no. 3, pp. 88–92, 2015.

[2] K.-. J. Neumärker, "Mortality and sudden death in anorexia nervosa," *The International Journal of Eating Disorders*, vol. 21, no. 3, pp. 205–212, 1997.

[3] J. Beatriz and I. Juregui, "Cardiovascular complications in eating disorders," *Relevant Topics in Eating Disorders. InTech;*-June 2012, http://www. http://intechopen.com/books/ relevant-topics-in-eating-disorders/ cardiovascular-complications-in-eating-disorders.

[4] L. Mont, J. Castro, B. Herreros et al., "Reversibility of cardiac abnormalities in adolescents with anorexia nervosa after weight recovery," *Journal of the American Academy of Child and Adolescent Psychiatry*, vol. 42, no. 7, pp. 808–813, 2003.

[5] E. Attia and B. T. Walsh, "Behavioral management for anorexia nervosa," *The New England Journal of Medicine*, vol. 360, no. 5, pp. 500–506, 2009.

[6] S. M. Solomon and D. F. Kirby, "The refeeding syndrome: a review," *Journal of Parenteral and Enteral Nutrition*, vol. 14, no. 1, pp. 90–97, 2016.

[7] M. R. Kohn, N. H. Golden, and I. R. Shenker, "Cardiac arrest and delirium: presentations of the refeeding syndrome in severely malnourished adolescents with anorexia nervosa," *Journal of Adolescent Health*, vol. 22, no. 3, pp. 239–243, 1998.

[8] G. J. Webb, K. Smith, F. Thursby-Pelham, T. Smith, M. A. Stroud, and A. N. Da Silva, "Complications of emergency refeeding in anorexia nervosa: case series and review," *Acute Medicine.*, vol. 10, no. 2, pp. 69–76, 2011.

[9] J. M. Isner, W. C. Roberts, S. B. Heymsfield, and J. Yager, "Anorexia nervosa and sudden death," *Annals of Internal Medicine*, vol. 102, no. 1, pp. 49–52, 1985.

[10] G. de Simone, L. Scalfi, M. Galderisi et al., "Cardiac abnormalities in young women with anorexia nervosa," *British Heart Journal*, vol. 71, no. 3, pp. 287–292, 1994.

[11] C. L. Birmingham and S. Gritzner, "Heart failure in anorexia nervosa: case report and review of the literature," *Eating and Weight Disorders - Studies on Anorexia, Bulimia and Obesity*, vol. 12, no. 1, pp. e7–e10, 2007.

[12] A. Davidson, P. C. Anisman, and E. Eshaghpour, "Heart failure secondary to hypomagnesemia in anorexia nervosa," *Pediatric Cardiology*, vol. 13, no. 4, pp. 241-242, 1992.

[13] A. P. Winston, C. P. Jamieson, W. Madira, N. M. Gatward, and R. L. Palmer, "Prevalence of thiamin deficiency in anorexia nervosa," *The International Journal of Eating Disorders*, vol. 28, no. 4, pp. 451–454, 2000.

[14] V. Fonseca and C. W. Havard, "Electrolyte disturbances and cardiac failure with hypomagnesaemia in anorexia nervosa," *BMJ*, vol. 291, no. 6510, pp. 1680–1682, 1985.

[15] J. Piza, R. Cespedes, L. Troper, J. H. Miller, and G. S. Berenson, "Myocardial lesions and heart failure in infantile malnutrition," *The American Journal of Tropical Medicine and Hygiene*, vol. 20, no. 2, pp. 343–355, 1971.

[16] M. Whitelaw, H. Gilbertson, P. Y. Lam, and S. M. Sawyer, "Does aggressive refeeding in hospitalized adolescents with anorexia nervosa result in increased hypophosphatemia?," *The Journal of Adolescent Health*, vol. 46, no. 6, pp. 577–582, 2010.

[17] G. J. Padfield, C. A. Escudero, A. M. De Souza et al., "Characterization of myocardial repolarization reserve in adolescent females with anorexia nervosa," *Circulation*, vol. 133, no. 6, pp. 557–565, 2016.

[18] J. Nedvidkova, I. Dostalova, V. Bartak, H. Papezov, and K. Pacak, "Increased subcutaneous abdominal tissue norepinephrine levels in patients with anorexia nervosa: an in vivo microdialysis study," *Physiological Research*, vol. 53, no. 4, pp. 409–413, 2004.

[19] H. Bonnemeier, G. Mall, and U. K. H. Wiegand, "Sudden cardiac death due to catecholamine cardiomyopathy in anorexia nervosa," *Resuscitation*, vol. 68, no. 1, pp. 9-10, 2006.

[20] C. Templin, J. R. Ghadri, J. Diekmann et al., "Clinical features and outcomes of Takotsubo (stress) cardiomyopathy," *New England Journal of Medicine*, vol. 373, no. 10, pp. 929–938, 2015.

[21] F. Santoro, I. J. Núñez Gil, T. Stiermaier et al., "Assessment of the German and Italian Stress Cardiomyopathy score for risk stratification for in-hospital complications in patients with Takotsubo syndrome," *JAMA Cardiology*, vol. 4, no. 9, pp. 892–899, 2019.

[22] T. Ono, S. Kasaoka, M. Fujita et al., "Complete recovery from severe myocardial dysfunction in a patient with anorexia nervosa," *Journal of Cardiology*, vol. 54, no. 3, pp. 480–484, 2009.

[23] N. H. Golden, D. K. Katzman, S. M. Sawyer et al., "Position paper of the Society for Adolescent Health and Medicine: medical management of restrictive eating disorders in adolescents and young adults," *The Journal of Adolescent Health*, vol. 56, no. 1, pp. 121–125, 2015.

[24] H. M. Mehanna, J. Moledina, and J. Travis, "Refeeding syndrome: what it is, and how to prevent and treat it," *BMJ*, vol. 336, no. 7659, pp. 1495–1498, 2008.

[25] J. Soar, J. P. Nolan, B. W. Böttiger et al., "European Resuscitation Council Guidelines for resuscitation 2015: section 3. Adult advanced life support," *Resuscitation*, vol. 95, pp. 100–147, 2015.

[26] S. G. Priori, C. Blomström-Lundqvist, A. Mazzanti et al., "2015 ESC guidelines for the management of patients with ventricular arrhythmias and the prevention of sudden cardiac death: the Task Force for the Management of Patients with Ventricular Arrhythmias and the Prevention of Sudden Cardiac Death of the European Society of Cardiology (ESC). Endorsed by: Association for European Paediatric and Congenital Cardiology (AEPC)," *European Heart Journal*, vol. 36, pp. 2793–2867, 2015.

[27] S. Zipfel, B. Lowe, D. L. Reas, H. C. Deter, and W. Herzog, "Long-term prognosis in anorexia nervosa: lessons from a 21-year follow-up study," *The Lancet*, vol. 355, no. 9205, pp. 721-722, 2000.

Noninvasive Recanalization of a Coronary Chronic Total Occlusion

Nikola Kos, Vjekoslav Radeljić, Nikola Pavlović, Krešimir Kordić, Kristijan Đula, Nikola Bulj, Tomislav Krčmar, Diana Delić Brkljačić, Ivan Zeljković, and Šime Manola

Department of Cardiovascular Diseases, University Hospital Centre Sestre Milosrdnice, Zagreb, Croatia

Correspondence should be addressed to Nikola Kos; nikolakos89@gmail.com

Academic Editor: Filippo M. Sarullo

Background. Spontaneous recanalization of a chronically occluded artery is rare and reported anecdotally. *Case Summary.* We report a case of a patient with a chronically occluded right coronary artery, found on a coronary angiography performed due to acute ST elevation myocardial infarction with an occluded circumflex artery as a culprit lesion. Three months later, a follow-up angiography was performed and a recanalization of the occluded right coronary artery was detected. *Discussion.* There is a possibility that intrinsic fibrinolytic mechanisms with the additional effect of standard antithrombotic drugs administrated after the acute coronary event led to the recanalization.

1. Introduction

Chronic total occlusion (CTO) of a coronary artery is defined as an occlusion > 6 weeks with well-developed collaterals which may provide flow equivalent to a flow obtained in an artery with 90-95% stenosis, preventing myocardial ischemia [1–4]. Although a spontaneous recanalization can occur in the acute myocardial infarction caused by a thrombotic event, it is a rare event in CTOs, especially in native coronary arteries occluded by a solid fibrocalcific plaque. We report a case of a female patient with a spontaneously recanalized CTO of the right coronary artery (RCA).

2. Case Report

A 67-year-old woman with a history of asthma presented to the Emergency Department (ED) with chest pain lasting 3 hours before admission. The 12-lead ECG revealed myocardial infarction with ST segment elevation (STEMI) (elevation present in the inferior and V5/V6 leads) (Figures 1(a)–1(c)). The patient was hemodynamically stable with normal blood pressure and Killip status I. After applying a bolus dose of acetylsalicylic acid (300 mg) and ticagrelor (180 mg) orally, an urgent coronary angiography was performed which showed a middle segment left circumflex artery (LCx) occlusion and a collateralized total occlusion of the proximal segment of RCA. Three drug-eluting stents (DES) were implanted in the LCx, and due to unsatisfactory postprocedural TIMI flow (TIMI I), GP IIb/IIIa inhibitor eptifibatide was applied after the procedure (180 mcg/kg as a IV bolus—15,3 mg, followed by a continuous infusion of 2 mcg/kg/min up to 75 mg of eptifibatide in total) (Figures 2–4). Postprocedural ECG revealed satisfactory ST segment resolution, and the patient had no chest pain. Laboratory tests revealed elevation of cardioselective markers (admission values: hsTI 51 ng/L and creatine kinase 106 U/L; peak values during hospitalization, 18 hours after the intervention: hsTI 24100 ng/L and creatine kinase 1348 U/L). Echocardiography during the first day after procedure showed a preserved left ventricular ejection fraction (50%) with a inferoposterior wall hypokinesis, with no other significant pathology. The patient was treated with beta blocker, ACE inhibitor, and statin permanently as well as with a 100 IU/kg dose of low-molecule heparin (enoxaparin) twice a day during the first 4 days. On the 5th day of the hospitalization, the patient reported nonspecific chest discomfort,

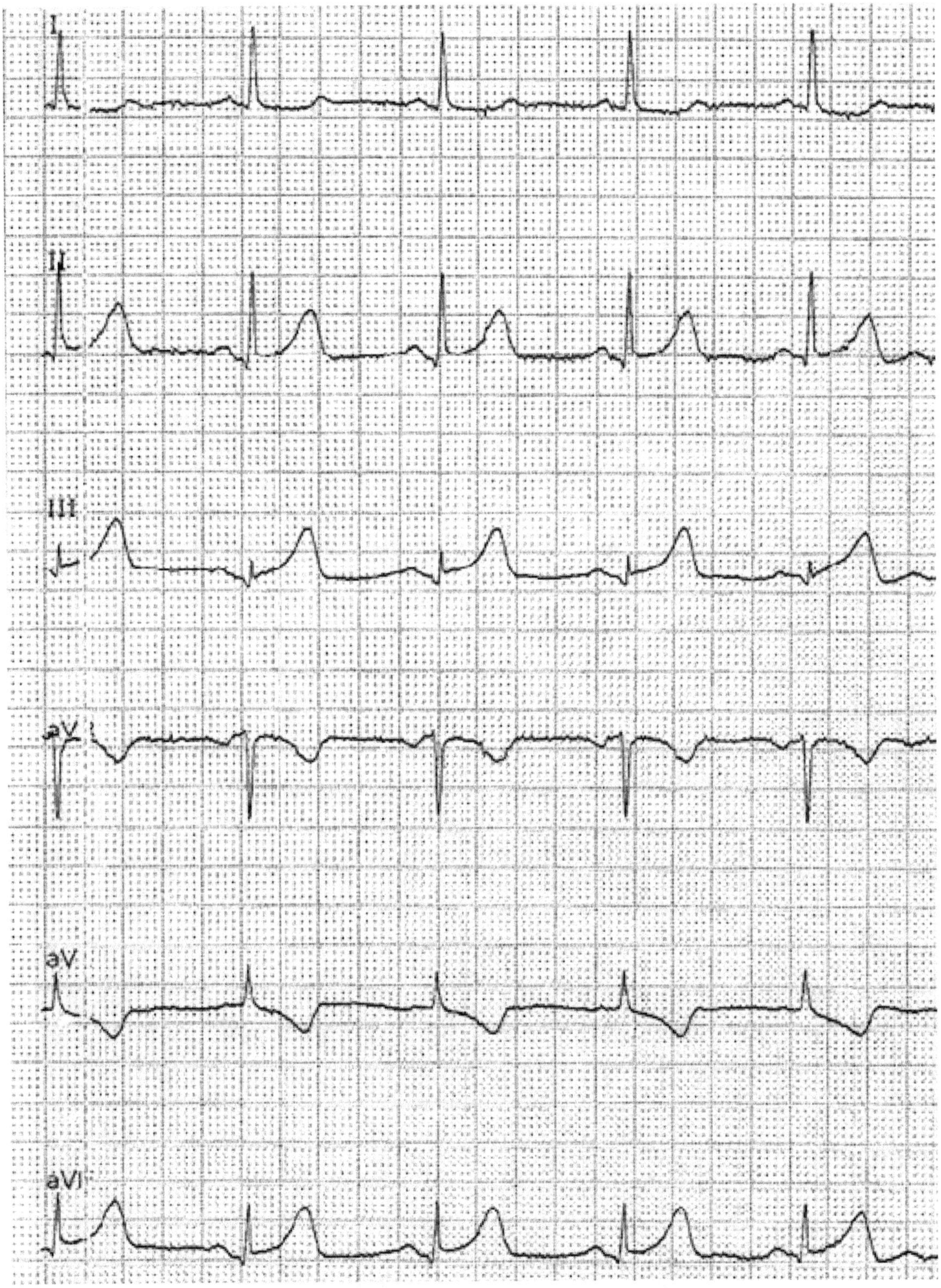

(a)

FIGURE 1: Continued.

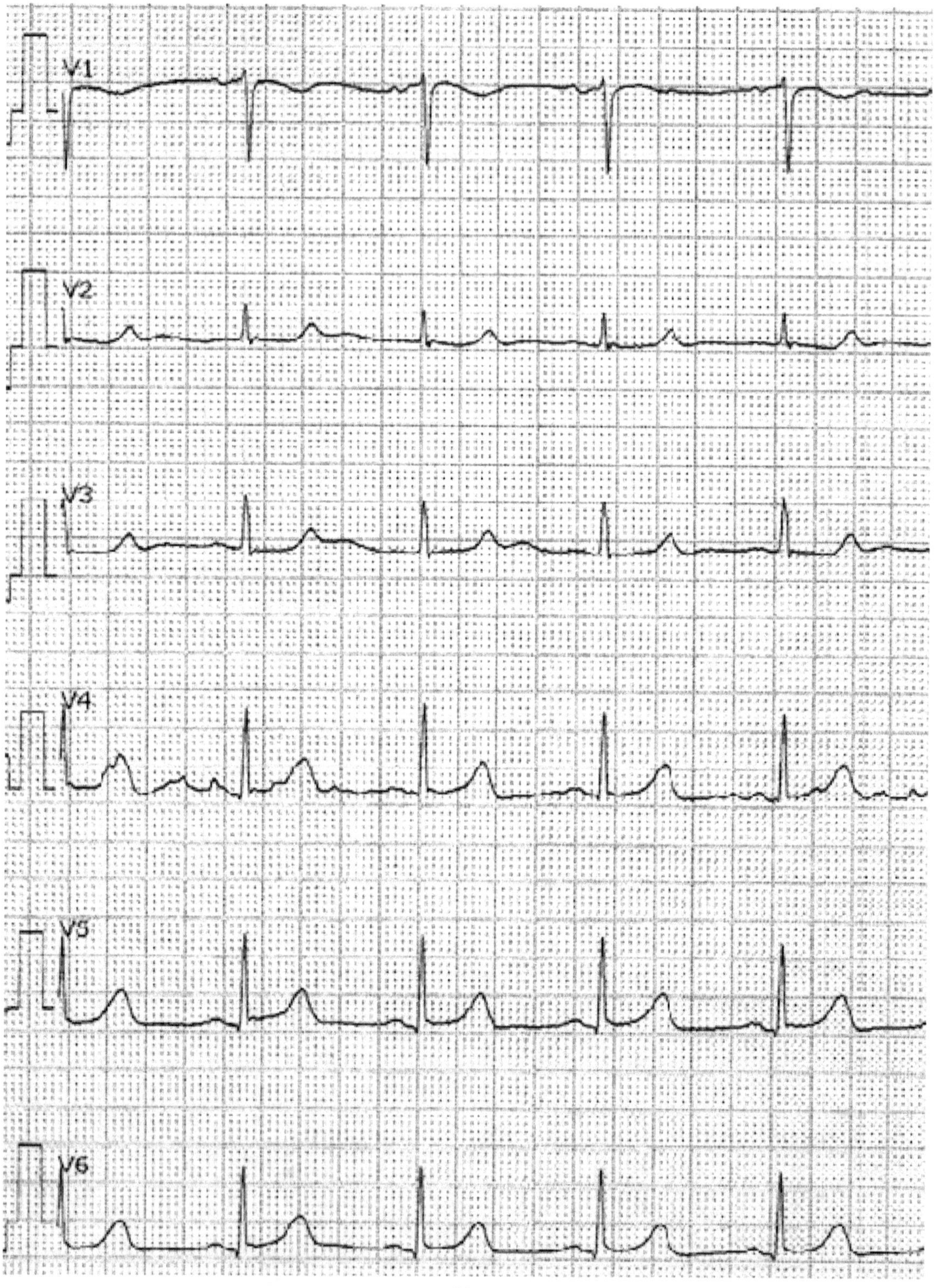

(b)

FIGURE 1: Continued.

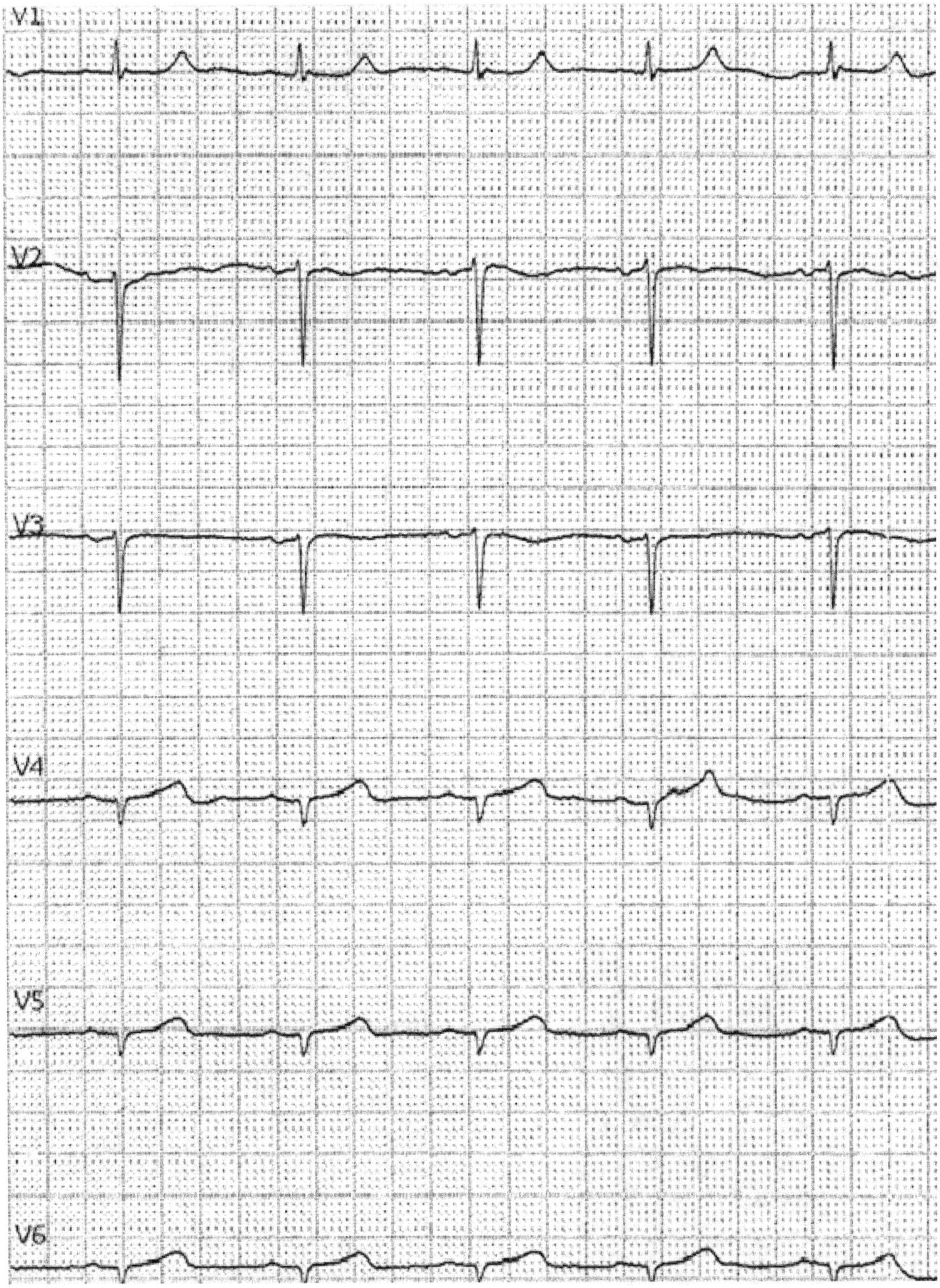

(c)

FIGURE 1: (a) ECG at admission (I, II, III, aVF, aVL, and aVF). (b) ECG at admission (V1-V6). (c) ECG at admission (right leads).

without cardioselective enzyme reelevation, but due to nonspecific changes in the inferior leads of the ECG, the new onset of the ischemia could not be excluded, so the coronary angiography was repeated. The second coronary angiography revealed CTO of the RCA and an in-stent thrombosis with occlusion of stents in LCx (Figure 5). Due to unsuccessful recanalization of the LCx using the guidewire and the TIMI I flow at the end of the first procedure, optimal anti-ischemic therapy was proposed including isosorbide-mononitrate, trimetazidine, ranolazine, in addition to ticagrelor,

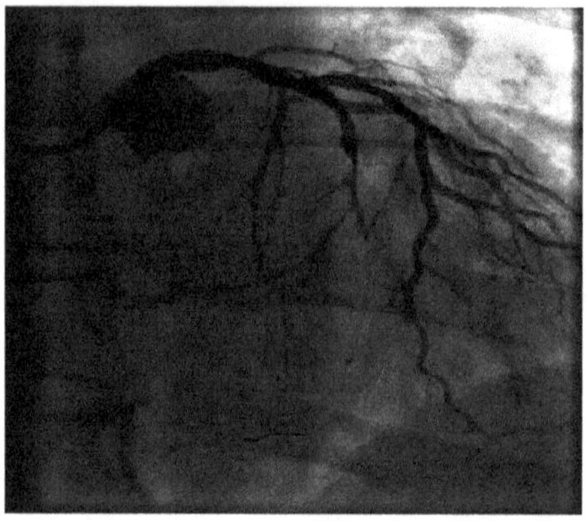

FIGURE 2: Occlusion of the middle segment of the left circumflex artery (LCx) (image after a partial recanalization with a guidewire).

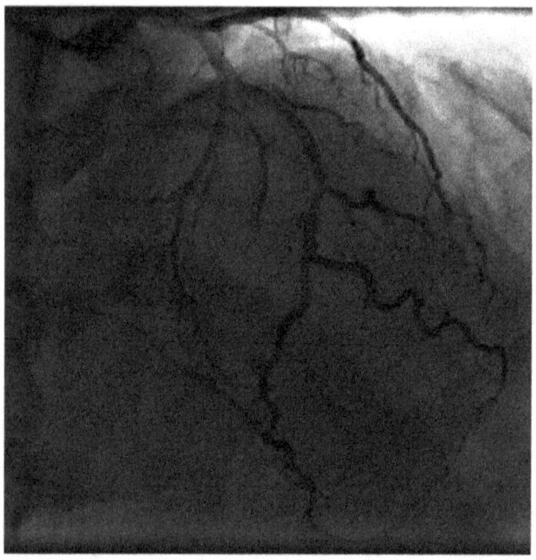

FIGURE 3: Left anterior descending artery (LAD) with collaterals to the right coronary artery (RCA).

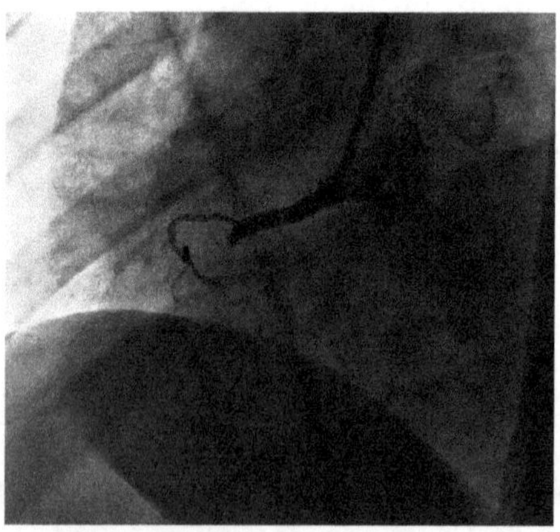

FIGURE 4: Chronic total occlusion (CTO) of the proximal right coronary artery (RCA) segment.

acetylsalicylic acid (ASA), nebivolol, ramipril, and atorvastatin. After the following four days of uneventful hospitalization, the patient was discharged with chronic therapy which included all the abovementioned medications. Three

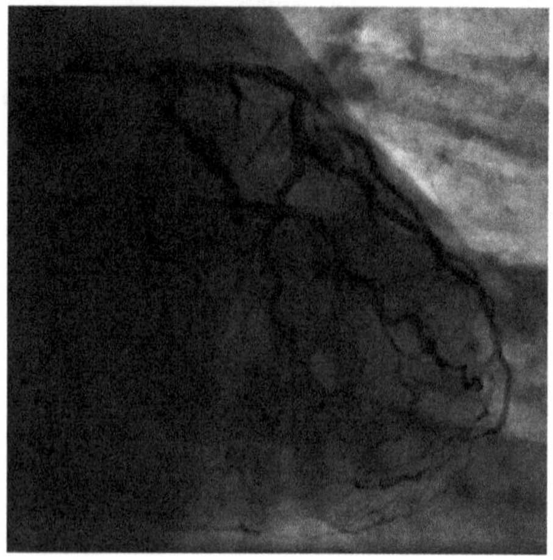

FIGURE 5: In-stent thrombosis of the left circumflex artery (LCx).

months later, at the planned outpatient follow-up visit, the patient presented with stable angina pectoris symptoms during moderate physical activity and a new coronary angiography was scheduled. After admission, coronary angiography was performed showing a spontaneous recanalization of the RCA, with a nonsignificant stenosis of the proximal-to-middle RCA segment, a 50% stenosis of the posterior descending artery, and no collaterals from left anterior descending artery (LAD) as well as persistent in-stent occlusion in the LCx with new collaterals from the first marginal artery (Figure 6). Dobutamine stress echocardiography was performed the day after the coronary angiography, showing no ischemia progression during testing in the RCA- and LCx-supplied myocardium. Due to stress echocardiography finding, no coronary intervention was indicated. Medical therapy was continued after dose optimization (80 mg of isosorbide-mononitrate daily instead of 40 mg and 1000 mg of ranolazine daily instead of 750 mg). Before discharge, an optimal ECG stress test was performed and no pain or ECG signs of ischemia were reported.

3. Discussion

We report a noninvasive CTO recanalization of the RCA. According to available data, a spontaneous recanalization of chronically occluded coronary arteries has been described anecdotally [5, 6]. All the cases (including ours) described CTO recanalization of the right coronary artery in the 60-year-old women. The majority of cases described CTO recanalization of carotid and peripheral arteries followed by discussion about the underlying mechanism [7–9]. In comparison to the reported cases with spontaneous CTO coronary artery recanalization, there are several specificities of our case. Firstly, no significant residual stenosis at the site of the previous CTO was noted, except a nonsignificant proximal-to-middle segment stenosis of the RCA [5, 6]. Secondly, the stimulation of the intrinsic fibrinolytic pathway by the anoxic tissue has been proposed as an underling mechanism of the discussed phenomenon [9]. In the reported case, acute therapy with low-molecule heparin and the GP IIb/IIIa inhibitor eptifibatide did not affect the

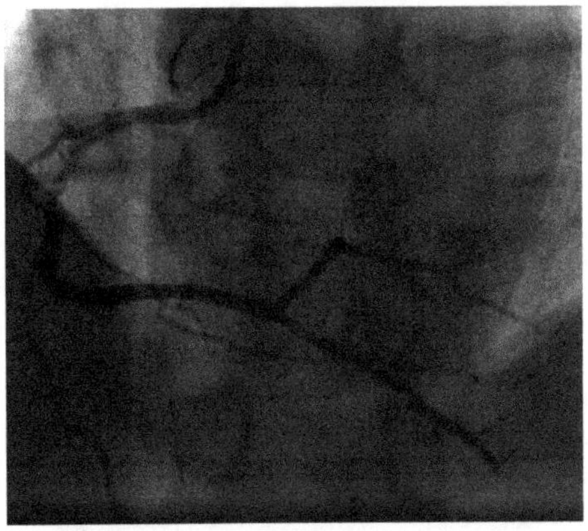

Figure 6: Recanalized right coronary artery (RCA) occlusion.

chronic occlusion which was confirmed by a control angiography performed 5 days after the acute infarction. However, the addition of dual antiplatelet therapy in a chronic setting may be added a synergistic effect to intrinsic mechanisms and led to the recanalization in less than three months. It raises the question why the CTO was recanalized and the stents remained occluded. The fact that stents are "foreign" objects in the coronary arteries with a chance of acute and chronic thrombosis supports the hypothesis that thrombosis activated intrinsic fibrinolytic pathways, but stents in the LCx encouraged the thrombosis or made it difficult to intrinsic fibrinolysis to make the artery patent again. Thirdly, there is a suspicion that the RCA was a culprit lesion of the acute infarction. However, there are few arguments against the RCA occlusion as a culprit infarction lesion: the initial ECG showed a inferolateral ST segment elevation with a slightly higher elevation in the 2nd standard lead (II) than in the 3rd lead, without a significant "mirror" ST segment denivelation in the 1st standard lead and without elevation in the right precordial leads (RV4) (Figures 1(a)–1(c)); no ischemic pain and satisfactory ST segment resolution were present after the acute intervention on the LCx occlusion; there were already existing collaterals from LAD to RCA; and no medically induced reperfusion of the RCA occlusion was obtained (confirmed by a control angiography 5 days after the index event) after applying ticagrelor, acetylsalicylic acid, eptifibatide, and low-molecule heparin in the acute setting. It is possible that excessive antithrombotic and anticoagulant therapy gave a "bite" to the chronic occlusion of the RCA, leading to the intrinsic fibrinolytic mechanism and medical thrombotic suppression to melt the chronic occlusion. On the other hand, stopping the heparin and GPII/IIIa therapy in a still acute prothrombotic milieu led to thrombosis of the three implanted stents in the LCx. Additionally, it remains unclear why the patient reported angina between two hospitalizations, especially after performing a stress echocardiography where no ischemia progression was found. There might be an angiographic undetectable underlying microvascular disease which symptoms' regression can be related to the therapy changes (control ECG stress test revealed no ECG signs of ischemia nor clinical AP symptoms). Although intravascular ultrasound (IVUS) would have provided useful information, we were not able to perform it due to the reimbursement issues. Magnetic resonance imaging with gadolinium could not have been performed due to unavailability of the method in our hospital as well as the contraindication of adenosine administration due to the patient's history of asthma. In addition, another option could explain this sequence of events—prolonged coronary artery spasm which was repeated during the first two coronary angiographies. There are several facts pointing to the unlikelihood of spasm: presence of occlusion on two consecutive angiographies with 5-day difference while the patient was on full anti-ischemic therapy including nitrates and presence of collaterals to RCA supplying territory, no evidence of dynamic component of stenosis in angiograms during two different angiographies, as well as no evidence of spasm tendency on the third angiography. However, acetylcholine or ergonovine test during the last angiography, when RCA was found patent, which could have revealed the possibility of coronary artery spasm, was unfortunately not done [10, 11]. Lamm et al. [6] suggested that CTO is not a definitive state and collateral formation is just a bypass to the natural occlusion resolution. Perhaps it happens more often than we know because CTO patients are often treated with medications and usually no control angiographies are performed routinely. We hope that our data will help other authors to understand better the patho(physio)logy of the described unusual finding and encourage new basic studies in this area.

Consent

The patient has signed the informed consent.

References

[1] G. W. Stone, D. E. Kandzari, R. Mehran et al., "Percutaneous recanalization of chronically occluded coronary arteries: a consensus document: part I," *Circulation*, vol. 112, no. 15, pp. 2364–2372, 2005.

[2] C. Di Mario, G. S. Werner, G. Sianos et al., "European perspective in the recanalisation of chronic total occlusions (CTO): consensus document from the EuroCTO Club," *EuroIntervention*, vol. 3, no. 1, pp. 30–43, 2007.

[3] G. S. Werner, U. Emig, O. Mutschke, G. Schwarz, P. Bahrmann, and H. R. Figulla, "Regression of collateral function after recanalization of chronic total coronary occlusions: a serial assessment by intracoronary pressure and Doppler recordings," *Circulation*, vol. 108, no. 23, pp. 2877–2882, 2003.

[4] C. Seiler, M. Stoller, B. Pitt, and P. Meier, "The human coronary collateral circulation: development and clinical importance," *European Heart Journal*, vol. 34, no. 34, pp. 2674–2682, 2013.

[5] J. D. Häner, G. C. M. Siontis, M. Stoller, and S. Gloekler, "Spontaneous recanalization of a chronically occluded right coronary artery — when nature is more successful than technology," *International Journal of Cardiology*, vol. 214, pp. 161-162, 2016.

[6] G. Lamm, J. Auer, R. Berent, and B. Eber, "Chronic total occlusion—a definite state?," *International Journal of Cardiology*, vol. 102, no. 1, pp. 155-156, 2005.

[7] S. Som and B. Schanzer, "Spontaneous recanalization of complete internal carotid artery: a clinical reminder," *Journal of Surgical Technique and Case Report*, vol. 2, no. 2, pp. 73-74, 2010.

[8] G. Camporese, F. Verlato, G. Salmistraro, R. Ragazzi, and G. M. Andreozzi, "Spontaneous recanalization of internal carotid artery occlusion evaluated with color flow imaging and contrast arteriography," *International Angiology*, vol. 22, no. 1, pp. 64–71, 2003.

[9] N. J. Gargiulo III, F. J. Veith, E. C. Lipsitz et al., "Spontaneous recanalization of arterial occlusions: an unusual mechanism for symptomatic improvement," *Journal of Vascular Surgery*, vol. 36, no. 6, pp. 1161–1166, 2002.

[10] M. J. Hung, P. Hu, and M. Y. Hung, "Coronary artery spasm: review and update," *International Journal of Medical Sciences*, vol. 11, no. 11, pp. 1161–1171, 2014.

[11] J. H. Oh, S. Song, C. Kim et al., "Effect of intracoronary adenosine on ergonovine-induced vasoconstricted coronary arteries," *Cardiology Journal*, 2018.

46

Brugada Phenocopy Type 1 Secondary to Synthetic Cannabinoids

Mohammad Amro,[1] Kelechukwu U. Okoro,[2] Kanaan Mansoor,[2] Ahmed Amro,[2] and Paul Okhumale[2]

[1]*School of Medicine, Misr University for Science and Technology, Cairo, Egypt*
[2]*Marshall University School of Medicine, Huntington, WV, USA*

Correspondence should be addressed to Ahmed Amro; amro@live.marshall.edu

Academic Editor: Ertugrul Ercan

Brugada phenocopies (BrP) are clinical entities that have EKG tracings similar to the congenital Brugada syndrome (BrS) but without ventricular tachyarrhythmias or sudden cardiac death. BrP is caused by various factors such as metabolic disturbances (electrolyte imbalance), drugs, mechanical compression of the mediastinum, and inflammatory conditions such as myocarditis or pericarditis. We present a very rare case of a young patient who had a Brugada phenocopy Type 1 suspected to be secondary to synthetic cannabinoids.

1. Introduction

BrS is an autosomal dominant genetic disorder that is associated with sudden cardiac death (SCD) secondary to ventricular tachyarrhythmia in the setting of a structurally normal heart [1]. It is characterized by three morphologic phenotypes. Type 1 is referred to as the coved pattern, Type 2 is referred to as the saddle-back pattern, and Type 3 demonstrates the characteristics of either Type 1 and/or 2 without meeting all the criteria for either Type 1 or 2.

BrP are clinical conditions that demonstrates classical Brugada pattern on ECG but do not lead to sudden cardiac death (SCD) from ventricular tachyarrhythmia [2]. Distinguishing between BrS and BrP is most important as the management is different for both diagnoses. The primary objective of BrS is prevention of SCD; thus, patients usually receive an implantable cardioverter defibrillator (ICD) once diagnosis is made. In patients with BrP, implantation of ICD is not indicated as these patients do not go onto develop SCD. Also, ECG changes in patients diagnosed with BrP are transient and secondary to an underlying clinical condition. Once the underlying condition is rectified, characteristic Brugada ECG changes resolve.

2. Case Presentation

A 33-year-old Caucasian gentleman was admitted to our facility after he was found unresponsive by his girlfriend after an unknown prolonged absence. The girlfriend could not arouse the patient despite multiple attempts. Paramedics arrived on the scene and administered 6 mg of Naloxone which was successful in resuscitating the patient. Upon initial interrogation, the patient reported that he had snorted heroin. There was also report that he has been using a form of impure heroin colloquially known as "Black Tar Heroin" due to its characteristic appearance which is similar to roofing tar. Despite this, his toxicology screen was negative for heroin, but it did return with a positive result for synthetic cannabinoids.

Serum chemistry demonstrated lactic acid of 7.2 mmol/L, bicarbonate 16 mmol/L, blood glucose 271 mg/dL, BUN 17 mg/dL, and serum creatinine 2.3 mg/dL. Initial troponin was 0.045 ng/dL but trended upwards to 0.926 ng/dL. Creatinine kinase was 506 u/L and peaked at 7804 u/L before trending downwards. The patient's initial EKG demonstrated coved ST elevations in V1 and V2 which are characteristic changes consistent with BrS Type 1 (Figure 1). Repeat EKG

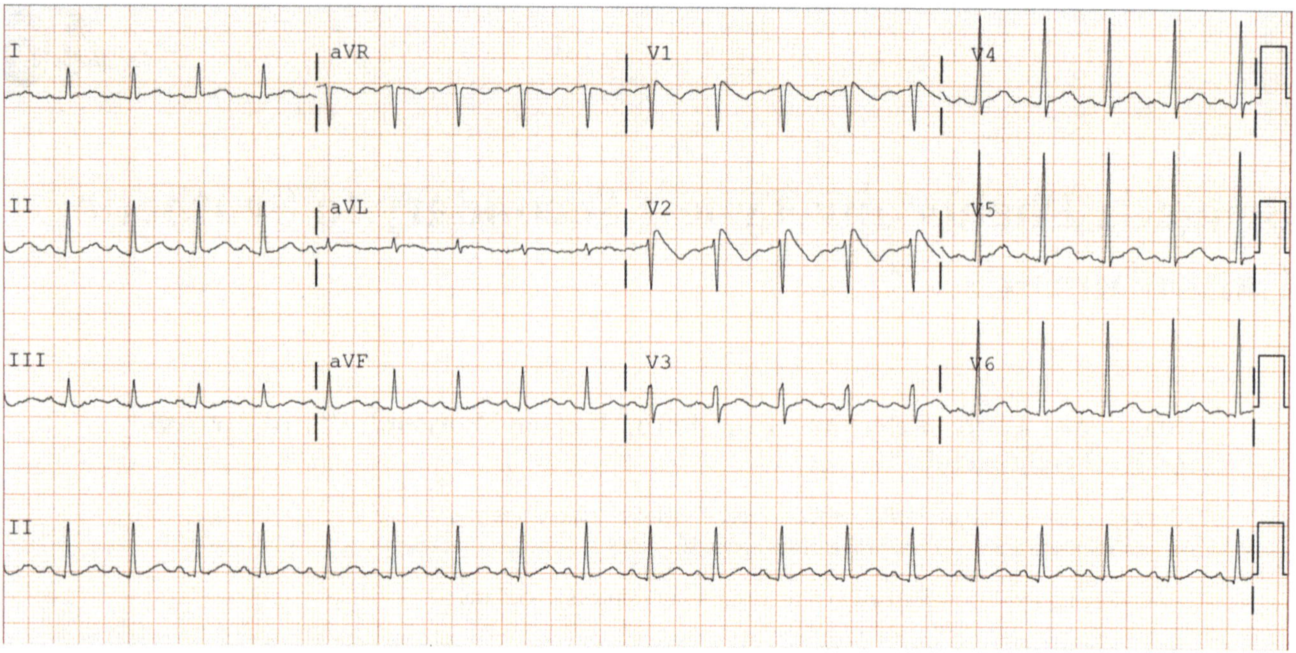

Figure 1: ECG on admission demonstrating characteristic Type 1 coved shaped ST segment elevation in leads V1 and V2.

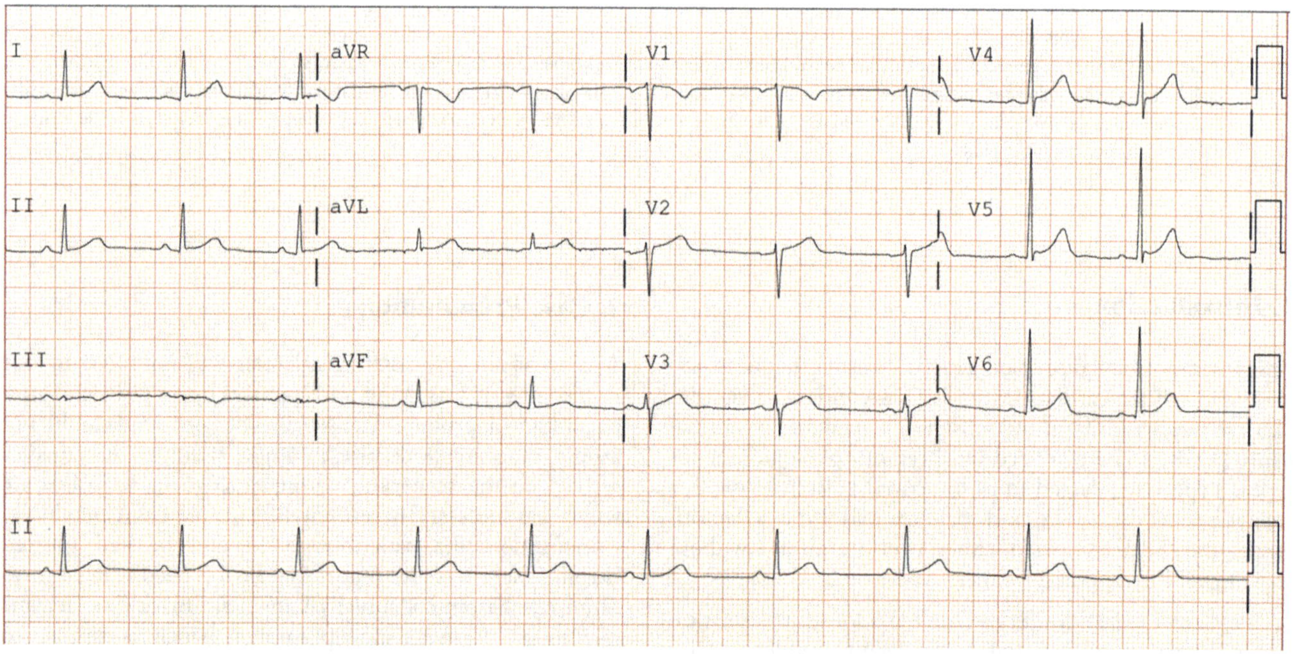

Figure 2: ECG two days after admission demonstrating absence of characteristic Brugada pattern.

after 1 day of admission demonstrated resolution of coved ST segment elevation (Figure 2). Electrophysiology (EP) service was consulted for implantation of ICD. The patient was evaluated and admitted for several occasions previously of loss of consciousness associated with drug overdose albeit he was not entirely certain. Due to reported history of multiple unclear episodes of loss of consciousness, we elected to proceed with EP study. Moving the EKG leads one rib space up which also failed to demonstrate the previously appreciated ECG changes. We proceeded with the Procainamide challenge. We administered Procainamide at 100 mg/min for 10 minutes till we achieved a maximum dose of 1 gm while continuously monitoring the patient's rhythm. We were unable to elicit symptoms or ECG changes consistent with BrS. As a result, the patient was diagnosed with BrP attributable to drugs of abuse which was synthetic cannabinoids based on toxicology screen which showed positive result for synthetic cannabinoids. The patient was diagnosed with BrP and discharged home.

TABLE 1: Patterns of ST abnormalities in leads V1-V3.

Feature	Type 1	Type 2	Type 3
J wave amplitude	≥2 mm	≥2 mm	≥2 mm
T wave	Negative	Positive or biphasic	Negative, positive, or biphasic
ST-T configuration	Coved	Saddle-back	Coved or saddle-back
Terminal portion of ST segment	Gradually descending	Elevated ≥1 mm	Gradually descending or elevated ≥1 mm

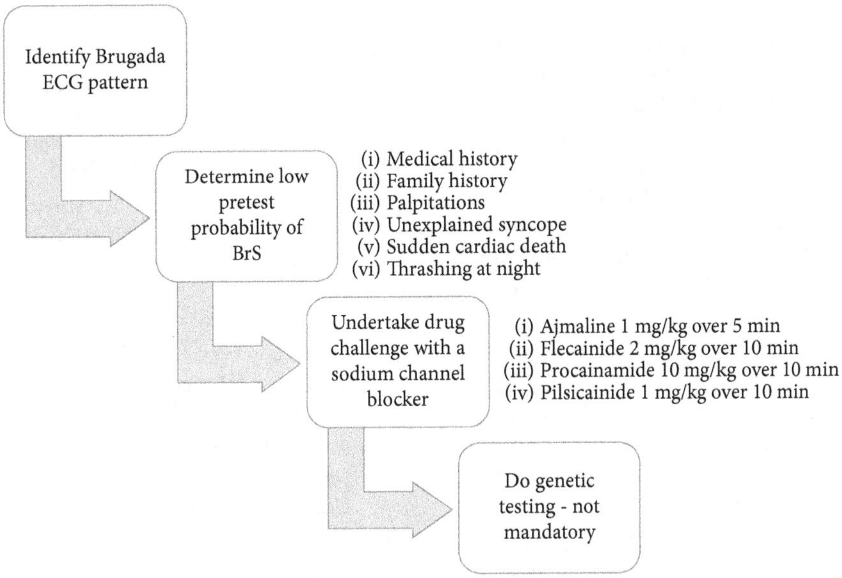

FIGURE 3: International Registry of Brugada Phenocopies proposed algorithm for appropriate diagnosis of Brugada phenocopies.

3. Discussion

BrS is an autosomal dominant genetic channelopathy that is associated with sudden cardiac death (SCD) secondary to ventricular tachyarrhythmia in the setting of a structurally normal heart [1–3]. It is inherited in an autosomal dominant pattern with variable penetrance with male predominance [4, 5]. The gene most associated with BrS is SCN5A which encodes for a cardiac sodium channel [5]. Mutations in this channel lead to unopposed potassium current in the RV epicardium through the I_{to} potassium channel. BrS is characterized by characteristic appearance on the ST segment and T wave in the anterior precordial leads [5, 6]. BrS is subclassified into three types depending on phenotypic appearance on the EKG (Table 1). Type 1 is referred to as the coved pattern, Type 2 is referred to as the saddle-back pattern, while Type 3 is a combination of both Types 1 and 2 without satisfying the criteria for either Type 1 or 2 [2–4, 7].

BrS ECG alterations can be dynamic, i.e., characteristic ECG patterns are absent at baseline but are "unmasked" due to derangements in homeostasis such as pyrexia and electrolyte abnormalities. Similar to BrS, BrP is also considered multifactorial [8, 9]. Patients with BrS are usually asymptomatic until they present with syncope or SCD [5]. Ventricular arrhythmia associated with BrS tends to occur nocturnally, in the setting of pyrexia particularly with children, or at rest especially after a large meal [3]. Adults usually succumb to either polymorphic VT or VF while the predominant arrhythmia in children is monomorphic VT. There is no medication that is indicated for management of BrS; rather individuals that receive a diagnosis of BrS require implantation ICD to prevent SCD.

BrP on the other hand is described as a selection of clinical disorders that demonstrate classic BrS ECG phenotypical appearance but lack the propensity to cause ventricular tachyarrhythmia and sudden death [2, 4, 10]. These disorders are classified by their etiological category which include metabolic imbalance, mechanical compression, ECG modulation, myocardial or pericardial disease, ischemia or pulmonary embolism, and miscellaneous causes.

It is important to properly identify unmasked BrS vs. BrP in patient who develops characteristic Brugada ECG pattern. The International Registry of Brugada Phenocopies have proposed an algorithm which allows for appropriate diagnosis of BrP (Figure 3) [11]. Of most importance in the algorithm is the provocation/challenge test with sodium channel blockers [1, 5]. These medications act by blocking predominantly sodium currents thus increasing the already-present ionic imbalance. This test should only be performed in a setting where continuous ECG monitoring is available and in the presence of health care providers who can provide management in the setting of an emergency. A positive result is connoted by the depiction of Brugada pattern [3]. The inability to demonstrate Brugada pattern constitutes a negative result and a diagnosis of BrP. The appearance of QRS widening, occurrence of frequent PVCs, or complex ventricular arrhythmias should lead to the cessation of the challenge. Isoprenaline infusion may be utilized to counteract the development of ventricular arrhythmias [3].

Once diagnosed, BrP is classified in the same vein as BrS, i.e., depending on the phenotypic appearance on ECG. A further subclassification is designated to BrP depending on the criteria met in the aforementioned algorithm. Class A represents cases in which all criteria were met, class B includes cases in which not all criteria are met but BrP is highly suspected, and class C are cases with unjustified provocative testing [1, 12]. The utilization of the algorithm is most important as it has been demonstrated that an experienced cardiologist cannot discern between BrP and BrS by ECG alone [1, 12, 13].

Our patient presented to the ED after drug overdose. It is unclear what he may have consumed as he was not forthcoming with details surrounding the events before his loss of consciousness. His toxicology screen demonstrated the presence of synthetic cannabinoids despite the fact he reported use of heroin multiple times in the past.

Drugs of abuse such as cannabinoids, heroin, and cocaine have been associated with BrP [14]. Changes in the ECG secondary to heroin such as QTc prolongation, torsades de pointes, and bradyarrhythmia are also well documented [15]. Ramsaroop et al. described a patient who required Naloxone to be resuscitated with positive toxicology screen for alcohol and opiates [15]. Ghovanloo et al. demonstrated that cannabinoids have a potential inhibitory effect on sodium channels under certain circumstances [16]. However, synthetic cannabinoids effect on sodium channels is not described in literature; also, our review of literature failed to demonstrate any reports or cases of synthetic cannabinoids leading to unmasked BrS or BrP.

The patient's EKG demonstrated Type 1 Brugada pattern which spontaneously resolved after several hours. Our patient also reported several episodes of loss of consciousness in the past. He was unclear what the etiology of his syncope was, but he believed it to be secondary to drug abuse although he was uncertain. As a result, we had to entertain the idea of a diagnosis of unmasked BrS vs. BrP. We proceeded with sodium channel provocation/challenge test. Procainamide was chosen as the challenge drug due to availability. Once it was ensured that all affairs were in order, we proceeded with the test. There was no QT prolongation, ventricular arrhythmia, PVC, or development of Type 1 Brugada pattern. The patient remained asymptomatic throughout the entirety of the examination.

4. Conclusion

Clinicians should be aware of the differentiation between BrS and BrP. Both conditions are distinct from each other as thus management is different. Early recognition of the presence of each disease can prevent misdiagnosis and inappropriate treatment.

References

[1] N. R. de Oliveira Neto, W. S. de Oliveira, F. Mastrocola, and L. Sacilotto, "Brugada phenocopy: mechanisms, diagnosis, and implications," *Journal of Electrocardiology*, vol. 55, pp. 45–50, 2019.

[2] S. F. M. Awad, R. Barbosa-Barros, L. de Sousa Belem et al., "Brugada phenocopy in a patient with pectus excavatum: Systematic review of the ECG manifestations associated with pectus excavatum," *Annals of Noninvasive Electrocardiology*, vol. 18, no. 5, pp. 415–420, 2013.

[3] C. Pappone, V. Santinelli, Arrhythmology Department et al., "Brugada syndrome: Progress in diagnosis and management," *Arrhythmia & Electrophysiology Review*, vol. 8, no. 1, pp. 13–18, 2019.

[4] D. D. Anselm, B. H. Gottschalk, and A. Baranchuk, "Brugada Phenocopy Is an Important Differential Diagnosis in Patients with Type 1 Brugada ECG Patterns," *The American Journal of Medicine*, vol. 128, no. 11, p. e33, 2015.

[5] A. A. M. Wilde, C. Antzelevitch, M. Borggrefe et al., "Proposed Diagnostic Criteria for the Brugada Syndrome," *European Heart Journal*, vol. 23, no. 21, pp. 1648–1654, 2002.

[6] A. R. Pérez-Riera, R. Barbosa Barros, R. Daminello-Raimundo, M. P. C. Resende Barbosa, and L. C. de Abreu, "Brugada phenocopy caused by a compressive mediastinal tumor," *Annals of Noninvasive Electrocardiology*, vol. 23, no. 3, p. e12509, 2018.

[7] A. B. de Luna, J. Brugada, A. Baranchuk et al., "Current electrocardiographic criteria for diagnosis of Brugada pattern: a consensus report," *Journal of Electrocardiology*, vol. 45, no. 5, pp. 433–442, 2012.

[8] S. Sreenivasan, M. Monaghan, and A. Baranchuk, "Multifactorial Brugada Phenocopy," *JAMA Internal Medicine*, vol. 178, no. 6, pp. 872-873, 2018.

[9] M. Heckle, S. Alsafwah, and M. Agarwal, "Multifactorial Brugada phenocopy—reply," *JAMA Internal Medicine*, vol. 178, no. 6, p. 873, 2018.

[10] G. Xu, B. H. Gottschalk, D. D. Anselm et al., "Relation of the Brugada phenocopy to hyperkalemia (from the International Registry on Brugada Phenocopy)," *The American Journal of Cardiology*, vol. 121, no. 6, pp. 715–717, 2018.

[11] Brugada Phenocopy Registry, http://www.brugadaphenocopy.com/.

[12] A. G. Carrizo, A. Goransky, and A. Baranchuk, "Brugada phenocopy during right coronary artery dissection," *Journal of Electrocardiology*, vol. 50, no. 6, pp. 969–971, 2017.

[13] B. H. Gottschalk, D. D. Anselm, J. Brugada et al., "Expert cardiologists cannot distinguish between Brugada phenocopy and Brugada syndrome electrocardiogram patterns," *Europace*, vol. 18, no. 7, pp. 1095–1100, 2016.

[14] A. Akinlonu, R. Suri, P. Yerragorla et al., "Brugada Phenocopy Induced by Recreational Drug Use," *Case Reports in Cardiology*, vol. 2018, 4 pages, 2018.

[15] K. Ramsaroop, R. Seecheran, V. Seecheran et al., "Suspected hyponatremia-induced Brugada phenocopy," *International Medical Case Reports Journal*, vol. 12, pp. 61–65, 2019.

[16] M. R. Ghovanloo, N. G. Shuart, J. Mezeyova, R. A. Dean, P. C. Ruben, and S. J. Goodchild, "Inhibitory effects of cannabidiol on voltage-dependent sodium currents," *The Journal of Biological Chemistry*, vol. 293, no. 43, pp. 16546–16558, 2018.

47

Large Device-Related Thrombus Detected following Symptoms of Transient Ischemic Attack

Osayi Lawani[1] and **Edward Baptista**[2]

[1]*University of Houston College of Medicine/HCA Houston Healthcare, USA*
[2]*Vital Heart & Vein, USA*

Correspondence should be addressed to Osayi Lawani; osayimd@gmail.com

Academic Editor: Luigi Sciarra

As an independent risk factor for stroke, atrial fibrillation has been shown to be associated with a fivefold increase in the cause of embolic stroke in comparison to healthy individuals without atrial fibrillation. This risk may be compounded by other factors; however, the main probable cause of stroke leading from atrial fibrillation is thrombus formation in the left atrial appendage. In patients for whom anticoagulation is contraindicated, left atrial appendage occlusion has become a leading alternative option for therapeutic prevention of thromboembolism and stroke in patients with this condition. Unfortunately, these devices (particularly the WATCHMAN) have been associated with a 3-6% incidence of intracardiac thrombus development postimplantation. Some risk factors for the development of device-related thrombus are high platelet count, permanent atrial fibrillation, resistance to clopidogrel, and prior transient ischemic attack or stroke. Despite following an anticoagulant regimen, thrombus formation was reported in 5.6% of participants of a randomized clinical trial, and further analysis showed that some of these patients continued to develop either ischemic stroke or thromboembolism five years later as compared to patients without initial thrombus development. We present a case of an elderly male with prior history of stroke and transient ischemic attack who developed a large device-related thrombus five months following WATCHMAN FLX™ implantation. Currently, there are no specific recommendations on the management of this rare complication; however, we discuss possible consideration of initially prolonging anticoagulation therapy following implantation for high-risk individuals, as there is an increased possibility for thrombus formation in this population. Management options should continue to be studied for therapeutic benefit in streamlining postprocedural therapy and improve future outcomes in the use of left atrial appendage occlusion devices, as well as continual thrombus prevention.

1. Introduction

The incidence and prevalence of atrial fibrillation (AF) have increased greatly in the past 20 years as the population of elderly individuals continues to grow, with 75 years being the median age of patients with AF [1]. Currently, there are greater than two million Americans and eight million Europeans that are affected with this condition and is likely underestimated due to lack of notable symptoms [2]. Since the first confirmation of a relationship between an electrocardiogram with AF and a clinical irregularly irregular pulse was published by a group of European physicians in 1909, there has been a continual attempt to find various methods to eliminate or manage this disorder [3]. Management in non-rheumatic AF patients with a $CHA_2DS_2-VASc\,score \geq 2$ consists of an antiarrhythmic agent along with common oral anticoagulants such as vitamin K antagonists, or direct oral anticoagulants via thrombin inhibition, or factor X_a inhibition as to prevent thrombosis [2, 4]. Additionally, in patients with a history of coronary artery disease and planned percutaneous coronary intervention, dual antiplatelet therapy with aspirin and a $P2Y_{12}$ receptor antagonist is included to prevent risk of thrombotic ischemic events and stent thrombosis [2].

In patients for whom anticoagulation is contraindicated, device implantation to close off the left atrial appendage

(LAA) is the next likely choice in intervention and has become a leading alternative option for therapeutic prevention of thromboembolism; several devices have been developed for this use (Table 1) [5]. Unfortunately, some of these devices have been associated with about a 3-6% incidence of intracardiac thrombus development postimplantation despite the use of anticoagulant therapy [6]. In this report, we present a case of an elderly male who was found to develop a large device-related thrombus in his left atrium five months following placement of a WATCHMAN device.

2. Case History

A 75-year-old male with a past medical history of paroxysmal atrial fibrillation, recent WATCHMAN FLX™ placement, coronary artery disease with three cardiac stents, hypertension, hyperlipidemia, bilateral carotid endarterectomies, recurrent transient ischemic attack (TIA), and two prior cerebrovascular accidents presented to our emergency department with complaints of left-sided numbness that began two hours prior to arrival.

Roughly eight months earlier, the patient experienced similar symptoms and was diagnosed with TIA. He had been taking apixaban 5 mg daily and clopidogrel 75 mg daily following previous cardiac stenting and asserted that he remained compliant with his prescriptions. A transthoracic echocardiogram (TTE) performed showed an ejection fraction of 55-60% and a mildly dilated left atrium. No defects or shunts were noted, and the foramen ovale was not patent. The patient was discharged home and advised to continue his prescriptions for apixaban and clopidogrel.

One month later, the patient returned to an emergency department with complaints of acute onset right-sided weakness and numbness. A magnetic resonance imaging (MRI) of the brain showed ischemic events in multiple territories, and a computed tomography (CT) angiogram of the neck vessels indicated a focal left (dominant) vertebral artery stenosis. Neurointerventional radiology was consulted, and a stenting of the left vertebral artery was performed. Telemetry showed atrial fibrillation with controlled ventricular response. The patient stated that he had remained compliant with taking apixaban and clopidogrel. A platelet $P2Y_{12}$ assay was performed to assess failure of therapy with clopidogrel and was negative. As there was no clear etiology to the diagnosed embolic stroke, a transesophageal echocardiogram (TEE) was ordered. The TEE was deferred to a later date due to patient preference. On discharge, apixaban was changed to rivaroxaban 20 mg daily, and the patient was instructed to continue taking clopidogrel and to follow-up out-patient with his primary cardiologist.

Exactly one month later, the patient was found to be in persistent AF during a follow-up appointment with his cardiologist. The patient also admittedly had several mechanical falls in the past few months. It was decided by his outpatient cardiologist that the patient would undergo implantation of a WATCHMAN FLX™ device for left atrial appendage closure under TEE guidance. The appendage, which was 22 mm in diameter, showed no clot within its interior prior to device implantation. A 27 mm device was ultimately placed more distally following a partial recapture after an initial attempt placed the device somewhat proximal to the opening. A tug test was satisfactory, and no leaks were noted. The patient was instructed to begin taking aspirin 81 mg daily, to continue taking clopidogrel and rivaroxaban, and to return in six weeks for a repeat TEE.

About two months later, the patient had a repeat TEE which showed a normal sized left atrium and a well-positioned WATCHMAN FLX™ without significant peri-device leak (<4 mm). No spontaneous echo contrast, new shunt, or evidence of thrombus was observed. As per protocol, the patient was instructed by his cardiologist to continue taking clopidogrel and aspirin daily, to discontinue use of rivaroxaban, and to follow-up within six months.

Over three months later, the patient presented to the emergency department at our hospital with complaints of left-sided numbness. It was the patient's first encounter at this facility as he was visiting family from out-of-town. Laboratory results at the time of admission were as follows: creatinine 1.2 mg/dL, calcium 8.6 mg/dL, rapid troponin 0.01 ng/ml, low-density lipoprotein 76.45 mg/dL, high-density lipoprotein 26 mg/dL, hemoglobin 14.7 g/dL, and a platelet count of 124×10^3/uL. Chest X-ray, head CT, brain MRI, and CT angiogram of the head and neck were unremarkable. The patient stated that he had been compliant with taking his prescribed clopidogrel and aspirin, as well as amlodipine 5 mg daily and carvedilol 6.25 mg twice a day. Causes of the patients' symptoms that may have mimicked a TIA (e.g., anxiety, seizure, migraine, and syncope) were unfounded following laboratory results and a bedside evaluation by neurology. As the etiology of the diagnosed TIA was unclear, cardiology was consulted, and a TEE was scheduled to reevaluate the positioning of his previously implanted WATCHMAN FLX™ device for leakage and to rule out any thrombus formation. The TEE showed an ejection fraction of 55-59%, a mildly dilated left atrium, and a well-positioned WATCHMAN FLX™ without peri-device leakage. Surprisingly, it was revealed that there was a large thrombus measuring 2.5 × 1.5 cm at the mouth of the LAA that was adherent to and covered the entire top of the WATCHMAN FLX™ device (Figures 1 and 2). No other structural cardiac defects were noted. The patient was promptly restarted on rivaroxaban and on discharge was instructed to follow-up out-patient with his cardiologist for continued management.

A little over two months later, the patient returned to his cardiologist for an outpatient follow-up. He denied any further complaints of stroke-like symptoms and continued to take rivaroxaban as prescribed. Another TEE was performed and showed a moderate to severely dilated left atrium. The WATCHMAN FLX™ device was noted in the LAA, as was a small mobile thrombus. The right atrium was also moderately dilated without evidence of thrombus. In comparison to the previous TEE performed over two months prior, the attached thrombus to the device was significantly smaller, but not completely dissolved (Figure 3). The patient was advised to continue rivaroxaban 20 mg daily and to follow-up with his cardiologist for continued surveillance.

Table 1: Devices for use in percutaneous left atrial appendage occlusion [5].

Device	Manufacturer	Design	Sizes (mm)	Sheath (F)	Approval status
Endocardial LAAO devices					
WATCHMAN	Boston Scientific	Single (lobe)	21, 24, 27, 30, 33	14	CE Mark (2005) FDA (2015)
WATCHMAN FLX			20, 24, 27, 31, 35	14	CE Mark (2019) FDA (2020)
Amplatzer Cardiac Plug	Abbot Vascular, formerly St. Jude Medical	Double (lobe and disc)	16, 18, 20, 22, 24, 26, 28, 30	9-13	CE Mark (2008)
Amplatzer Amulet			16, 18, 20, 22, 25, 28, 31, 34	12-14	CE Mark (2013)
WaveCrest	Biosense Webster, Inc. (Johnson and Johnson company)	Single (lobe)	22, 27, 32	12	CE Mark (2013)
Occlutech	Occlutech International AB	Single (lobe)	15, 18, 21, 24, 27, 30, 33, 36, 39	12, 14	CE Mark (2016)
LAmbre	Lifetech Scientific Co., Ltd.	Double (umbrella and cover)	16, 18, 20, 22, 24, 26, 28, 30, 32, 34, 36	8-10	CE Mark (2016); CFDA (2017)
Sideris transcatheter patch	Custom Medical Devices	Frameless, bioabsorbable, balloon-deliverable device	15-25	13	Undergoing clinical evaluation
Ultraseal	Cardia, Inc.	Double (bulb and sail)	16, 18, 20, 22, 24, 26, 28, 30, 32	10-12	CE Mark (2016)
SeaLA	Hangzhou Valued Medtech Co., Ltd.	Double (dual disc)	16, 18, 20, 22, 24, 26, 28, 30, 32, 34, 36	9-12	Undergoing clinical evaluation
LeFort	Lepu Medical Technology (Beijing) Co., Ltd.	Single (lobe)	21-33	—	Undergoing clinical evaluation
Pfm device	Pfm Medical	Single (disc), dual anchor	—	10-12	Undergoing clinical evaluation
Epicardial LAAO devices					
Lariat	SentreHeart, Inc.	Endoepidcardial	40 (W), (45 [W] lariat +) x 20 (H) x 70 (L)	12	CE Mark (2015); FDA 510(k) (2006), surgical use only
Sierra	Aegis Medical Innovations Inc.	Epicardial	Single size	20	Undergoing clinical evaluation

LAAO: left atrial appendage occlusion; CE Mark: Comformité Europëenne Mark; CFDA: China Food and Drug Administration; FDA: United States Food and Drug Administration; W: width; H: height; L: length.

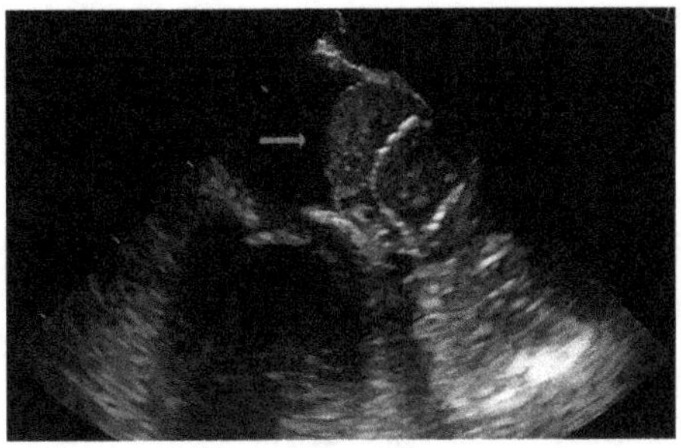

FIGURE 1: Transesophageal echocardiogram indicating a large thrombus located at the opening of the left atrial appendage covering an implanted WATCHMAN FLX™ device.

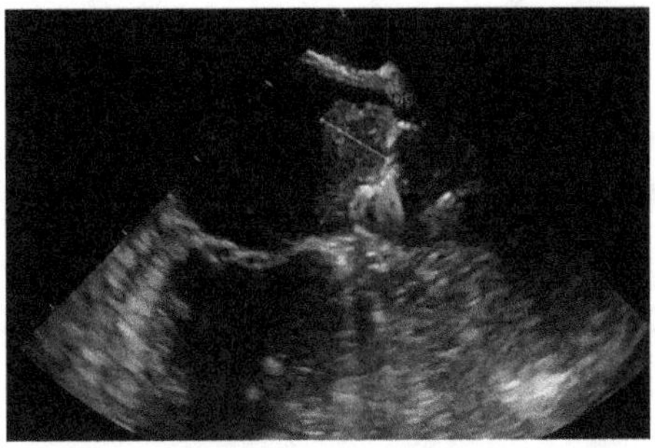

FIGURE 2: Transesophageal echocardiogram measuring a large thrombus within the left atrium atop an implanted WATCHMAN FLX™ device.

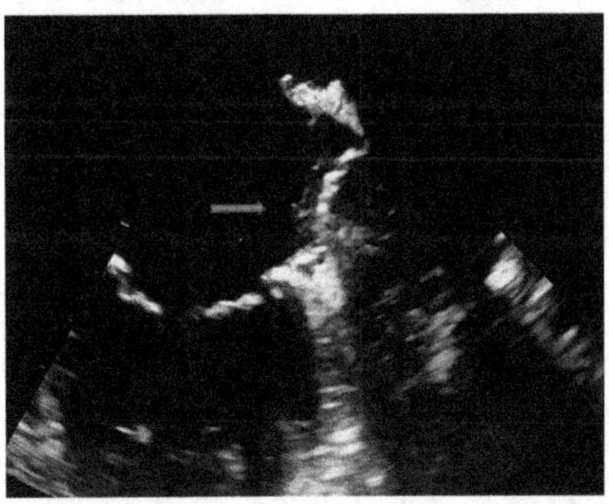

FIGURE 3: Repeat transesophageal echocardiogram showing a decrease in clot formation on a WATCHMAN FLX™ device within the left atrial appendage.

3. Discussion

As the left atrium dilates from continued fibrillation, there is more stasis and thrombus formation within the LAA [7]. Since the 1990s, interest in treating the LAA in AF patients increased with the advancement of the maze procedure, common use of TEE, and the development of percutaneous occlusion devices [8]. Left atrial appendage occlusion (LAAO) has been the primary method of stroke prevention in AF patients who have a contraindication to anticoagulation therapy, which includes increased risk for fall, lack of patient compliance, discontinuation of anticoagulants due to gastrointestinal bleed or recent stroke, or difficulty in maintaining a therapeutic window (as seen with warfarin use) [7, 8]. Based on both the PROTECT-AF and PREVAIL studies, the WATCHMAN has continually been a popular choice in AF treatment, as it was shown that using this device was not inferior to being on oral anticoagulation to prevent thromboembolism in AF [8].

Changes in the second version of the WATCHMAN FLX in comparison to its predecessor were evaluated during the PINNACLE FLX study and indicated that there was indeed a decreased incidence of complications and increased evidence of effective LAA closure at one year [9]. Device-related thrombosis (DRT) was only found in 3.7% of patients after 12 months of follow-up; however, it was attributed to both the change in the structure of the device and possibly the change in the 6-week postimplantation anticoagulation course regimen from warfarin and aspirin used in the PROTECT-AF and PREVAIL trials, to use of direct oral anticoagulants and aspirin [9]. It was also noted that the new antithrombotic regimen showed an absence of DRT in patients who were compliant with taking these medications [9]. This was not the case for the individual in this report, although his DRT could have had a multifactorial cause.

It is important to mention that although the patient in this report was discovered to have a DRT following a TIA, thrombus is not always associated with an embolic event and is usually an incidental finding. Risk factors for the development of DRT are high platelet count, resistance to clopidogrel, an elevated $CHADS_2$ and CHA_2DS_2-VASc score, decreased left ventricular ejection fraction, permanent AF, prior TIA or stroke, or device-specific issues (large mean device size or deep implantation) [10]. With regards to this case, the patient met at least three risk factors for thromboembolism formation. The pathophysiology of DRT can be directly related to elderly individuals with prior history of stroke, elevated CHA_2DS_s-VASc score, and vascular disease, all of which are indicated in an increased prothrombotic state [11]. DRT may also be induced by incomplete or deep implantation of the device by exposing areas of trabeculations [11]. Large devices also increase the risk for DRT due to having an increased fabric surface area [11]. The patient in this case had his device implanted deeply on a second attempt and also had a device placed that was 5 mm larger than the diameter of his LAA.

The most common cause of DRT has been noted to occur following the discontinuation of oral anticoagulant therapy [6]. At this time, there is no indication of which oral anticoagulant is preferred as one retrospective study suggested that there was no significant difference in developing DRT with the initial use of either vitamin K antagonists or direct oral anticoagulants [11]. What is known is that a recent analysis showed that after five years, about 25% of patients who were diagnosed with DRT from the PROTECT-AF and PREVAIL studies later developed either ischemic stroke or thromboembolism compared to patients without DRT, and that there was also a temporal association [11]. Although the incidence of DRT is about 3-7%, it is associated with a threefold increase in stroke risk [11].

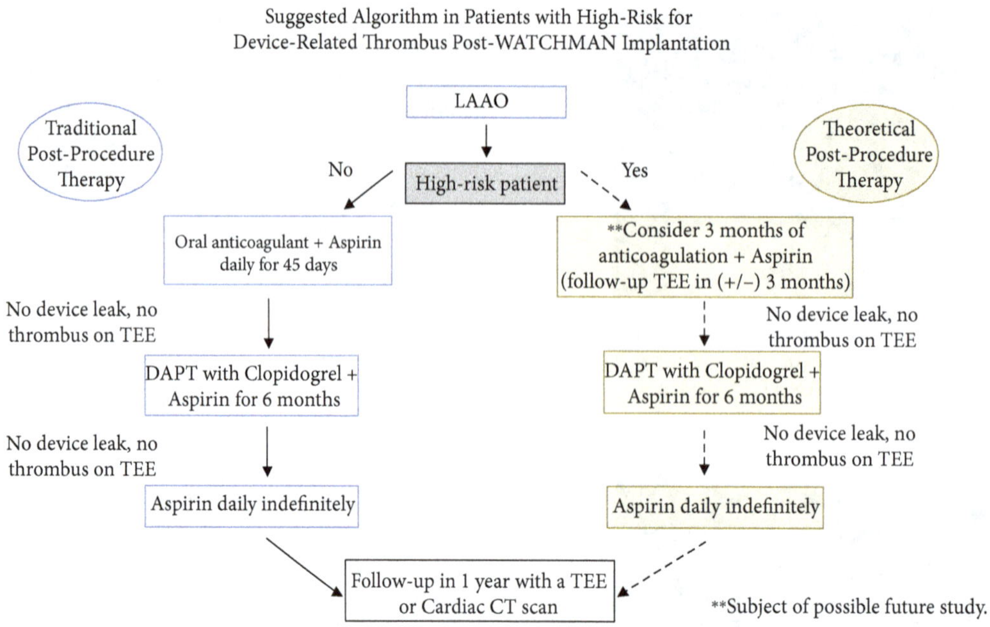

FIGURE 4: Suggested algorithm for assessment and treatment of a patient post-WATCHMAN placement who may be high risk for DRT. LAAO: left atrial appendage occlusion; TEE: transesophageal echocardiogram; DAPT: dual antiplatelet therapy; DRT: device-related thrombus; CT: computed tomography [11].

Furthermore, as there is usually resolution of DRT with the use of direct oral anticoagulation, there have been several accounts of recurrent DRT after anticoagulation was discontinued [12]. Consequently, more thoughtful consideration should be placed for patients that qualify for an LAAO device and have a significant history of stroke or thromboembolism.

For high-risk patients prior to LAAO device placement, it is proposed that anticoagulation continue for >45 days following implantation, then a repeat TEE is performed at a later date, and the patient can start dual antiplatelet therapy followed by aspirin indefinitely if there is no evidence of peri-device leaks or DRT [13]. Future studies should focus on an optional length of time a high-risk patient should stay on anticoagulation postimplantation as this is presently undetermined (Figure 4) [11].

Duration of use and choice of anticoagulant and antiplatelet regimen should be tailored for high-risk patients. In addition, it may be worth investigating whether $P2Y_{12}$ inhibitors other than clopidogrel should be used for patients who are prone to thromboembolism as they have better platelet aggregation inhibition during the device sealing process [13]. Previously, a DRT score based on predictors was suggested to assist in identifying individuals that would be at a high risk for thrombus development postdevice implantation. This would be helpful as it would potentially lead to finding whether factors related to anticoagulation, the patient, or the actual procedure contributed to the formation of DRT [12]. At this time, treatment strategies for high-risk individuals who may develop DRT have not been clinically proven and should be treated on a case-by-case basis.

4. Conclusion

Although the incidence of DRT following WATCHMAN implantation is relatively low, it does have a significant impact on how high-risk patients are viewed and considered for treatment. As the results of the ASAP-TOO trial will indicate whether anticoagulation is needed overall after device implantation, the incidence of DRT should continue to be further investigated, particularly for high-risk individuals. Prolonging anticoagulation or change in antiplatelet regimen should also continue to be studied for therapeutic benefit. One study suggested possible coating of the device in an antithrombotic agent to help in decreasing the risk of DRT development [12]. Integration of these changes into clinical practice will likely assist in streamlining postprocedural therapy as to keep up with achieving continual promising outcomes with the use of LAAO devices, as well as continual thrombus prevention.

Authors' Contributions

Osayi Lawani participated in conceptualization, data curation, investigation, visualization, and creation, review, and editing of the original draft. Edward Baptista provided supervision, methodology, validation, resources, and editing of original draft.

Acknowledgments

The authors would especially like to thank Dr. Justin Saunders, Patricia Dottery, Saadia Farehan, and Amanda Posada for their support.

References

[1] S. S. Chugh, J. L. Blackshear, W.-K. Shen, S. C. Hammill, and B. J. Gersh, "Epidemiology and natural history of atrial fibrillation: clinical implications," *Journal of the American College of Cardiology*, vol. 37, no. 2, pp. 371–378, 2001.

[2] D. Capodanno, H. Huber, R. Mehranet al. et al., "Management of Antithrombotic Therapy in Atrial Fibrillation Patients Undergoing PCI:," *Journal of the American College of Cardiology*, vol. 74, no. 1, pp. 83–99, 2019.

[3] T. Fazekas, "The concise history of atrial fibrillation," *Orvostörténeti Közlemények*, vol. 53, no. 3-4, pp. 37–68, 2007.

[4] O. de Backer, S. Arnous, N. Ihlemann et al., "Percutaneous left atrial appendage occlusion for stroke prevention in atrial fibrillation: an update," *Open Heart*, vol. 1, no. 1, article e000020, 2014.

[5] L. Asmarats and J. Rodes-Cabau, "The spectrum of devices for percutaneous left atrial appendage occlusion," *Cardiac Interventions Today*, vol. 12, no. 3, pp. 34–39, 2018.

[6] B. Hannawi, F. Beg, M. Valderrabano, and K. Kurrelmeyer, "Device-related thrombus: a reason for concern?," *Methodist Debakey Care*, vol. 15, no. 1, pp. 77–80, 2021.

[7] J. Romero, I. E. Perez, A. Krumerman, M. J. Garcia, and R. J. Lucariello, "Left atrial appendage closure devices," *Clinical Medicine Insights: Cardiology*, vol. 8, pp. CMC.S14043–CMC.S14052, 2014.

[8] S. Chatterjee, J. C. Alexander, P. J. Pearson, and T. Feldman, "Left atrial appendage occlusion: lessons learned from surgical and transcatheter experiences," *The Annals of Thoracic Surgery*, vol. 92, no. 6, pp. 2283–2292, 2011.

[9] S. Kar, S. K. Doshi, A. Sadhu et al., "Primary outcome evaluation of a next-generation left atrial appendage closure device," *Circulation*, vol. 143, no. 18, pp. 1754–1762, 2021.

[10] S. R. Dukkipati, S. Kar, D. R. Holmes et al., "Device-related thrombus after left atrial appendage closure," *Circulation*, vol. 138, no. 9, pp. 874–885, 2018.

[11] M. Turagam, V. Y. Reddy, and S. Dukkipati, "Device-related thrombus: understanding and managing the "Achilles heel" of LAA closure," in *American College of Cardiology*, 2018, June 2021, https://www.acc.org/latest-in-cardiology/articles/2018/09/14/09/54/device-related-thrombus.

[12] M. Alkhouli and D. R. Holmes, "Remaining challenges with transcatheter left atrial appendage closure," *Mayo Clinic Proceedings*, vol. 95, no. 10, pp. 2244–2248, 2020.

[13] P. Garot, B. Cormier, and J. Horvilleur, "Device-related thrombus after left atrial appendage closure," *International Cardiology Review*, vol. 14, no. 1, pp. 42–44, 2019.

48

Interruption of the Right Pulmonary Artery in a Neonate

Mohammadreza Khalilian,[1] **Taraneh Faghihi Langroudi**,[2] **Ali Dabbagh**,[3] **Ramin Baghaei Tehrani**,[4] **and Tahmineh Tahouri**[1]

[1]*Department of Pediatrics, School of Medicine, Shahid Beheshti University of Medical Sciences, Tehran, Iran*
[2]*Radiology Department, Shahid Modarres Hospital, Shahid Beheshti University of Medical Sciences, Tehran, Iran*
[3]*Cardiac Anesthesia, Anesthesiology Research Center, Shahid Beheshti University of Medical Sciences, Tehran, Iran*
[4]*Cardiac Surgery, Shahid Modarres Educational Hospital, School of Medicine, Shahid Beheshti University of Medical Sciences, Tehran, Iran*

Correspondence should be addressed to Tahmineh Tahouri; tahmineh.tahouri@hotmail.com

Academic Editor: Christopher Snyder

Interruption of the right pulmonary artery is a very rare anomaly which can be associated with other congenital heart lesions or can occur in isolation. Clinical presentations of the unilateral interruption of a pulmonary artery are varied including pulmonary hypertension, recurrent infection, dyspnea, exercise intolerance, hemoptysis, and chest pain. Less commonly, patients may be asymptomatic. Diagnosis of this anomaly is made by echocardiography and CT angiography as well as cardiac MRI. Treatment options are medical versus surgical management and often recommended in symptomatic patients with pulmonary hypertension, recurrent infection, and hemoptysis. Herein, we describe a very rare case of right pulmonary artery originating from the right subclavian artery in a 12-day-old neonate.

1. Introduction

Normally, the pulmonary artery originates from the right ventricle and bifurcates into the right and left pulmonary artery branches (1). Anomalous origin of the right and left pulmonary arteries is a rare congenital anomaly which is usually accompanied by other congenital heart diseases; however, it can occur in isolation. Interruption of the right pulmonary artery is one of the extremely rare branch pulmonary artery anomalies which occur due to abnormal development of the proximal part of the sixth primitive aortic arch. In this condition, perfusion of the right lung is through collateral arteries arising from the systemic circulation (2). Needless to say, the right and left pulmonary arteries are nonconfluent, and the left pulmonary artery is normally connected to the right ventricle and thus receives the entire cardiac output (3, 4).

Herein, we describe a very rare case of an isolated right pulmonary artery originating from the right subclavian artery in a 12-day-old neonate.

2. Case Presentation

A 12-day-old newborn girl was referred to our hospital, Shahid Modarres Educational Hospital, located in Tehran, Iran, from a district hospital for further evaluation of pulmonary hypertension. She was delivered by cesarean section at term gestation in a twin pregnancy and had APGAR scores of 9/10 and a birth weight of 2100 g. Shortly after birth, she developed tachypnea and was consequently transferred to the neonatal intensive care unit. The second twin was healthy. The parents were Pakistani. The mother of the patient did not take any medications during pregnancy. The pregnancy was uneventful, and there was no relevant familial history of consanguinity or congenital heart defects. The patient was diagnosed with pulmonary hypertension, and medical treatment was initiated with sildenafil. She was discharged after 11 days in stable condition.

After discharge, the patient was referred to our Pediatric Cardiology Clinic in a tertiary center. Physical examination

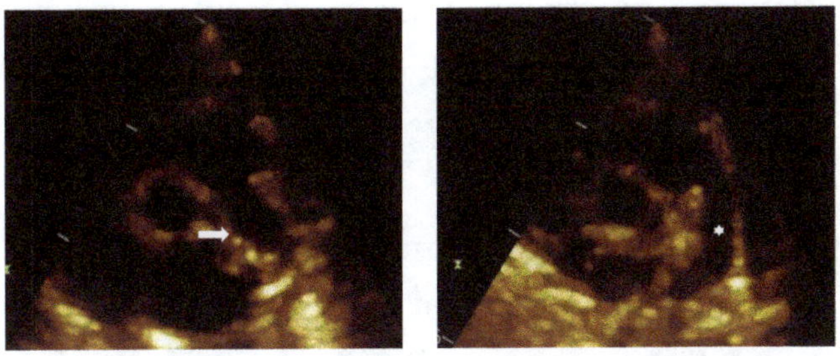

(a) (b)

FIGURE 1: Cross-sectional echocardiogram (parasternal short axis view) showing (a) the LPA at its typical location (arrow) and absence of the RPA and (b) large left side PDA (asterisk). LPA: left pulmonary artery. RPA: right pulmonary artery.

on admission revealed a respiratory rate of 45 cycle/minute, BP of 85/50 mmHg, and heart rate of 120 beat/minute. She had no respiratory distress, and oxygen saturation was 94% in room air. Cardiac auscultation revealed a systolic murmur on the left upper sternal border. Examination of other body system was normal. Electrocardiogram (ECG) showed normal sinus rhythm and right axis deviation. Chest X-ray indicated mild cardiomegaly with mild increase in pulmonary vascular markings suggestive of pulmonary hypertension.

An echocardiogram was notable for mild right atrial and right ventricular enlargement. The main pulmonary artery was mildly dilated, and the typical bifurcation of the pulmonary artery was not detectable; instead, only the left pulmonary artery was seen at its expected location, and the right pulmonary artery was absent. The pulmonary valve was normal. A large PDA with bidirectional shunt was noted with a typical insertion to the LPA (Figure 1). There was a mild tricuspid regurgitation and estimated a systolic pulmonary artery pressure of 50 mmHg above right atrial pressure. There was mild right ventricular diastolic dysfunction on M-mode and tissue Doppler evaluation. Otherwise, echocardiogram was normal with no other cardiac anomaly except for a small patent foramen ovale which had a bidirectional shunt too. Since we could not see the right pulmonary artery on the echocardiogram, cardiac CT angiography was performed which demonstrated an isolated right pulmonary artery arising from the right subclavian artery (Figure 2). Since the patient was mildly symptomatic, she was discharged from the hospital with no medications and a plan for monthly follow-up. At the age of 3 months, the patient underwent angiography and catheterization. At cardiac catheterization, the left pulmonary artery pressure was 80/50 mmHg versus an aortic pressure of 90/50 mmHg. There was a significant step up from the right ventricle at 82% to the left pulmonary artery at 99%. Aortogram subsequently revealed a large left tubular patent ductus arteriosus. The origin of the right pulmonary artery was demonstrated from the right subclavian artery with a significant proximal stenosis at the origin from the right subclavian artery (Figure 3). The size of the right pulmonary artery was within normal ranges while the left pulmonary artery was significantly dilated.

The patient subsequently underwent surgical PDA ligation (Figure 4). It was felt that the proximal RPA stenosis reduced the risk of arterial hypertension in the right lung, so no intervention was performed on the right pulmonary artery at that time. The postoperative course was uneventful, and she was discharged after 6 days with a recommendation for continued follow-up. She was also started on medical therapy with sildenafil and furosemide which in the months that followed was discontinued. At present, the patient is 8 months old and remains asymptomatic with an estimated pulmonary artery pressure of 20 mmHg on echocardiography and normal growth and development.

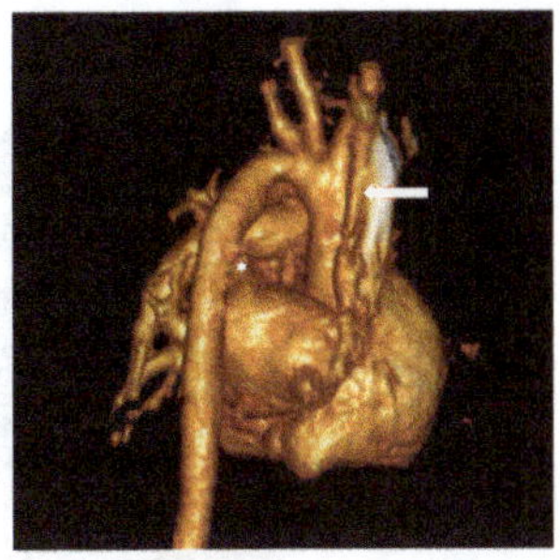

FIGURE 2: 3D reconstruction CT imaging from right posterior view shows the origin of the right pulmonary artery from the right subclavian artery (white arrows) and the left-sided PDA (asterisk). The stenosis of the RPA is also seen.

3. Discussion

Interruption of the right pulmonary artery is a very rare anomaly with a prevalence of 1 : 200,000 to 1 : 300,000 in adult, which was first described in 1868 by Frantzel O. Angeborener. This anomaly has been described in literature as unilateral absence of the pulmonary artery; however, the distal intrapulmonary network is usually intact in these cases and perfused by collateral vessels. Therefore, the term "interruption" rather than "absence" is the preferred term (5, 6). To our best knowledge, the case herein represents the fourth definite diagnosis of neonatal isolated interrupted right pulmonary artery reported in literature. The three other cases refers to a two-day-old female presenting with a murmur, a one-day-old neonate presenting with severe cyanosis, and a two-day-old neonate presenting with cyanosis and oxygen saturation of 80% (5, 7).

Interruption of the right pulmonary artery is commonly associated with other congenital heart defects such as truncus arteriosus and tetralogy of Fallot. In isolated forms which mostly concerns the right pulmonary artery, it often involves

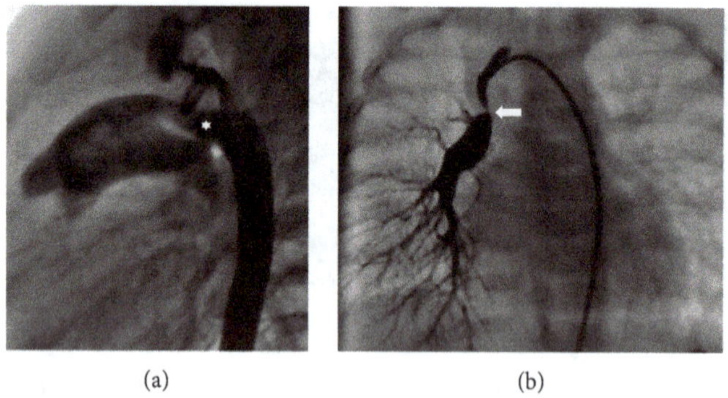

FIGURE 3: Angiogram showing (a) a large size patent ductus arteriosus (asterisk), and (b) the right pulmonary artery originates from the right subclavian artery with a significant stenosis at the origin point (arrow).

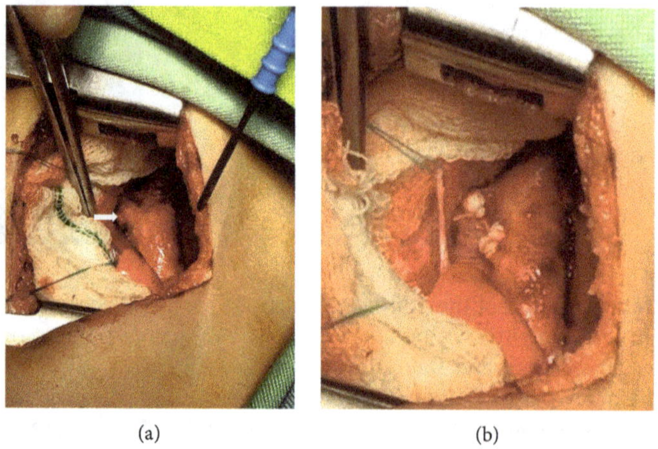

FIGURE 4: Intraoperative images: (a) large size patent ductus arteriosus was obvious (arrow); (b) ligation of the PDA was performed.

the pulmonary artery branch contralateral to the aortic arch (5, 8).

Review of the literature revealed that abnormal right pulmonary artery origin can be of three types. In the first type, the right or left pulmonary artery arises from the ascending aorta; in the second type, the proximal portion of the left or right pulmonary artery is absent, and the distal part is supplied by a patent ductus arteriosus, and the last type is absence of left or right pulmonary artery, and the supply of distal pulmonary artery branch is through aortopulmonary collaterals (9). Our patient had interruption of the right pulmonary artery, and the origin of the distal part was from the right subclavian artery which can be placed in the second category.

Clinical presentations of the unilateral interruption of a pulmonary artery can be varied. Pulmonary hypertension, dyspnea, recurrent pulmonary infections or chest pain, exercise intolerance, and hemoptysis in older patients have been reported. However, in rare condition, patients can be asymptomatic and remain undiagnosed until adulthood (10). At the time of our patient's presentation, she had signs and symptoms of pulmonary hypertension. Indeed, the patient's main pulmonary artery seemed mildly dilated in both echocardiography and CT angiography, and her oxygen saturation was decreased to 92%. The cause of pulmonary hypertension, which can be present in about 40-45% of unilateral absence of a pulmonary artery cases, is the fact that the entire cardiac output is directed to the contralateral lung leading to endothelial injury and vasoconstrictor mediator release (11).

Currently, there is no consensus as to the treatment of unilateral interruption of a pulmonary artery. Treatment is often recommended in symptomatic patients with pulmonary hypertension, recurrent infection, or hemoptysis. Medical treatment with pulmonary vasodilators or surgical management, including total or staged pulmonary artery anastomosis partial or complete pneumonectomy, has been suggested. Basically, in the presence of an isolated pulmonary artery branch, if the size of intrapulmonary branches is within normal range, an anastomosis with the central pulmonary artery is the best surgical approach. In the patients with small intrapulmonary arteries, a modified Blalock-Taussig shunt is recommended before the anastomosis to aid with vessel growth prior to unifocalization. In asymptomatic patients who have no cardiopulmonary dysfunction, clinical follow-up may be reasonable (12, 13). Our patient had pulmonary hypertension; therefore, PDA ligation was performed in hopes of decreasing the pulmonary artery pressure. The right pulmonary artery was normal in size, and there was no significant reduction in perfusion of the right lung on the chest X-ray. On the other hand, there was a significant stenosis at the origin of the right pulmonary artery which limits the blood flow from the subclavian and therefore reduces the risk of pulmonary hypertension in the right lung. Accordingly, our pediatric cardiology team decided not to perform any intervention on the right pulmonary artery. Accordingly, the patient's follow-up at regular intervals showed that she was asymptomatic. However, since the connection between the right subclavian artery and the right pulmonary artery, which allows degrees of left to right shunt, remains, it seems necessary to measure left ventricular volume over times.

In conclusion, since the isolated interruption of the right pulmonary artery is a very rare congenital anomaly, it can be difficult to diagnose. Early diagnosis in neonatal period and treatment, if necessary, will hopefully prevent significant morbidity and mortality in these patients.

Consent

Informed consent was obtained from the parent of the child to publish this case report. The consent form is available upon request.

Authors' Contributions

All authors contributed toward data gathering and compilation, drafted and critically revised the paper, gave final approval of the version to be published, and agreed to be accountable for all aspects of the work.

References

[1] B. W. Carter, J. P. Lichtenberger, and C. C. Wu, "Congenital abnormalities of the pulmonary arteries in adults," *American Journal of Roentgenology*, vol. 202, no. 4, pp. W308–W313, 2014.

[2] J. Bueno, L. Flors, and M. Mejía, "Congenital anomalies of the pulmonary arteries: spectrum of findings on computed tomography," *Radiologia (English Edition)*, vol. 59, no. 3, pp. 209–217, 2017.

[3] S. Agati, C. G. Sousa, F. D. Calvaruso et al., "Anomalous aortic origin of the pulmonary arteries: case series and literature review," *Pediatric Cardiology*, vol. 12, no. 3, pp. 248–253, 2019.

[4] P. Garg, S. Talwar, S. S. Kothari et al., "The anomalous origin of the branch pulmonary artery from the ascending aorta," *Interactive cardiovascular and thoracic surgery*, vol. 15, no. 1, pp. 86–92, 2012.

[5] A. Raymond, E. Pedretti, G. Privitera, C. Cicero, and G. Biasucci, "Neonatal diagnosis of isolated absence of the right pulmonary artery: a case report and review of the literature," *Italian Journal of Pediatrics*, vol. 44, no. 1, p. 27, 2018.

[6] S. H. Anand, A. Jasper, S. E. Mani, E. Joseph, and J. Mathai, "Proximal interruption of the pulmonary artery: a case series," *Journal of Clinical and Diagnostic Research: JCDR*, vol. 9, no. 12, pp. TD04–TD06, 2015.

[7] M. Kardos, M. Kaldararova, and M. Ondriska, "Double ductus arteriosus and anomalous origin of the right pulmonary artery from the right-sided duct," *Journal of Cardiology Cases.*, vol. 10, no. 3, pp. 97–99, 2014.

[8] E. C. Cortinas, N. R. Jiménez, M. B. Zurita, P. M. Haro, and L. G. Silva, "Unusual distal right pulmonary artery origin from right ductus arteriosus with uncommon left-sided aortic arch," *Revista Colombiana de Cardiología*, vol. 26, no. 5, pp. 300–303, 2019.

[9] P. A. Penkoske, A. R. Castañeda, D. C. Fyler, and R. Van Praagh, "Origin of pulmonary artery branch from ascending aorta," *The Journal of Thoracic and Cardiovascular Surgery*, vol. 85, no. 4, pp. 537–545, 1983.

[10] D. W. Reading and U. Oza, "Unilateral absence of a pulmonary artery: a rare disorder with variable presentation," *In Baylor University Medical Center Proceedings*, vol. 25, no. 2, pp. 115–118, 2012.

[11] L. Saladi, S. Roy, and G. Diaz-Fuentes, "Unilateral pulmonary artery agenesis: an unusual cause of unilateral ARDS," *Respiratory Medicine Case Reports*, vol. 23, no. 23, pp. 148–151, 2018.

[12] A. Y. Weldetsadik, Y. M. Asfaw, and A. M. Tekleab, "Isolated absence of right pulmonary artery in a 4-year old child: a case report," *International Medical Case Reports Journal*, vol. 11, no. 11, pp. 297–301, 2018.

[13] A. K. Singhi, E. Francis, and R. K. Kumar, "Isolated absence of right pulmonary artery," *Annals of Pediatric Cardiology*, vol. 3, no. 2, pp. 119–122, 2010.

49

Unusual Cardiac Presentation of COVID-19 and use of Convalescent Plasma

William R. Hartman[1] **Aaron S. Hess,**[1,2] **and Joseph P. Connor**[2]

[1]*Department of Anesthesiology, University of Wisconsin-Madison School of Medicine and Public Health, USA*
[2]*Department Pathology and Laboratory Medicine, University of Wisconsin-Madison School of Medicine and Public Health, USA*

Correspondence should be addressed to William R. Hartman; wrhartman@wisc.edu

Academic Editor: Kuan-Rau Chiou

COVID-19 infection caused by the SARS-CoV-2 virus has been associated with cardiac abnormalities, including conduction abnormalities. Convalescent plasma is emerging as a potentially safe and effective treatment option for patients severely or critically ill with COVID-19. Here, we describe a case of a COVID-19 patient with new-onset cardiac ectopy who had near resolution of his cardiac sequelae following convalescent plasma transfusion.

1. History of Presentation

A 62-year-old man with history of moderate persistent asthma, sinus bradycardia, COPD, and chronic pain was admitted to a tertiary health care center with laboratory-confirmed COVID-19 after 5 days of increased cough and shortness of breath. He had been taking 20 mg of prednisone daily for four days prior to admission as well as three doses of an old prescription of amoxicillin-clavulanate. He had not taken any hydroxychloroquine. Proper ethical guidelines have been followed, and the patient has documented consent to be part of a research study as well as have his case used in future publications.

2. Differential Diagnosis

(i) COPD Exacerbation

(ii) Asthma Exacerbation

(iii) Bacterial pneumonia

(iv) COVID-19 pneumonia.

3. Investigations

His admission D-dimer was 0.73 mcg/mL, and his C-reactive protein (CRP) was 0.8 mg/dL. His baseline heart rate was between 40 and 50 bpm but fell as low as 30 bpm overnight. His SpO2 remained >92% on room air. He was admitted for monitoring and remained clinically stable until hospital day 2 when he developed new tachycardia, worsening cough, and shortness of breath. His telemetry revealed frequent premature atrial contractions (PACs) as well as new premature ventricular contractions (PVCs) and apparent trigeminy (Figure 1). He was placed on 2 L/min oxygen by nasal cannula. His troponin was negative. Repeat D-dimer was 1.35 mcg/mL, CRP was 5.7 mg/dL, ferritin was 188, and potassium was 4.1 mEq/L.

4. Management

Based on his sudden deterioration, this patient was consented for and received 217 mL of COVID-19 convalescent plasma. No other interventions were made at the time. 24 hours later, his heart rate had improved to the 60-70 bpm with less

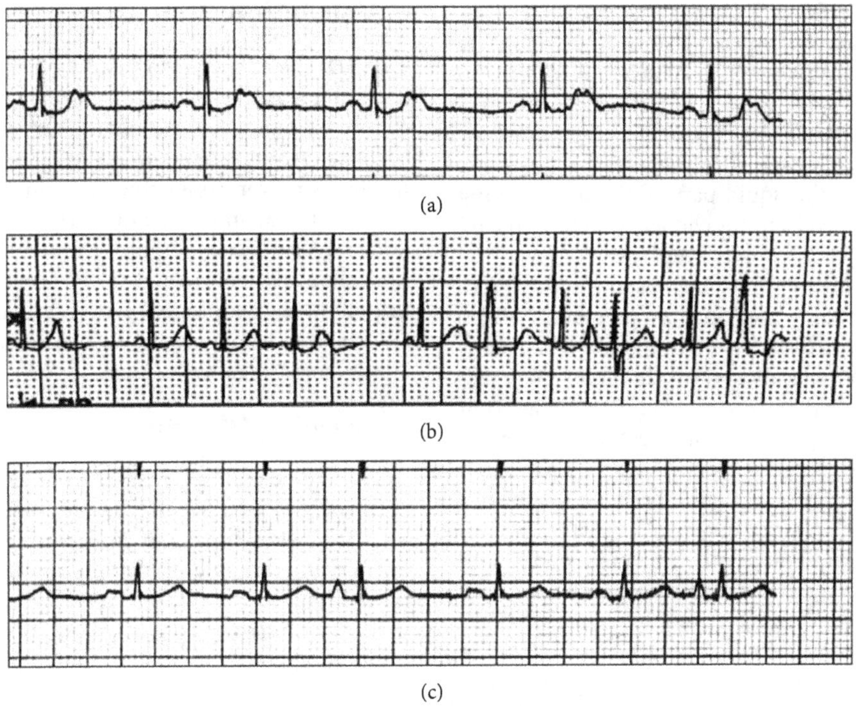

FIGURE 1: Representative lead II ECG tracings. ECG from day 1 (a), prior to convalescent plasma treatment (b), and after convalescent plasma treatment (c). The ectopy that presented during hospitalization was nearly resolved following treatment with convalescent plasma.

frequent PACs and PVCs and he was breathing comfortably on room air. His CRP decreased to 5.3 mg/dL and ferritin to 168. He was able to pass a 6-minute walk test with saturations of 94% and greater, and he competed evaluations with occupational and physical therapy. 36 hours after transfusion, the patient was discharged from the hospital reporting that he felt improved, although still with cough and subjective shortness of breath with activity similar to his baseline COPD symptoms.

5. Discussion

At the end of 2019, a novel coronavirus was identified as the cause of a cluster of pneumonia cases in Wuhan, China. The virus rapidly spread, resulting in a global pandemic with a devastating impact on populations and the global economy. While most infections remain asymptomatic or recover as outpatients from milder variations of the disease, a subset of individuals are hospitalized with some requiring intensive care unit admission both with or without mechanical ventilation. Although fever and respiratory symptoms are the most common manifestations of disease in admitted patients, some patients present with chest palpitations or other cardiac-related symptoms including chest pain. Patients presenting with cardiac-related symptoms have been estimated to be approximately 7% of cases [1]. In Wuhan, China, abnormal cardiac conduction/arrhythmia was seen in 17% of hospitalized patients in general care but was seen in twice as many (44%) of the patients require intensive care unit admission [2]. COVID-19 has been associated with cardiac morbidity and mortality, with individuals having evidence of cardiac damage as defined by an increased troponin level having a worse outcome than those without elevated troponin [3].

In a study of myocardial injury in COVID-19 patients in Wuhan, China, patients with myocardial injury had higher leukocyte ($P < .001$), lower lymphocyte ($P < .001$), and lower platelet counts ($P < .001$) [4]. A retrospective study from another Wuhan hospital demonstrated that patients with high troponin-T levels had leukocytosis ($P < .001$), increased neutrophils ($P < .001$), and decreased lymphocytes ($P = .01$) [5]. Our patient had an elevated leukocyte count but a normal lymphocyte count and elevated neutrophils. While his troponin-T level was not elevated, he did have an elevated creatinine kinase and D-dimer.

The pathophysiology of COVID-19-associated cardiac disease and the conduction abnormalities described is complex; however, it is thought to most likely be secondary to excessive systemic inflammation leading to myocardial damage [6]. Previous reports of COVID-19-associated acute myocardial injury suggest that cardiovascular sequalae are secondary to a high systemic inflammatory response and the associated excessive cytokine release [7, 8]. Other contributing factors that have been reported include the presence of preexisting cardiac disease, primary cardiac myocyte damage by direct viral infection, and the increased and often overwhelming demand brought on by hypoxia associated with severe infection and respiratory failure [9].

Cardiac conduction abnormalities were also observed during the original SARS-CoV outbreak (2002–2003). *In vitro* studies demonstrated that the angiotensin-converting enzyme 2 (ACE2) was responsible for viral uptake into host cells via spike protein and that the ACE2 receptor is abundant in cardiac myocytes [10]. Autopsy studies of mice and rabbits infected with SARS-CoV demonstrated a direct viral RNA inclusion in myocytes of specimens with cardiac injury and conduction system disease [11]. ACE2 is also the viral receptor for SARS-CoV2 [12].

Convalescent plasma (CP) is an emerging treatment for COVID-19 infection, and early data suggests that it is safe. Convalescent plasma is the liquid part of blood containing antibodies and is collected from individuals who have recovered from a viral infection. It has been used for over 100 years in treatment of other viral pandemics in which no vaccine was available including the "Spanish" influenza, SARS, MERS, Argentine hemorrhagic fever, and Ebola. The results from using convalescent plasma as a treatment for these diseases remain somewhat uncertain. While convalescent plasma has become recognized as the treatment of choice for Argentine hemorrhagic fever, convalescent plasma use in Ebola, while safe, has not proven efficacious. Published reports of convalescent plasma use in other coronaviruses including MARS and SERS are limited to case reports and case series or retrospective nonrandomized analyses which are difficult to draw conclusions from [13]. An early randomized study of convalescent plasma in COVID-19 patients was underpowered and terminated early, but failed to establish effectiveness as a therapy for COVID-19 disease [14]. Convalescent plasma is currently being studied as a potential therapy for hospitalized patients suffering from COVID-19 infection [15].

CP has not been reported as a treatment for patients with cardiac symptoms. We present the case of a man admitted with COVID-19 who developed severe worsening of his baseline arrythmia and recovered after CP administration [16]. Here, we report the case of a 62-year-old male with COVID-19-associated arrythmias that improved following administration of COVID-19 convalescent plasma. Of particular interest is that the abnormal conduction episodes documented were not in the setting of hydroxychloroquine administration. This patient developed palpitations associated with new-onset PACs and PVCs. There were laboratory markers of severe disease, but not myocardial injury. Following convalescent plasma administration, he had rapid improvement in his symptoms and electrocardiogram findings and was discharged shortly thereafter.

We do not know by what mechanism convalescent plasma might have aborted this patient's ectopy and led to clinical improvement. It is possible that donor anti-SARS-CoV-2 antibodies may have contributed to rapid inactivation of viral particles and so reduced myocardial irritation. Although this is only a hypothesis to explain the temporal association between treatment and improvement, no other medications were administered concurrently, and he only was hydrated with oral water and electrolyte drinks. This represents the first reported case of COVID-19-associated cardiac ectopy being treated and apparently terminated after administration of COVID-19 convalescent plasma. While purely speculative, we postulate that convalescent plasma might be used effectively in infected individuals who display signs of cardiac conduction system abnormalities and not only those with primary pulmonary presentations.

6. Conclusion

COVID-19 has been associated with cardiac conduction system abnormalities. Patients with confirmed COVID-19 should be monitored closely for changes from their cardiac baseline including new-onset PACs and PVCs. Potential viral mechanisms for conduction system abnormalities include myocardial inflammation or direct viral infiltration. Convalescent plasma, an emerging treatment for COVID-19 infection, should be considered as an early therapy when patients present with symptoms of myocardial irritability. Further studies are clearly needed to help delineate the safety and effectiveness of this treatment.

7. Learning Objective

COVID-19 manifests itself in a variety of ways in different patients. A less common, but serious complication of this virus is new cardiac conduction abnormalities. With no cure for the disease, Convalescent plasma was attempted as a way to neutralize the virus and quell the cardiac ectopy. In this patient, convalescent plasma therapy was able to return him to his baseline.

Acknowledgments

This study was funded by the University of Wisconsin-Madison Institute for Clinical and Translational Research, Madison, Wisconsin.

References

[1] S. A. Glantz, "It is all in the numbers," *Journal of the American College of Cardiology*, vol. 21, no. 3, pp. 835–837, 1993.

[2] F. Zhou, T. Yu, R. du et al., "Clinical course and risk factors for mortality of adult inpatients with COVID-19 in Wuhan, China: a retrospective cohort study," *Lancet*, vol. 395, no. 10229, pp. 1054–1062, 2020.

[3] W. Wang, Y. Xu, R. Gao et al., "Detection of SARS-CoV-2 in different types of clinical specimens," *JAMA*, vol. 323, no. 18, pp. 1843-1844, 2020.

[4] H. C. Sullivan and J. Roback, "Convalescent plasma: therapeutic hope or hopeless strategy in the SARS-CoV-2 pandemic," *Transfusion Medicine Reviews*, vol. 23, 2020.

[5] S. Shi, M. Qin, B. Shen et al., "Association of cardiac injury with mortality in hospitalized patients with COVID-19 in Wuhan, China," *JAMA Cardiology*, vol. 5, no. 7, pp. 802–810, 2020.

[6] G. Lippi, C. J. Lavie, and F. Sanchis-Gomar, "Cardiac troponin I in patients with coronavirus disease 2019 (COVID-19): evidence from a meta-analysis," *Progress in Cardiovascular Diseases*, vol. 63, no. 3, pp. 390-391, 2020, [Epub ahead of print].

[7] E. Driggin, M. V. Madhavan, B. Bikdeli et al., "Cardiovascular considerations for patients, health care workers, and health systems during the coronavirus disease 2019 (COVID-19) pandemic," *Journal of the American College of Cardiology*, vol. 75, no. 18, pp. 2352–2371, 2020.

[8] A. N. Kochi, A. P. Tagliari, G. B. Forleo, G. M. Fassini, and C. Tondo, "Cardiac and arrhythmic complications in patients with Covid-19," *Journal of Cardiovascular Electrophysiology*, vol. 31, no. 5, pp. 1003 1008, 2020.

[9] W. Wang, L. Ye, L. Ye et al., "Up-regulation of IL-6 and TNF-alpha induced by SARS-coronavirus spike protein in murine macrophages via NF-kappaB pathway," *Virus Research*, vol. 128, no. 1-2, pp. 1–8, 2007.

[10] P. Cheng, H. Zhu, R. M. Witteles et al., "Cardiovascular risks in patients with COVID-19: potential mechanisms and areas of uncertainty," *Current Cardiology Reports*, vol. 22, no. 5, p. 34, 2020.

[11] Y. Y. Zheng, Y. T. Ma, J. Y. Zhang, and X. Xie, "COVID-19 and the cardiovascular system," *Nature Reviews Cardiology*, vol. 17, no. 5, pp. 259-260, 2020.

[12] L. K. Alexander, B. W. Keene, J. D. Small, Yount B Jr, and R. S. Baric, "Electrocardiographic changes following rabbit coronavirus-induced myocarditis and dilated cardiomyopathy," *Coronaviruses*, vol. 342, pp. 365–370, 1994.

[13] G. Y. Oudit, Z. Kassiri, C. Jiang et al., "SARS-coronavirus modulation of myocardial ACE2 expression and inflammation in patients with SARS," *European Journal of Clinical Investiagtion*, vol. 39, no. 7, pp. 618–625, 2009.

[14] M. Donoghue, H. Wakimoto, C. T. Maguire et al., "Heart block, ventricular tachycardia, and sudden death in ACE2 transgenic mice with downregulated connexins," *Journal of Molecullar and Cellular Cardiology*, vol. 35, no. 9, pp. 1043–1053, 2003.

[15] L. Li, W. Zhang, Y. Hu et al., "Effect of convalescent plasma therapy on time to clinical improvement in patients with severe and life-threatening COVID-19: a randomized clinical trial," *JAMA*, vol. 324, no. 5, pp. 460–470, 2020.

[16] T. Guo, Y. Fan, M. Chen et al., "Cardiovascular implications of fatal outcomes of patients with coronavirus disease 2019 (COVID-19)," *JAMA Cardiology*, vol. 5, no. 7, pp. 811–818, 2020.

Permissions

All chapters in this book were first published by Hindawi Publishing Corporation; hereby published with permission under the Creative Commons Attribution License or equivalent. Every chapter published in this book has been scrutinized by our experts. Their significance has been extensively debated. The topics covered herein carry significant findings which will fuel the growth of the discipline. They may even be implemented as practical applications or may be referred to as a beginning point for another development.

The contributors of this book come from diverse backgrounds, making this book a truly international effort. This book will bring forth new frontiers with its revolutionizing research information and detailed analysis of the nascent developments around the world.

We would like to thank all the contributing authors for lending their expertise to make the book truly unique. They have played a crucial role in the development of this book. Without their invaluable contributions this book wouldn't have been possible. They have made vital efforts to compile up to date information on the varied aspects of this subject to make this book a valuable addition to the collection of many professionals and students.

This book was conceptualized with the vision of imparting up-to-date information and advanced data in this field. To ensure the same, a matchless editorial board was set up. Every individual on the board went through rigorous rounds of assessment to prove their worth. After which they invested a large part of their time researching and compiling the most relevant data for our readers.

The editorial board has been involved in producing this book since its inception. They have spent rigorous hours researching and exploring the diverse topics which have resulted in the successful publishing of this book. They have passed on their knowledge of decades through this book. To expedite this challenging task, the publisher supported the team at every step. A small team of assistant editors was also appointed to further simplify the editing procedure and attain best results for the readers.

Apart from the editorial board, the designing team has also invested a significant amount of their time in understanding the subject and creating the most relevant covers. They scrutinized every image to scout for the most suitable representation of the subject and create an appropriate cover for the book.

The publishing team has been an ardent support to the editorial, designing and production team. Their endless efforts to recruit the best for this project, has resulted in the accomplishment of this book. They are a veteran in the field of academics and their pool of knowledge is as vast as their experience in printing. Their expertise and guidance has proved useful at every step. Their uncompromising quality standards have made this book an exceptional effort. Their encouragement from time to time has been an inspiration for everyone.

The publisher and the editorial board hope that this book will prove to be a valuable piece of knowledge for researchers, students, practitioners and scholars across the globe.

List of Contributors

George Joy
Cardiology Department, St Bartholomew's Hospital, West Smithfield, London EC1A 7BE, UK

Hany Eissa
Cardiology Department, Queen Elizabeth Queen Mother Hospital, St Peter's Rd, Margate CT9 4AN, UK

Oreoluwa Oladiran and Rashmi Dhital
Reading Hospital, Tower Health System, West Reading, Pennsylvania, USA

Ifeanyi Nwosu
Leighton Hospital NHS Trust, Crewe, Cheshire, UK

Gbujie Ezioma
Saint Peter's University, New Brunswick, New Jersey, USA

Aniket S. Rali, Andrew Sauer and Zubair Shah
Department of Cardiovascular Medicine, The University of Kansas Health System, USA

Farhad Sami
Department of Internal Medicine, The University of Kansas Health System, USA

Noura Ayoubi and Zaydi Javeed
Morsani College of Medicine, University of South Florida, Tampa, Florida, USA

Raymond Cutro
Department of Cardiology, James A. Haley Veterans' Hospital, Tampa, Florida, USA

Brooke T. Baldwin
Department of Dermatology, James A. Haley Veterans' Hospital, Tampa, Florida, USA

Maria Silvia Negroni, Alessandro Tayar, Simone Persampieri and Stefano Carugo
Division of Cardiology, San Paolo Hospital, Department of Health Sciences, University of Milan, Via A. Di Rudini 8, Milan, Italy

Arianna Marengo, Patrizia Rubiolo and Maria Laura Colombo
Department of Drug Science and Technology, Università degli Studi di Torino, Via Pietro Giuria 9, Turin, Italy

Donatella Caruso, Flavio Giavarini, Enrico Sangiovanni and Mario Dell'Agli
Department of Pharmacological and Biomolecular Sciences, Università degli Studi di Milano, Via Balzaretti 9, Milan, Italy

Franca Davanzo
Poison Control Centre of Milan, Niguarda Ca' Granda Hospital, Milan, Italy

Raed Aqel
National Center for Diabetes, Endocrinology and Genetics Center, Amman, Jordan

Muawiyah Elqadi and Ahmad Hammouri
Al-Quds University, Faculty of Medicine, Jerusalem, State of Palestine

Mohammad S. Alqadi
Al-Ahli Hospital, Hebron, State of Palestine

Andres Cordova Sanchez
Department of Medicine, SUNY Upstate Medical University, Syracuse, NY 13210, USA

Mostafa Vasigh, Oluwateniola Olatunde and Debanik Chaudhuri
Division of Cardiology, SUNY Upstate Medical University, Syracuse, NY 13210, USA

Sohab S. Radwan and Owen G. Schwartz
Department of Internal Medicine, Med Star Washington Hospital Center, USA

Zeid Nesheiwat, Marcel Ghanim, Joseph Eid, Neha Patel and Cameron Burmeister
Department of Internal Medicine, The University of Toledo Medical Center, Toledo, Ohio, USA

Ehab Eltahawy
Department of Cardiology, The University of Toledo Medical Center, Toledo, Ohio, USA

Rishi Raj and Aasems Jacob
University of Kentucky, Lexington, KY, USA

Dileep Unnikrishnan, Amulya Prakash and Ajay Shah
Monmouth Medical Center, Long Branch, NJ, USA

Kumar Ashish
Crozer-Chester Medical Center, Upland, PA, USA

A. van Broekhoven and H. W. M. Niessen
Department of Pathology, Amsterdam UMC, Vrije Universiteit, Amsterdam, Netherlands
Amsterdam Cardiovascular Sciences, Amsterdam, Netherlands
Department of Cardiac Surgery, Amsterdam UMC, Vrije Universiteit, Amsterdam, Netherlands

Moumita Naidu, Robby Singh and Marcel Zughaib
Providence Hospital-Michigan State University, USA

P. A. J. Krijnen
Department of Pathology, Amsterdam UMC, Vrije Universiteit, Amsterdam, Netherlands
Amsterdam Cardiovascular Sciences, Amsterdam, Netherlands

A. B. A. Vonk
Amsterdam Cardiovascular Sciences, Amsterdam, Netherlands
Department of Cardiac Surgery, Amsterdam UMC, Vrije Universiteit, Amsterdam, Netherlands

Kristin Stawiarski, Asiya Mamhut, Elenita Kanin and Stuart Zarich
Yale New Haven Health Heart and Vascular Center, Bridgeport Hospital, Bridgeport, CT, USA

Makio Muraishi and Masahiko Noguchi
Department of Cardiology, Tokyo Bay Urayasu Ichikawa Medical Center, Urayasu, Japan

Kosuke Maeda and Takuya Okada
Department of Cardiology, Yokosuka General Hospital Uwamachi, Yokosuka, Japan

Osayi Lawani
HCA Houston Healthcare, Kingwood, USA
University of Houston College of Medicine/HCA Houston Healthcare, USA

Rick Ganim
Vital Heart & Vein, HCA Houston Healthcare, Kingwood, USA

Jason R. Stuck
Pinnacle Health Cardio Vascular Institute, 1000 North Front Street, Wormleysburg, PA 17043, USA

Amgad N. Makaryus
Donald and Barbara Zucker School of Medicine at Hofstra/Northwell, Department of Cardiology, North Shore University Hospital, 300 Community Drive, Manhasset, NY 11030, USA
Department of Cardiology, Nu Health, Nassau University Medical Center, 2201 Hempstead Turnpike, East Meadow, NY 11554, USA

Nicholas Peterman and Bradley Kaptur
Carle Illinois College of Medicine, University of Illinois Urbana-Champaign, Champaign, IL, USA

Naveed Adoni
Carle Illinois College of Medicine, University of Illinois Urbana-Champaign, Champaign, IL, USA
Carle Foundation Hospital, Urbana, IL, USA

Simon G. Findlay and Nicholas M. Child
North Tees and Hartlepool NHS Trust, Stockton-on-Tees, UK

Douglas F. Muir
The James Cook University Hospital, Middlesbrough, UK

Muhammad Ajmal, Amitoj Singh and Saad Kubba
Division of Cardiology, Department of Internal Medicine, USA

Michelle Hershman
Department of Medical Imaging, University of Arizona College of Medicine, Tucson, USA
Banner University Medical Center, Tucson, USA

Tushar Acharya
Division of Cardiology, Department of Internal Medicine, USA
Department of Medical Imaging, University of Arizona College of Medicine, Tucson, USA
Banner University Medical Center, Tucson, USA

Nobunari Tomura, Masashi Fujino, Yu Kataoka, Shuichi Yoneda and Teruo Noguchi
Department of Cardiovascular Medicine, National Cerebral and Cardiovascular Center, 6-1 Kishibe-Shimmachi, Suita, Osaka, Japan

Hiroaki Sasaki
Department of Cardiovascular Surgery, National Cerebral and Cardiovascular Center, 6-1 Kishibe Shimmachi, Suita, Osaka, Japan

Valerie R. Ramiro, Jezreel L. Taquiso, Stephanie Martha O. Obillos, Charlene F. Agustin, Jose Donato A. Magno and Eric Oliver D. Sison
Section of Cardiology, Department of Medicine, University of the Philippines-Philippine General Hospital, Philippines

Abdul-Subulr Yakubu
Tamale Teaching Hospital, Tamale, Ghana

Xiaoqiang Zhang
Chengdu 2nd People Hospital, China

Bin Zhang
Second Division of the Cardiology Department, Guangdong Cardiovascular Institute, Guangdong General Hospital, Guangdong, China

Miguel Rodriguez-Guerra and Manoj Bhandari
BronxCare Health System, New York, USA

Mayank Yadav, Jonathan N. Bella and Eduard Sklyar
BronxCare Health System, New York, USA
Icahn School of Medicine at Mount Sinai, New York, USA

Archna Sinha
St. Charles Hospital, Port Jefferson, New York, USA

Ana Rita Pereira, Alexandra Briosa, Rita Miranda, Sofia Sequeira Almeida, Luís Brandão and Hélder Pereira
Cardiology Department, Hospital Garcia de Orta, Avenida Torrado da Silva, 2805-267 Almada, Portugal

Alexis Javier Atuesta-Rodriguez, Yimy F. Medina-Velasquez, Orfa Motta, Maria Isabel Narvaez-Reyes and Federico Rondon-Herrera
Rheumatology Unit, National University of Colombia, Colombia

Akihiro Kobayashi, Yoshimori Araki, Takafumi Terada and Osamu Kawaguchi
Department of Cardiac Surgery, Toyota Kosei Hospital, Ibobara 500-1, Jousui-cho, Toyota, Aichi 470-0396, Japan

Matthew T. Lee and Ayush Mohan
Central Michigan University College of Medicine, USA

Jenna E. Lee and Daniel T. Lee
McLaren Bay City Regional Medical Center, USA

Tommaso La Macchia
Department of Clinical and Experimental Medicine, Unit of Cardiology, University of Messina, Via C. Valeria, 98125 Messina, Italy

Remo Albiero
Interventional Cardiology Unit-Sondrio Hospital, Via Stelvio, 25, 23100 Sondrio, Italy

Tommaso Invernizzi
Ophthalmology Unit-Sondrio Hospital, Via Stelvio, 25, 23100 Sondrio, Italy

Giorgia Ceravolo
Department of Human Pathology and Evolutive Age "Gaetano Barresi", University of Messina, Via C. Valeria, 98125 Messina, Italy

Ida Ceravolo
Department of Clinical and Experimental Medicine, University of Messina, Via C. Valeria, 98125 Messina, Italy

Thalia Bekelaar, Frederic De Roeck and Steven Haine
Department of Cardiology, Antwerp University Hospital, University of Antwerp, Edegem, Belgium

Gervais Nougon and Marc Peters
Department of Emergency Medicine, Sint-Jozef Hospital, Malle, Belgium

Dirk Ysebaert
Department of Hepatobiliary-Transplantation-Endocrine Surgery, Antwerp University Hospital, University of Antwerp, Edegem, Belgium

Maarten Spinhoven
Department of Radiology, Antwerp University Hospital, University of Antwerp, Edegem, Belgium

Philippe G. Jorens, Rudi De Paep and Frederik Lahaye
Intensive Care Medicine, Antwerp University Hospital, University of Antwerp, Edegem, Belgium

Mark Coyle, Mark Wilkinson and Mark Sheehy
Department of Medicine, Midlands Regional Hospital Mullingar, Longford Road, Robinstown, Mullingar, Westmeath, Ireland

Muhammad Talha Ayub, Dinesh Kalra, Melissa Tracy and Anupama K. Rao
Division of Cardiovascular Medicine, RUSH University Medical Center, Chicago IL, USA

Allison Zimmerman
Department of Medicine, RUSH University Medical Center, Chicago IL, USA

Wajeeha Rasool
Department of Medicine, Amita Health Presence St Francis Hospital, Evanston IL, USA

Rongfeng Xu, Jiandong Ding, Lijuan Chen, Yi Feng and Genshan Ma
Department of Cardiology, Zhongda Hospital, Medical School of Southeast University, Nanjing, 210009 Jiangsu, China

Md Mashiul Alam
Jahurul Islam Medical College Hospital, Bhagalpur, Bajitpur, Kishoregonj, Bangladesh

Md Fakhrul Islam Khaled
University Cardiac Center, Bangabandhu Sheikh Mujib Medical University, Room No-418, D Block, Dhaka, Bangladesh

Lu Zhang, Ming Bai, Ji-zhe Xu, Ga-xue Jiang, Ai-yun Deng and Zheng Zhang
Department of Cardiology, The First Hospital of Lanzhou University, China
Gansu Provincial Clinical Research Center for Cardiovascular Diseases and Gansu Provincial Key Laboratory of Cardiovascular Disease, China
National Project of Improving the Diagnosis and Treatment Ability of Cardiovascular and Cerebrovascular Diseases, The First Hospital of Lanzhou University, China

Nabil Braiteh
United Health Services Hospitals, Wilson Medical Center, Department of Cardiology, 30 Harrison St, Johnson City, NY, USA

Wajeeh Rehman
United Health Services Hospitals, Wilson Medical Center, Department of Internal Medicine, 33-57 Harrison St, Johnson City, NY, USA

Wajiha Ali
American University of Antigua College of Medicine, USA

Owais Ahmed
United Health Services Hospitals (Heart & Vascular Institute), Wilson Medical Center, Department of Cardiology, 30 Harrison St, Johnson City, NY 13790, USA

Y. Khalid
Department of Cardiology, The Wright Center for Graduate Medical Education, Scranton, PA, USA

N. Dasu
Department of Gastroenterology, Jefferson Health New Jersey, Cherry Hill, NJ, USA

M. Daneshvar and P. Jang
Department of Internal Medicine, Jefferson Heath New Jersey, Stratford, NJ, USA

A. Patel
Department of Internal Medicine, St. Mary's Medical Center, Langhorne, PA, USA

K. Dasu
Department of Biomedical Sciences and Professional Studies, Drexel University, Philadelphia, PA, USA

A. Shah
Department of Cardiology, University of Pittsburgh Medical Center, Pittsburgh, PA, USA

Connor Charles Kerndt
Michigan State University College of Osteopathic Medicine, East Lansing, MI 48824, USA

Alexander Michael Balinski
Oakland University William Beaumont School of Medicine, Rochester, MI 48309, USA

Hayk Vahe Papukhyan
Department of Internal Medicine, Henry Ford Macomb Hospital, Clinton Township, MI 48038, USA

Kojiro Toda and Kota Murai
Department of Cardiovascular Medicine, National Cerebral and Cardiovascular Centre, Suita, Japan

Gregory Scott Troutman
Sidney Kimmel Medical College at Thomas Jefferson University, Philadelphia, PA, USA

Jason Salamon
Department of Medicine, Division of Cardiology, Morristown Medical Center, Atlantic Medical Group, Morristown, NJ, USA

Matthew Scharf
Department of Medicine, Division of Sleep Medicine, Robert Wood Johnson University Hospital, New Brunswick, NJ, USA

Jeremy A. Mazurek
Department of Medicine, Division of Advanced Heart Failure and Transplant Cardiology, Hospital of the University of Pennsylvania, Philadelphia, PA, USA

Arthur Cicupira Rodrigues de Assis, Gustavo Andre Boeing Boros, Thiago Luis Scudeler and Paulo Cury Rezende
MASS Research Unit, Instituto do Coração (InCor), Hospital das Clínicas da Faculdade de Medicina da Universidade de São Paulo, São Paulo, Brazil

Lea Maria Macruz Ferreira Demarchi
Pathology Department, Instituto do Coração (InCor), Hospital das Clínicas da Faculdade de Medicina da Universidade de São Paulo, São Paulo, Brazil

Rony Shammas, Prasanna Sengodan and Assad Movahed
Division of Cardiology, Vidant Medical Center-East Carolina University at Brody School of Medicine, Greenville, NC, USA

Bashar Khiatah
Department of Internal Medicine, Community Memorial Hospital, 147 N Brent St, Ventura, CA 93003, USA

Jonathan Dukes
Electrophysiology, Cardiology Associate Medical Group, USA

Christina Desai
Internal Medicine, Community Memorial Hospital, USA

Amanda Frugoli
GME Department, Community Memorial Hospital, USA

Jasna Čerkez Habek, Tea Friščić, Jozica Šikić, Marko Perčić and Dean Strinić
Department of Cardiology, Clinic of Internal Medicine, "Sveti Duh" University Hospital, School of Medicine, University of Zagreb, Zagreb, Croatia

Daria Ljubas Perčić
Department of Neonatology, Clinic of Gynecology and Obstetrition, "Sveti Duh" University Hospital, School of Medicine, University of Zagreb, Zagreb, Croatia

Daniela Waddell, Felix Meincke, Samer Hakmi, Hendrick van der Schalk, Niklas Schenker, Jonas Hahn, Anna Moschner, Mintje Bohné, Da-Un Chung, Stephan Willems and Edda Bahlmann
Department of Cardiology, Asklepios Clinic St. Georg, Hamburg, Germany

Dietmar Kivelitz
Department of Radiology, Asklepios Clinic St. Georg, Hamburg, Germany

Nikola Kos, Vjekoslav Radeljić, Nikola Pavlović, Krešimir Kordić, Kristijan Đula, Nikola Bulj, Tomislav Krčmar, Diana Delić Brkljačić, Ivan Zeljković and Šime Manola
Department of Cardiovascular Diseases, University Hospital Centre Sestre Milosrdnice, Zagreb, Croatia

Mohammad Amro
School of Medicine, Misr University for Science and Technology, Cairo, Egypt

Kelechukwu U. Okoro, Kanaan Mansoor, Ahmed Amro and Paul Okhumale
Marshall University School of Medicine, Huntington, WV, USA

Edward Baptista
Vital Heart & Vein, USA

Mohammadreza Khalilian and Tahmineh Tahouri
Department of Pediatrics, School of Medicine, Shahid Beheshti University of Medical Sciences, Tehran, Iran

Taraneh Faghihi Langroudi
Radiology Department, Shahid Modarres Hospital, Shahid Beheshti University of Medical Sciences, Tehran, Iran

Ali Dabbagh
Cardiac Anesthesia, Anesthesiology Research Center, Shahid Beheshti University of Medical Sciences, Tehran, Iran

Ramin Baghaei Tehrani
Cardiac Surgery, Shahid Modarres Educational Hospital, School of Medicine, Shahid Beheshti University of Medical Sciences, Tehran, Iran

William R. Hartman
Department of Anesthesiology, University of Wisconsin-Madison School of Medicine and Public Health, USA

Joseph P. Connor
Department Pathology and Laboratory Medicine, University of Wisconsin-Madison School of Medicine and Public Health, USA

Aaron S. Hess
Department of Anesthesiology, University of Wisconsin-Madison School of Medicine and Public Health, USA
Department Pathology and Laboratory Medicine, University of Wisconsin-Madison School of Medicine and Public Health, USA

Index

www.ingramcontent.com/pod-product-compliance
Lightning Source LLC
LaVergne TN
LVHW082155200926
848484LV00008B/2166